PROGRESS IN *IN VITRO* TOXICOLOGY

ALTERNATIVE METHODS IN TOXICOLOGY
VOLUME 6

PROGRESS IN *IN VITRO* TOXICOLOGY

Editor
ALAN M. GOLDBERG

Editorial Assistant
MARILYN L. PRINCIPE

Mary Ann Liebert, Inc. publishers • New York

ALTERNATIVE METHODS IN TOXICOLOGY SERIES

Volume 1
Product Safety Evaluation

Volume 2
Acute Toxicity Testing: Alternative Approaches

Volume 3
In Vitro Methods in Toxicology

Volume 4
A Critical Evaluation of Alternatives to Acute Ocular Irritation Testing

Volume 5
In Vitro Toxicology: Approaches to Validation

Volume 6
Progress in *In Vitro* Toxicology

ISBN: 0-913113-16-6

Printed in the United States of America

Preface

This volume contains the proceedings of the fifth symposium held by the Johns Hopkins Center for Alternatives to Animal Testing since its inception in September of 1981.

Judging by the size of the audience in attendance and the papers encompassed in this volume, both as platform presentations and as poster presentations, it is apparent that the field of *in vitro* toxicology has reached definition and has matured scientifically. The audience in attendance at the meeting was truly international. The poster and platform sessions were no longer reviews of the past, but the cutting edge of science. The thinking of the participants, as displayed by the questions asked, was indicative of the progress made in the field and, more importantly, it demonstrated the extent of self-examination and identification of the problems to be faced. From the discussions at the meeting, I wish to focus on just two issues. The first of these is to define the barriers to progress in the development of alternatives, and the second is to look at the areas in need of future development.

If one measures progress by the number of publications in the field, *in vitro* toxicology is becoming most successful. However, with the burgeoning numbers of publications, there is clearly a lack of conceptual progress as to what is required for validation and the transfer of technology from development laboratory to useful, practical, reproducible, reliable tests. This transfer of technology, the conversion of scientific observation to usable methodology, has yet to be achieved. Clearly, there are several reasons for this. The field is so new and the methods so close to the cutting edge that there has not been time for refinement, development, and the necessary testing of these methods by a large segment of the scientific community to reach consensus that they will be predictive of the human experience. However, a second and equally significant barrier has been the lack of developmental funds necessary to manage the transfer of the technology and the refinement of the methodologies. The many small validations and correlative studies that have been attempted to date, although useful as first studies, have not been well designed, have not been coordinated, and have not attempted to transfer the technology. Individual laboratories have made significant progress, but again were hampered by the lack of a structured validation program against which to test their model. The Center has sought funding to provide this necessary structure; however, it has been unsuccessful. Validation and acceptance of methodology will happen, but if the process is more appropriately managed and funded, it will happen more quickly and more efficiently than has occurred to date.

In the area of dermal testing, a different phenomenon appears. Here, the development of methodology is at the most complex forefront of science. The science associated with skin and keratinocytes has been combined with private commercial interests for the development of skin "equivalents" and the use of these preparations in toxicity testing. One can anticipate that testing strategies using artificially derived skin will soon occur. The papers included in this volume clearly attest that routine *in vitro* methodology will be available in the near future.

The last part of the symposium focused on the problems of the future; that is, how does one test species-specific proteins, either human or animal, in species that are immunologically incapable of responding or that respond inappropriately to compounds from a different species. One answer, and clearly not the only one, is the use of appropriate cells *in vitro*. In the case of human-specific proteins, it will become necessary to use human cells as the models and systems on which we test these products. Bioengineering has reached a most significant stage, and it is necessary for us to provide methodology that will look at the efficacy and toxicity of an unbelievable number of compounds expected to be marketable over the next five to ten years, not only in the area of drugs but also in the area of food and food additives, cosmetic products, and other commercial products. The challenge is not how or if we will use *in vitro* systems in testing for the products of biotechnology, but when.

In a recent editorial in the November 6, 1987 issue of *Science*, Daniel Koshland, Jr. states, "de Toqueville noted that the public will choose to believe a simple lie in preference to a complicated truth. Sometimes we must face the fact that a situation is so complex that we cannot extract the causes immediately and devise simple solutions. In other cases the causes will be sufficiently understood by experts so that certain courses of action are more likely to have good outcomes than others. Issues such as the danger of microorganisms in the environment, . . . and the use of animals in research are some of the complex dilemmas in which some people are better at predicting the future than others. A track record in real prophecies that proved to be correct may help us select those who have a true vision of the future from those formally describing the past."

De Toqueville's commentary has been restated by many in all fields of science. Inappropriate rushing of unfinished methods into acceptance will only delay the further development of truly acceptable *in vitro* methodology. We must progress with deliberate speed, but in doing so we must not compromise our ability to predict safety.

Alan M. Goldberg, Ph.D.
January 20, 1988

Contents

Part 2. Poster Presentations

Acknowledgments

This Symposium and the Center's programs are made possible by funding from the following companies:

Sponsors
Abbott Laboratories
Amoco Corporation
Avon Products, Inc.
Bristol-Myers Company
The Cosmetic, Toiletry and Fragrance Association, Inc.
The Geraldine R. Dodge Foundation
Exxon Corporation

Patrons
Allied-Signal Inc.
The Clorox Company
E.I. du Pont de Nemours & Company
Health Industry Manufacturers Association (HIMA)
Hoffmann-LaRoche, Inc.
ICI Americas, Inc.
S.C. Johnson & Son, Inc.
Pfizer Inc.
Sterling-Winthrop Research Institute

Benefactors
Boyle-Midway
Chesebrough-Pond's Inc.
Maybelline
The Procter & Gamble Company
Shell Companies Foundation

Corporate Contributors
Alza Corporation
BDF Beiersdorf Inc.
Beecham Cosmetics Inc.
Best Foods, a Division of CPC International Inc.

The Coca-Cola Company
Hershey Foods Corporation
Johnson & Johnson Baby Products Company
The Mennen Company
Parfums Christian Dior
ROC, S.A.
Taconic Farms Inc.
Walgreens

Corporate Friends
Allergan Pharmaceuticals
Bonne Bell, Inc.
Houbigant, Inc.
The Andrew Jergens Company
Lion Corporation Biological Science Laboratories
MEM Company, Inc.
Yves Rocher Inc.
West Cabot Cosmetics Associates

Contributing Authors

Michael D. Aleo
State University of New York at Buffalo, Department of Pharmacology and Therapeutics and Toxicology Research Center, Buffalo, NY 14214

Harvey Babich
Laboratory Animal Research Center, The Rockefeller University, 1230 York Avenue, New York, NY 10021-6399

Daniel M. Bagley, Ph.D.
Department of Pharmacology and Toxicology, Research and Development, Colgate-Palmolive Company, 909 River Road, Piscataway, NJ 08854

Eugene Bell, Ph.D.
Organogenesis, Inc., 83 Rogers Street, Cambridge, MA 02142

H.C. Bergman
National Testing Corporation, 888 Research Drive, Palm Springs, CA 92262

Michael G. Bird, Ph.D.
Exxon Biomedical Sciences, Inc., East Millstone, NJ 08873-0802

Marie-Noëlle Blaude
Laboratoire de Biochimie Toxicologique et Cancérologique, Université Catholique de Louvain, 73 Av. Mounier, B-1200 Bruxelles, Belgium

Ellen Borenfreund, Ph.D.
Laboratory Animal Research Center, The Rockefeller University, 1230 York Avenue, New York, NY 10021-6399

Steven T. Boyce, Ph.D.
Department of Surgery, University of California San Diego Medical Center, Box H640C, 225 Dickinson Street, San Diego, CA 82103

K. Brendel
Department of Pharmacology and Toxicology, University of Arizona, Tucson, AZ 85724

Daniel Calp
Department of Pharmacology, The Hebrew University–Hadassah Medical School, P.O.B. 1172, 91010 Jerusalem, Israel

Andrew Cohen
Department of Surgery, University of Connecticut School of Medicine, Farmington, CT 06032

D. Deboyser
Laboratoire de Biochimie Toxicologique et Cancérologique, Université Catholique de Louvain, 73 Av. Mounier, B-1200 Bruxelles, Belgium

Vincent A. DeLeo, M.D.
Columbia University, College of Physicians & Surgeons, Department of Dermatology, 630 West 168 Street, New York, NY 10032

Janis Demetrulias, Ph.D.
The Dial Corporation, Dial Technical Center, Scottsdale, AZ 85254

Salvatore J. De Salva, Ph.D.
Department of Pharmacology and Toxicology, Research and Development, Colgate-Palmolive Company, 909 River Road, Piscataway, NJ 08854

Norman H. Dubin, Ph.D.
Department of Gynecology/Obstetrics, Johns Hopkins University School of Medicine, 601 North Wolfe Street, Park Building—Room B202, Baltimore, MD 21205

J. Dunnigan
L'Institut de l'Amiante, Division Santé et Environnement, Université de Sherbrooke, Sherbrooke, Québec, Canada J1K 2R1

Salwa A. Elgebaly, Ph.D.
Department of Surgery, School of Medicine, University of Connecticut, Farmington, CT 06032-9984

Ben Eng
Laboratory Animal Research Center, The Rockefeller University, 1230 York Avenue, New York, NY 10021-6399

John L. Farber, M.D.
Department of Pathology, Thomas Jefferson University, 11th & Walnut Streets, Philadelphia, PA 19107

Dennis K. Flaherty, Ph.D.
Environmental Health Laboratory, Monsanto Agricultural Company and the Environmental Health Department, Monsanto Company, 645 South Newstead Street, St. Louis, MO 63110

T.W. Fofonoff
Organogenesis, Inc., 83 Rogers Street, Cambridge, MA 02142

L. Fouquette
Laboratoire de Caractérisation de L'Amiante Département de Biologie, Faculte des Sciences, Université de Sherbrooke, Sherbrooke, Québec, Canada J1K 2R1

John M. Frazier, Ph.D.
Department of Environmental Health Sciences, The Johns Hopkins University School of Hygiene and Public Health, 615 North Wolfe Street, Baltimore, MD 21205

A. Jay Gandolfi, Ph.D.
Department of Pharmacology and Toxicology, University of Arizona, Tucson, AZ 85724

Vincent F. Garry, M.D.
Environmental Pathology Laboratory, Department of Laboratory Medicine and Pathology, University of Minnesota, Minneapolis, MN

R.J. Gay, Ph.D.
Organogenesis, Inc., 83 Rogers Street, Cambridge, MA 02142

R.B. Ghodgaonkar
Department of Gynecology/Obstetrics, Johns Hopkins University School of Medicine, 601 North Wolfe Street, Park Building—Room B202, Baltimore, MD 21205

Fabienne Goethals, Ph.D.
Laboratoire de Biochimie Toxicologique et Cancérologique, Université Catholique de Louvaine, 73 Av. Mounier, Box 73.69, B-1200 Bruxelles, Belgium

Alan M. Goldberg, Ph.D.
The Johns Hopkins University School of Hygiene and Public Health, 615 North Wolfe Street, Baltimore, MD 21205

Lowell A. Goldsmith, M.D.
University of Rochester, School of Medicine and Dentistry, 601 Elmwood Avenue, Rochester, NY 14642

Concepcion González
Laboratoire de Biochimie Toxicologique et Cancérologique, Université Catholique de Louvain, 73 Av. Mounier, B-1200 Bruxelles, Belgium

Virginia C. Gordon, Ph.D.
National Testing Corporation, 888 Research Drive, Palm Springs, CA 92262

Yale Gressel, Ph.D.
Avon Products, Inc., Division Street, Suffern, NY 10901

H.B. Haimes, Ph.D.
Organogenesis, Inc., 83 Rogers Street, Cambridge, MA 02142

John F. Hansbrough, M.D.
Department of Surgery, University of California San Diego Medical Center, Box H640C, 225 Dickinson Street, San Diego, CA 82103

Jacqueline Hong
Department of Dermatology, Columbia University, New York, NY 10032

Izumi Ishii
Biochemical Research Laboratory, Nihon Menado Cosmetic Corporation, Gifu 505, Japan

D.T. Kagan
Organogenesis, Inc., 83 Rogers Street, Cambridge, MA 02142

P.D. Kemp, Ph.D.
Organogenesis, Inc., 83 Rogers Street, Cambridge, MA 02142

Betty M. Kong, Ph.D.
Department of Pharmacology and Toxicology, Research and Development, Colgate-Palmolive Company, 909 River Road, Piscataway, NJ 08854

Hiroaki Konishi
Biochemical Research Laboratory, Nihon Menado Cosmetic Corporation, Gifu 505, Japan

Paul J. Kostyniak, Ph.D.
State University of New York at Buffalo, Department of Pharmacology and Therapeutics and Toxicology Research Center, Buffalo, NY 14214

Robert A. Kreiger, Ph.D.
Health Risk Assessment Section, Minnesota Department of Health, 717 S.E. Delaware Street, P.O. Box 9441, Minneapolis, MN 55440

C.L. Krumdieck
Department of Nutritional Science, University of Alabama, Birmingham, AL 35294

Gerald S. Lazarus, M.D.
Department of Dermatology, University of Pennsylvania School of Medicine, 229 Medical Education Building, 36th & Hamilton Walk, Philadelphia, PA 19104-6065

Philip W. Ledger
ALZA Corporation, 950 Page Mill Road, P.O. Box 10950, Palo Alto, CA 94303-0802

V.S. Mason
Organogenesis, Inc, 83 Rogers Street, Cambridge, MA 02142

James P. McCulley, M.D.
Department of Ophthalmology, Southwestern Medical School, Dallas, TX 75235

Fathia Metwally
Department of Surgery, University of Connecticut School of Medicine, Farmington, CT 06032

Dale R. Meyer, Ph.D.
Department of Ophthalmology, Southwestern Medical School, Dallas, TX 75235

Denis Nadeau
Laboratoire de Caractérisation de l'Amiante, Département de Biologie, Faculte des Sciences, Université de Sherbrooke, Sherbrooke, Québec, Canada J1K 2R1

Osamu Nikaido
Pharmaceutical Sciences, Kanazawa University, Kanazawa 920, Japan

David A. Norris, M.D.
Department of Dermatology, University of Colorado Health Sciences Center, Denver, CO

Helen North-Root, Ph.D.
The Dial Corporation, Dial Technical Center, Scottsdale, AZ 85254

Daniel Paradis
Laboratoire de Caractérisation de l'Amiante, Département de Biologie, Faculte des Sciences, Université de Sherbrooke, Sherbrooke, Québec, Canada J1K 2R1

N.L. Parenteau, Ph.D.
Organogenesis, Inc., 83 Rogers Street, Cambridge, MA 02142

D.V. Parke
Surrey University, Guilford, Surrey, UK

T.H. Parmley
Department of Gynecology/Obstetrics, Johns Hopkins University School of Medicine, 601 North Wolfe Street, Park Building—Room B202, Baltimore, MD 21205

M.E. Prevo
ALZA Corporation, 950 Page Mill Road, P.O. Box 10950, Palo Alto, CA 94303-0802

Perveen Y. Rizvi
Colgate-Palmolive Company, 909 River Road, Piscataway, NJ 08854

Marcel Roberfroid
Laboratoire de Biochimie Toxicologique et Cancérologique, Université Catholique de Louvain, 73 Av. Mounier, B-1200 Bruxelles, Belgium

Edward F. Rossomando
Department of Biostructure and Function, University of Connecticut School of Medicine, Farmington, CT 06032

Una S. Ryan, Ph.D.
Department of Medicine (R58), University of Miami, School of Medicine, P.O. Box 016960, Miami, FL 33101

Robert A. Scala, Ph.D.
Exxon Biomedical Sciences, Inc., Mettlers Road, East Millstone, NJ 08873-2350

Sara Scheide
Department of Dermatology, Columbia University, New York, NY 10032

Paul L. Sherman
Monsanto Agriculture Company, 645 South Newstead Street, St. Louis, MO 63110

Charles Shopsis, Ph.D.
Department of Chemistry, Adelphi University, Garden City, NY 11530

Raymond E. Stoll, Ph.D.
Sandoz Research Institute, Building 404, Room 442, 59 Route 10, East Hanover, NJ 07936

Tsutomu Sugahara
Health Research Foundation, Kyoto 606, Japan

Keiji Suzuki
Division of Radiation Biology, School of Medicine, Yokohama City University, Yokohama 236, Japan

M. Swiderek, M.A.
Organogenesis, Inc., 83 Rogers Street, Cambridge, MA 02142

D.A. Swisher
ALZA Corporation, 950 Page Mill Road, P.O. Box 10950, Palo Alto, CA 94303-0802

Ruy Tchao, Ph.D.
Department of Pathology, Medical College of Pennsylvania, 3300 Henry Avenue, Philadelphia, PA 19129

James M. Vann
Department of Medicine, University of Miami School of Medicine, Miami, FL 33101

Pierre Vossen
Laboratoire de Biochimie Toxicologique et Cancérologique, Université Catholique de Louvain, 73 Av. Mounier, B-1200 Bruxelles, Belgium

Peter Ward, M.D.
Department of Pathology, University of Michigan Medical School, 1315 Catherine Road, Ann Arbor, MI 48109

Kimiko Watanabe
Division of Radiation Biology, School of Medicine, Yokohama City University, Yokohama 236, Japan

Masami Watanabe
Division of Radiation Biology, School of Medicine, Yokohama City University, Yokohama 236, Japan

Paul T. Wegener
Clonetics Corporation, San Diego, CA 92123

Peggy A. Winzenburger
Monsanto Agricultural Company, 645 South Newstead Street, St. Louis, MO 63110

G. Witz
UMDNJ Robert Wood Johnson Medical School, Piscataway, NJ

G.H.I. Wolfgang
Department of Pharmacology and Toxicology, University of Arizona, Tucson, AZ 85724

Uri Wormser, Ph.D.
Department of Pharmacology, The Hebrew University—Hadassah Medical School, P.O.B. 1172, 91010 Jerusalem, Israel

Gerhard Zbinden, M.D.
Institut fur Toxicologie, der Eidgenossischen Technischen Hochschule und der Universitat Zurich, Schorenstrasse 16, CH8603 Swerzenbach, Switzerland

Part 1

Symposium Presentations

A. Epidermal Toxicity

A1

Skin Toxicity

LOWELL A. GOLDSMITH

University of Rochester
School of Medicine and Dentistry
601 Elmwood Avenue
Rochester, NY 14642

ABSTRACT:

The epidermis contains several cell types including keratinocytes, melanocytes and Langerhans cells. Knowledge of the biochemistry of the cytoskeleton, cell envelope and keratinocyte lipids is growing rapidly allowing the toxicologist to critically examine the applicability of in vitro epidermal systems to the problem of epidermal toxicity.

INTRODUCTION:

Skin toxicity is related to a set of integrated and synergistic reactions involving several cell types within the epidermis and dermis. The epidermis is the initial site of interaction between chemicals and the envirnoment; a few minutes will be spent describing epidermal structure and function and the integration of epidermal function with the rest of the skin.

A simple model will be presented since even the most sophisticated of minds can sometimes use a model; the model is that of the skin as a shopping mall.

Why is the skin like a shopping mall? It is a shopping mall because there are multiple independent businesses in the skin with multiple independent functions. Each of these businesses has its individual profit and loss statement, and just like a shopping mall, there is frequently a major business e.g. a department store in the mall; one of the major businesses in the skin mall are the keratinocytes.

These are chain stores, stores distributed in other sites in the body, in addition to the skin, the melanocytes and Langerhans cells, cells of the immune system; there are little, individual boutiques in the skin. In the epidermis there is the Merkel cell boutique and thy-one positive immune cells, another boutique.

Why are the cells together? There is a profit or advantage from being together. Maybe it's the use of common parking lot analogous to the blood supply or there may be advantages of integrating function and developing efficient function by being close together. Those of you who have started to invest in real estate now that the stock market has melted down know that in real estate, it's location, location, location which is extremely important. In the skin location is a critical variable.

It is interesting that in our epidermal shopping mall there is very even spacing of various immigrant cell populations like the Langerhans cells and the melanocytes; one of the major questions in epidermal biology is the nature of the factors controlling that spacing and how these populations of immigrant cells are integrated. We know that even among epidermal keratinocytes there are differences in their membrane structure, basement membrane zones, and even their mitotic capability depending upon where they are located within epidermis.

DISCUSSION:

One of the questions to be addressed in the next decade is how the various patterns and interrelationships between the different cell populations develop. There has been major efforts in the past decade looking at individual cell types and their physiological and pathological functions. Certainly one of our challenges, and one I think it's going to be very important for understanding various toxicities, is understanding how the various cells inter-react, e.g. how metabolic changes or products e.g. interleukins from the keratinocytes affect the Langerhans cell.

The keratinocyte is a cell which lives to die. The cells and intercellular lipids of the stratum corneum, which we think of as normally dead cells, fulfill the function of the stratum corneum. They can't multiply but because of their programmed pattern of cell death and the relationships between structural proteins, cell envelope proteins and lipids they are the major regulator of water and small molecule transport through the epidermis. There has been tremendous progress in the past decade defining the various structural protein inside the cells, the keratins, the filaggrins which is the new name for the keratohyalin matrix proteins of the keratinocytes and cross-linked proteins of the cell envelope, the very protease-resistant structure inside the epidermal cells.

Over the past decade the cytoskeleton of epithelial cells has been precisely defined. Epithelial cells have extremely organized cytoskeletons, the cytokeratins (1). The cytokeratins have important genetic and structural relationships with other intermediate filament proteins, the lamins of the cell nucleus, vimentin of the fibroblast and the smooth muscle protein, desmin.

There are different genes controlling the keratins and these genes are frequently organized into coordinatedly controlled gene families. Vitamin A is a major modulator of these epidermal keratins and when investigating cellular toxicity cells in the various artificial systems discussed today, the amount and role of Vitamin A in the <u>in vitro</u> system my be a critical feature controlling or modulating toxic effect. Vitamin A is an agent that we need to know more about since it profoundly affects epidermal differentiation (2,3).

The cytoskeletal system because of its presumed function, because of the intrinsic beauty of many of the patterns formed by its molecules is the subject of intense study. Although we know a lot about various structural and biochemical features of the cytokeratins, their functional characteristics are still incompletely understood.

We've learned during the past decade that keratins are part of a superfamily of molecules with different types of intermediate filament proteins. Intermediate filaments, including the cytokeratins, follow a very orderly organization (4). The molecules have an N-terminal region of random conformation; there's a long, regular run of α-helix, and then there is a more random sections at the C-terminus. They all have the same central rod domain of a very fixed length and N terminal and C terminal domains. Keratins may react with each other through the helical regions and with other molecules in the cells through the non-helical N and C-terminal portions of the molecule.

Cytokeratins can be separated into two families of proteins: one of basic and one of acidic charge (1). These proteins constitute about 70% of the epidermal cell mass. Combined isoelectric focusing and SDS-electrophoresis can be used to identify the individual cytokeratins. The proteins are products of individual genes under individual yet coordinate control. Henry

SKIN AS A SHOPPING MALL

Multiple independent businesses
Individual profit-loss statements
Major businesses and function
  Keratinocytes
Chains: Melanocytes, immune system
Boutiques: Merkel cells, Thy-1 cells

Profit being together-parking lots: blood supply

Location/ Location/ Location

KERATINOCYTE BIOLOGY

Lives to Die

Function in Dead Cells

Structural Proteins and Lipids

Keratins

Filaggrin (Keratohyalin)

Cell Envelope

KERATINS

Epithelial cells - cytoskeleton

Suprafamilies - IF - lamins, vimentins,

Neurofilaments, desmin

Individual coordinately controlled genes

Organized into gene families

Vitamin A

FILAGGRINS
Matrix Proteins
Terminal differentiation marker
Large precursor
Post-translational modifications
Phosphorylation, dephosphorylation,
Proteolysis, histidine deamination
Produces free amino acids, urocanic acid, PCA

Sun, who was at Hopkins and is now at NYU, has shown that the keratins follow a very orderly set of patterns during differentiation. Simple epithelia tend to have lower molecular weight keratins and as epithelia stratify in the skin higher molecular weight keratins are synthesized. As we hear about various in vitro systems, the ability of those systems to mimic various aspects of differentiation with respect to keratin patterns which are found within the normal epidermis, should be carefully delimited.

Filaggrins are matrix proteins and are important marker of terminal differentiation. They are synthesized as a large molecular weight precursor which has a variety of post-translational changes including phosphorylation, dephosphorylation, proteolysis and deamination (5). The majority of the free amino acid pool of stratum corneum comes from this protein; water holding capabilities of epidermis are related to these free amino acid pools. The ability to produce a fully formed normal stratum corneum is potentiated by having normal amounts filaggrin and this molecule will be very important to follow as one examines in vitro systems for their relevance to the in
state of the epidermis.

The cell envelope is intracellular, highly cross-linked and very insoluble structure resistant to various proteolytic enzymes and is thought to have protective functions within the stratum corneum cells (6). It is cross-linked by enzymes called tranglutaminases, several precursor proteins are incorporated into this cell envelope. There is a debate whether there are specific precursors going to this cell envelope or whether a protein mixture ends up in the envelope as a kind of a dust bin in which whatever proteins may be around at a particular point in time and location just may be swept up into this cell envelope. This an important and interesting area for the toxicologist to follow since this cell envelope ends up to be a major protective element inside cells.

Lipids are incredibly important for the functional characteristics of the epidermis. Most of the permeability pathways in cells function via lipids (7). Lipids are present between the cells in the stratum corneum. There is an intracellular lipid-containing organelle, the keratinosome, in the lower layers of the epidermis. Late in differentiation its contents are expelled intercellularly.

CELL ENVELOPE

Cross-linked insoluble

Transglutaminases

Dust-bin vs. specific precursors

Involucrin

MEMBRANE LIPIDS

Keratinsome precursor

Late in differentiation

Intracellular/extracellular transition

Cholesterol Sulfate

Alkanes

Acylglucosylceramide

Nutritional effects

MACROORGANIZATION OF THE MALL

Even spacing of immigrant cells

Differences in structure and mitotic

Capability depending on location in ridge pattern

Communication pathway

Development of patterns and interrelationships

BASEMENT MEMBRANE ZONE

Origin and integration

Epidermal origin for many components

Transport and Metastases

Communication

Lipids such as cholesterol sulfate which seem to have a major role in binding cells together and also various acylglucosylceramides which form major water holding lipids and the water barrier in the skin are among the lipids, in the intracellular space of the stratum corneum. They contain linoleic acid, 16 to 30 carbon lipids and sphingosine. One of the questions that we'll ask our speakers is the role of lipids in their system?

Lipid nutrition can affect skin lipids, and with many people altering dietary lipids for anti-inflammatory and anti-cholesterol effects, alterations of the skin lipids may have effects on toxicity.

Finally is the basement membrane zone, a critical area between the epidermis and the dermis, contains a variety of structural molecules that are made by epidermal and dermal cells, secreted and transported and then are integrated into a zone that is very important for transport, wound healing, metastases and for communication between the epidermis and dermis (8).

REFERENCES

1. Cooper, D., Schermer A., and Sun, T-T. (1985). Biology of Disease. Classification of human epithelia and their neoplasms using monoclonal antibodies to keratins: strategies, applications, and limitations. Lab. Invest. 52:243.

2. Tseng, S.C.G., Hatchell, D., Tierney, N., Huang, J.W., and Sun, T-T. (1984). Expression of specific keratin markers by rabbit corneal, conjunctival, and esopahageal epithelia during vitamin A deficiency. J. Cell Biol. 99:2279.

3. Eckert R.L., and Green, H. (1984). Cloning of cDNAs specifying vitamin A-responsive human keratins. Proc. Natl. Acad. Sci. (USA) 81:4321.

4. Marchuk, D., McCrohon, S., and Fuchs, E. (1984). Remarkable conservation of structure among intermediate filament genes. Cell 39:491.

5. Haydock, P.V., and Dale, B.A. (1986). The repetititve structure of the profilaggrin gene as deomonstrated using epidermal profilaggrin cDNA. J. Biol. Chem. 261:12520.

6. Simon, M., and Green, H. (1985). Enzymatic cross-linking of involucrin and other proteins by keratinocyte particulates in vitro. Cell 40:677.

7. Long, S.A., Wertz, P.W., Strauss, J.S., and Downing D.T. (1985). Human stratum corneum polar lipids and desquamation. Arch. Dermatol. Res. 277:284.

8. Terranova, V.P., Hujanen, E.S., and Martin, G.R. (1986). Basement membrane and invasive activity of metastatic tumor cells. JNCI 77:311.

A2

Proteinase Biology in Keratinocyte Culture: Possible Utility as a Model for Toxicological Testing

GERALD S. LAZARUS

Department of Dermatology
University of Pennsylvania School of Medicine
Philadelphia, PA 19104

Culture of human skin cells may provide opportunities to evaluate the toxic effects of agents. Culture of human: keratinocytes, fibroblasts, endothelial cells and mast cells may provide alternate means for testing of cutaneous toxins. Investigators are now defining indicators of cellular activation and damage in cell culture systems which may be useful in predicting toxicological effects of pertinent molecules.

Proteinases are enzymes which hydrolyze peptide bonds and cleave the backbone of protein molecules. They are quite specific in their activities because they recognize well-defined sequences of amino acids around the site of cleavage. Because of this specificity they play a major role in biological control. Proteinases degrade proteins and peptides which are taken into the cell. Protein synthesis uses single amino acids and proteinases cleave protein molecules to their constituitive amino acids. Proteinases are the machinery that rids the cells of damaged subcellular organelles such as ribosomes, mitochondria, etc. Recently it has become clear that the specific cleavage of protein molecules is very important in the control of their biological activity (1). Proteolytic cleavage appears to be a means by which the organism targets biologically important molecules to the appropriate site of action. Collagen is synthesized as a precursor molecule procollagen which does not easily form fibrils and fibers. Cleavage of the precursor molecule procollagen to collagen is important at the appropriate site in the formation of connective tissue structure. Many hormones are made as precursor molecules which are biologically inactive. Activation of the precursor hormone to the active hormone, at the site of action is produced by proteolytic cleavage; an example is the activation of proinsulin to insulin. Many proteinases are made as inactive precursor zzymogen molecules. Often, proproteinases are activated by other proteinases. Many metabolic processes involve hydrolysis of proteins; proteinases subserve these very important actions. Proteinases are intimately related to cell division and movement of cells through tissue is closely coupled to activation of proteolytic processes. It appears that activation of proteinases in malignant cells is important in spread through tissue and metastases. Cellular adhesion is profoundly affected by proteinase metabolism and studies of pemphigus have substantial biological importance because they address the issue of how cells adhere within a tissue (2). One of the most dramatic examples of programmed catabolism in nature is differentiation during keratinization. The rapid loss of cellular organelles as cells reach the stratum corneum is an extraordinary example of highly precise proteolytic activation. Another very exciting new area of investigation is the role of proteinases as biologically important mediators in inflammation. The complement, clotting and fibrinolytic cascade are a series of highly regulated proteolytic events.

Activation of C1 and production of the biologically active complement fragments of C3A and C5A are products of proteolytic activity. Bradykinin is activated by proteolytic cleavage and a number of biologically important factors in the clotting and fibrinolytic cascade are proteolytic fragments. Consequently, proteinases are extremely important in the pathophysiology of inflammation. Proteinases function in the induction of the inflammatory process by cleaving molecules and producing mediators. They play a central role in recruiting inflammatory cells and the movement of cells themselves, and finally proteinases are the factors which destroy tissue. The most obvious example is the role of the proteinase collagenase in the degradation of collagen. There are certain disease states which demonstrate the pivotal role of proteinases in disease process. Rheumatoid arthritis characterized by dissolution of joints and inflammation is clearly related to the synthesis and production of proteolytic enzymes. The lack of the alpha-1 proteinase inhibitor is associated with destruction of lung tissue in certain genetically determined varieties of pulmonary disease. There is preliminary evidence that oxidation of proteinase inhibitors in the lung by cigarette smoke allows proteinases to function without inhibition which is involved in the tissue destruction of lungs of chronic smokers. The work of Eisen and Bauer with epidermolysis bullosa suggests that the dystrophic form of this disease is related to abnormalities in collagenase metabolism.

Plasminogen activators are enzymes which specifically activate the inactive precursor enzyme plasminogen to the broad specificity proteinase plasmin (3). Plasminogen activator itself has a very narrow spectrum of action, but plasmin has a broad specificity and it can induce multiple degradative events in the extracellular millieu. Plasminogen activator is a serine proteinase operative at physiological or neutral pH. There are two absolutely distinctive plasminogen activators. The first is tissue type. This is a molecule of 72,000 MW which is secreted to the extracellular environment. It has a fibrin binding site so that it will target to a fibrin clot within the circulation. This is the enzyme being used in the therapy of coronary artery disease and it has extremely potent fibrinolytic activity. Under normal circumstances epidermis does not make tissue plasminogen activator. The second plasminogen activator is urokinase type. This enzyme is made in epidermal cells. It has a lower molecular weight, 55,000, and it lacks a binding site for fibrin. It can bind to a cell receptor on the outside of the cell surface, and decorates the plasma membrane so it can function in the immediate extracellular environment around cells.

Many cells can produce both types of plasminogen activator. The process of selection begins when DNA encodes for a specific messenger RNA which instructs the ribosomes to make the appropriate plasminogen activator. The presence of the specific messenger RNA provides a unique opportunity to measure the very beginning of the sequence in enzyme production. In the case of urokinase the enzyme is made as an inactive precursor zymogen which is secreted and can then bind itself on to a specific cell surface receptor. At this site it is difficult to measure the urokinase enzymatically because methods of detection require enzymatic activity. The urokinase bound to the cell is then activated by proteolytic cleavage - which now permits the enzyme to cleave plasminogen to plasmin. By contrast, tissue plasminogen activator is exported from the cell; it is also made as an inactive precursor which also requires proteolytic activation. The same cells can also make inhibitors of plasminogen activator. In epidermis this is primarily of the placental type (4). This is a control step so that when plasminogen activator is activated in the extracellular environment it can be inhibited at an appropriate time. In tissue there are other important control mechanisms. Ten per cent of the protein in serum is various proteinase inhibitors. These inhibitors can leak out of the vessel and also inhibit proteinases. Once enzyme is bound to inhibitors, complexes are cleared from the circulation. The complexities involved in measuring enzyme activity are now clear. That is why measurement of specific MRNA's is important to investigate proteinase systems. Over the years we have investigated the role of plasminogen activator in epidermal biology. Our studies of human keratinocytes treated with pemphigus antibody can be adapted to study potentially toxic agents. Pemphigus is an autoimmune disease characterized by cutaneous blisters and erosions and the presence of an antibody to specific epithelial cell surface constituents (5).

Bellone and Leone (6) first reported that organ cultures of human skin exposed to pemphigus antisera developed acantholysis (blistering in vitro). Subsequently, Michel and collaborators exploited the organ culture model to investigate the pathophysiology of pemphigus (7). We demonstrated that keratinocyte cultures were an intriguing method to study acantholysis in vitro and suggested that proteinases were involved in acantholysis (8). In a series of publications we demonstrated that pemphigus antibodies bound to keratinocytes in culture and induced the synthesis of plasminogen activator (8). We have also shown that acantholysis induced by pemphigus antibody in organ cultures can be blocked by inhibition of PA directly with antibodies to urokinase or with inhibitors of the plasmin system (5). Recent studies of PA inhibitors occurring in normal human keratinocytes also support the role for plasminogen activator in acantholysis. In our most recent work we have also observed that within three hours of incubating human keratinocytes with pemphigus antibody there are increases of messenger RNA for urokinase (9). The observation that binding of antibody to cell surface of keratinocytes induces synthesis and secretion of PA suggests that this biological event may have a somewhat broader applicability. Becker, Ossowski and Reich (10) incubated cell lines with cell surface antibodies and were able to induce PA synthesis and secretion. Our laboratory demonstrated that incubation of melanoma cells with anti-cell surface melanoma antibodies also increased the synthesis and secretion of plasminogen activator (11). These observations indicate that a variety of cell types will respond in a similar fashion to membrane perturbation with alterations in proteinase activity.

Proteinases play a major role in physiology and pathophysiology. Proteinase metabolism can be studied in human keratinocyte culture, and this model can be used to simulate a disease state. Indeed, addition of pemphigus immunoglobulin to human keratinocytes in culture does induce activation of the plasminogen activator system which appears to play a significant role in the cell separation or acantholysis which is characteristic of this disease. The metabolism of plasminogen activators is complicated, but tools are available by which the various components of the system can be quantitatively determined. It seems reasonable to consider the possibility that alterations in proteinase metabolism in cell cultures can be used to evaluate the effects of agents on epithelial biology. Such systems could provide tools which might be of use in toxicology generally and cutaneous toxicology specifically.

REFERENCES

1. OGAWA, H., LAZARUS, G.S. and HOPSU-HAVU, V.K., (1985), The Biological Role of Proteinases and Their Inhibitors in Skin. University of Tokyo Press.

2. SINGER, K. H., HASHIMOTO, K., JENSEN, P.J., MORIOKA, S. and LAZARUS, G.S., (1985), Pathogenesis of autoimmunity in pemphigus. Ann Rev Immunol 3:87.

3. DANO, K., ANDREASEN, P.A., GRONDAHL-HANSEN, J., KRISTENSEN, P., NIELSEN, L.S. and SKRIVER, L. (1985), Plasminogen activators, tissue degradation, and cancer. Adv Cancer Res 44:139.

4. HASHIMOTO, K., WUN T-C., BAIRD, J., MORIOKA, S., LAZARUS, G.S. and JENSEN, P.J., Keratinocyte inhibitors of plasminogen activator: Characterization and ability to prevent pemphigus IgG induced acantholysis. submitted.

5. JENSEN, P.J., MORIOKA, S., HASHIMOTO, K., SINGER, K.H. and LAZARUS, G.S., (1988) Chapter 37 - Pemphigus: An auto-antibody-mediated dermatosis. In - Inflammation: Basic Principles and Clinical Correlates, J.I. Gallin, I.M. Goldstein, Snyderman, R. (Eds) Raven Press, New York, 695-702.

6. BELLONE, A.G. and LEONE, V., (1956), Richerche sull influenza esercitata da sieri di soggetti san o affetti da pemfigo su pelle umans normale e pemfigosa coltivata in vitro. G Ital Dermatol Sifilol 2:97.

7. MICHEL, B. and KO, C.S., (1977), An organ culture model for the study of pemphigus acantholysis. Brit J Dermatol 96:295.

8. HASHIMOTO, K., SHAFRAN, K.M., WEBBER P.S., LAZARUS, G.S. and SINGER, K.H., (1983), Anti-cell surface pemphigus autoantibody stimulates plasminogen activator activity of human epidermal cells. J Exp Med 157:259.

9. HASHIMOTO, K., JENSEN, P.J., BAIRD, J. and LAZARUS, G.S., (1987), Pemphigus antibody induces synthesis of mRNA for urokinase type plasminogen activator in cultured human epidermal cells. Clin Res 35:690A.

(10) BECKER, D., OSSOWSKI, L. and REICH, E, (1981), Induction of plasminogen activator synthesis by antibodies. J Exp Med 154:385.

(11) SINGER, K.H., HASHIMOTO, K., STUHLMILLER, G.M. and LAZARUS, G.S., (1982), Antibody-induced release of cellular proteinases. J Immunol 128:1321.

A3

Testskin: A Hybrid Organism Covered by a Living Human Skin Equivalent Designed for Toxicity and Other Testing

E. BELL, N.L. PARENTEAU, H.B. HAIMES, R.J. GAY, P.D. KEMP, T.W. FOFONOFF, V.S. MASON, D.T. KAGAN, and M. SWIDEREK

Organogenesis, Inc.
83 Rogers Street
Cambridge, MA 02142

ABSTRACT

A hybrid organism, TESTSKIN (TM), has been fabricated to serve as a biotest system to evaluate the actions of substances brought into contact with the skin. It consists of a living integument that surrounds a core through which a circulation passes. The under surface of the dermis is separated physically from the outer surface of the stratum corneum of the epidermis, so that a substance applied to the latter can reach the dermis and the circulation only by passing through the skin. The integument is an adaptation of the Living Skin Equivalent constituted from cells and intercellular matrix molecules. Morphology and biosynthetic capabilities resemble those of skin and it exhibits long term viability in vitro. It has been grafted successfully to experimental animals and on grafting functions like full thickness skin. It has been used as a model system to study psoriasis and responses of skin to various substances.

INTRODUCTION

The need for a source of viable human skin to test substance toxicity, irritation and allergenicity, to determine the rate of entry of substances into the body through the skin, to test and develop cosmetic and pharmaceutical agents, and to study skin diseases and their treatment modalities has long been apparent. A large body of experimental data based on the use of excised human skin [1-3], and on the use of human skin in situ in volunteers [4-7] covering certain aspects of toxicity and other testing, exists.

The references cited are exemplary only and are not meant to be inclusive. It is clear, however, from the broad experience analyzed, that major problems are encountered with skin obtained from a cadaver or from a plastic surgery patient. Such skin is moribund at the outset since autolytic processes are triggered by removal; thus the life span of the tissues is necessarily short, and, more importantly, their exact state of health is difficult to assess. An equally critical shortcoming is the lack of availability of skin from these sources for testing. Similarly, the usefulness of the volunteer is severely limited. Most substances cannot be tested on human volunteers and individual differences among volunteers may be great enough to rule out the significance of the data obtained. TESTSKIN (TM) has been designed to meet the need for standardized viable human skin for a broad range of test requirements. It is an adaptation of Living Skin Equivalent (LSE) developed at MIT as a skin replacement [8-13] and as a skin biotest system [14-17].

<u>TESTSKIN (TM) a Hybrid Organism</u>: An organism is a complex structure of interdependent and subordinate elements whose relations and properties are largely determined by their function in the whole. We report here in prototype form a hybrid organism that is constituted with heterogeneous elements, in this instance, some living and some synthetic. We have given the name TESTSKIN (TM) to the organism which has a synthetic skeleton and a synthetic circulatory system, but is covered by a full thickness LSE and will serve as a skin biotest system. TESTSKIN (TM) is the subject of this symposium report.

<u>Living Skin Equivalent</u>: The properties and uses of the LSE have been reported on [8-17]; however, this symposium provides an opportunity to present an updated review of the LSE, as well as to unveil TESTSKIN (TM).

<u>Fabricating the LSE</u>: The LSE is made with normal human cells derived from a biopsy. The LSE consists of a dermis covered by a multilayered epidermis. The dermis is made up of dermal fibroblasts and a combination of matrix molecules normally present in the extracellular spaces of the tissue. In actual skin, the extracellular matrix molecules are the secreted biosynthetic products of the dermal fibroblasts; in reconstituted skin, they are obtained from other sources and combined with the appropriate cells. However, the cells of the resulting dermal equivalent are biosynthetically active and secrete products that enrich the extracellular matrix provided by the fabricator. Thus, the extracellular matrix of the dermal equivalent is a biosynthetic hybrid containing the secretory products of resident cells as well as the matrix molecules derived from other sources, added at the time of initial fabrication.

When the dermal fibroblasts, the matrix molecules and the nutrients are combined and poured into a mold, the mixture gels, taking on the geometry of the mold that is preserved as the cells interact with the matrix polymers and condense them [18]. The volume of the cell matrix mixture diminishes at the expense of fluid that is expressed from it (Fig. 1a). Microscopically, the cells play the key role of collecting and organizing the extracellular collagen fibrils whose concentration per unit volume may be increased as much as 30-fold. The net effect of this activity is also a comparable increase, per unit volume, of the number of cells and other formed elements

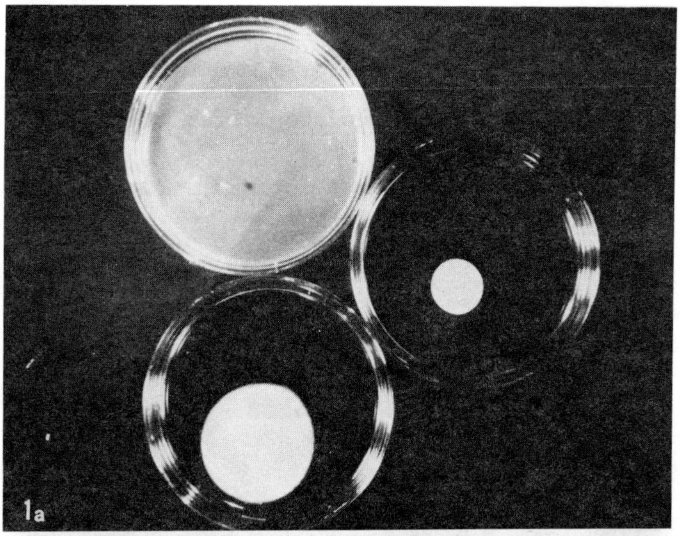

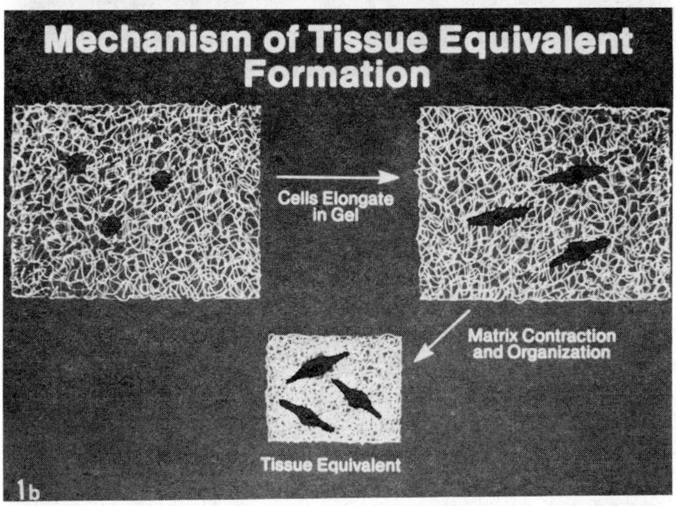

Fig. 1--a-Condensation of Dermal Equivalent as a function of time. Volume decrease observed over a four day period. An equilibrium size is attained by the end of four days. b- Schematic representation of events leading to tissue condensation. When the cell-matrix mixture is poured into a mold, the collagen polymerizes into a random network of fibrils. Fibroblasts, originally spherical, after removal from a culture plate by trypsin, elongate and extend filopodia that interact with, collect and compact the collagen fibrils. This activity causes fluid to be expressed from the forming tissue leading to a decrease in volume and increased concentration of cells and intercellular matrix constituents.

(Fig. 1b). While the volume of an unconstrained tissue decreases uniformly in all dimensions, a tissue such as the dermis cast around a core, can be constrained to condense in the thickness mode only. Once the dermis has contracted, it serves as an accommodating substrate for the proliferation of keratinocytes. Cells plated onto the dermal surface divide and differentiate forming a continuous multilayered epidermis (Fig. 2). The combined dermis and epidermis make up the LSE that continues to develop in vitro.

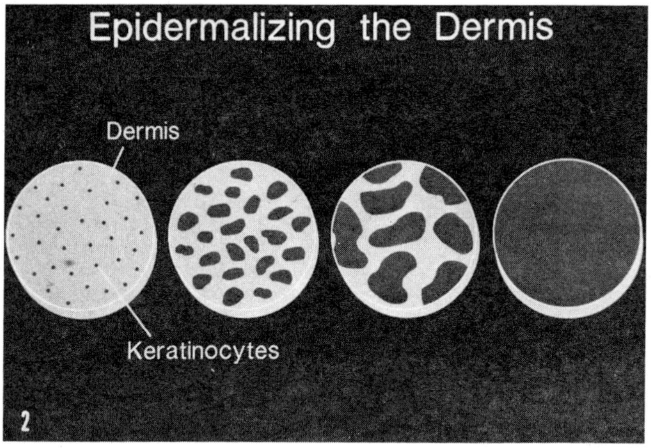

Fig. 2 -- Schematic showing second step in LSE formation. Keratinocytes are plated onto the surface of the dermal equivalent. They divide, spread and differentiate vertically providing a multilayered epidermis that completely covers the dermal equivalent.

<u>TESTSKIN</u> (TM): TESTSKIN (TM) is a hybrid organism designed for toxicity testing and other tests that require a patch of human skin. TESTSKIN (TM) incorporates the LSE that is cast around a hollow or porous core that serves several functions: the core provides a skeleton which determines the final shape of TESTSKIN (TM); it provides an internal circulation in contact with the dermal equivalent; and it insures that the internal living surface of TESTSKIN (TM) is isolated physically from its outer surface. While the inner surface of TESTSKIN (TM) is bathed by a circulating fluid, the outer surface is in contact with the ambient atmosphere. The prototype of the chamber within which TESTSKIN (TM) is cast is shown in Fig. 3. It contains a hollow core on a stem through which incurrent and excurrent elements of the circulation pass. Circulating fluid can be introduced by pumping or by gravity feed. The excurrent flow can be fraction collected or recirculated. To dermalize TESTSKIN (TM) the ingredients required for the fabrication of a dermal equivalent are introduced aseptically into the casting chamber. As the cell-matrix components become compacted, fluid is expressed and the developing dermis condenses around the core (Fig. 4). When the process of condensation reaches equilibrium, the dermis consists of a tissue

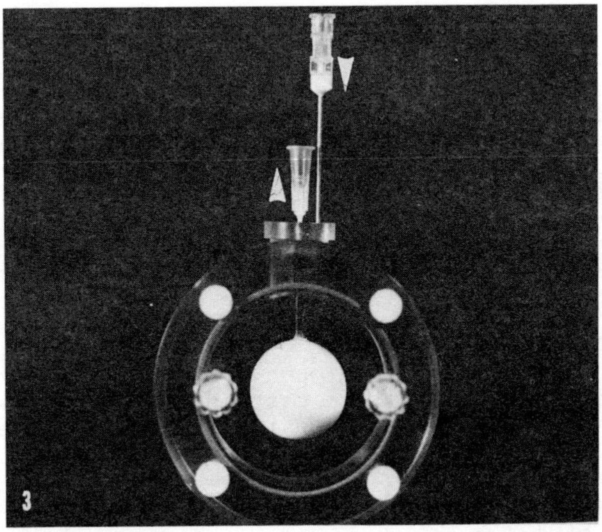

Fig. 3 -- Prototype chamber or casting mold in which TESTSKIN (TM) is cast. It contains a hollow or porous core through which fluid can flow. The fluids supply nutrients to the LSE cast around the core and leave through an exit port. Arrows show direction of flow.

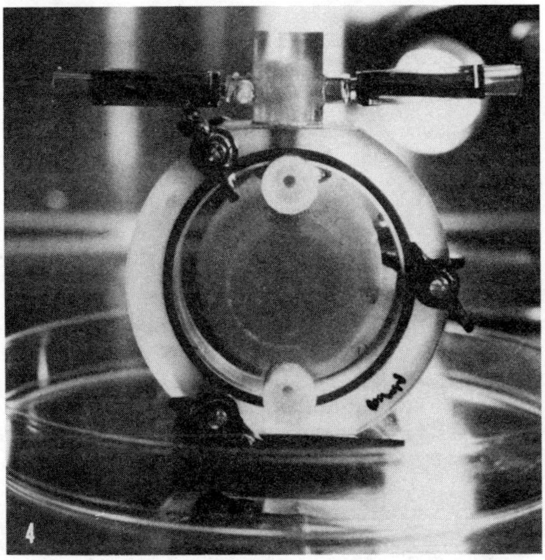

Fig. 4 -- The casting mold is filled with the constituents of the dermal equivalent, that is, the cell-matrix mixture that gels and condenses around the core. The process has begun in the illustration shown and fluid expressed from the contracting tissue is seen in the periphery of the chamber.

approximately 1.0mm in thickness and is ready for epidermalization. Keratinocytes in suspension are applied to the outer surface of the dermal equivalent at a rate of 1 x 10(5) cells/cm(2) and by four days after epidermalization it is covered by a stratified epidermis; the fabrication of TESTSKIN (TM) is then complete. Differentiation of the epidermis and biosynthesis of products for secretion by keratinocytes and dermal fibroblasts are ongoing events. TESTSKIN (TM) becomes self-contained in four to five days after it is epidermalized, that is, fluid circulating through it internally will not leak out. The complete physical separation of the inner dermal surface of TESTSKIN (TM) and its outer epidermal surface is insured since TESTSKIN (TM) bonds itself to the neck of the core in the course of its formation.

Fluid can be pumped through TESTSKIN (TM) through a closed circulatory loop (Fig. 5) or, to test the passage of a substance through TESTSKIN (TM), a substance is applied to the epidermalized surface of the hybrid organism and its entry into the internal circulation of TESTSKIN (TM) may then be monitored by collecting fractions of medium passing out of the excurrent arm of the circulatory system.

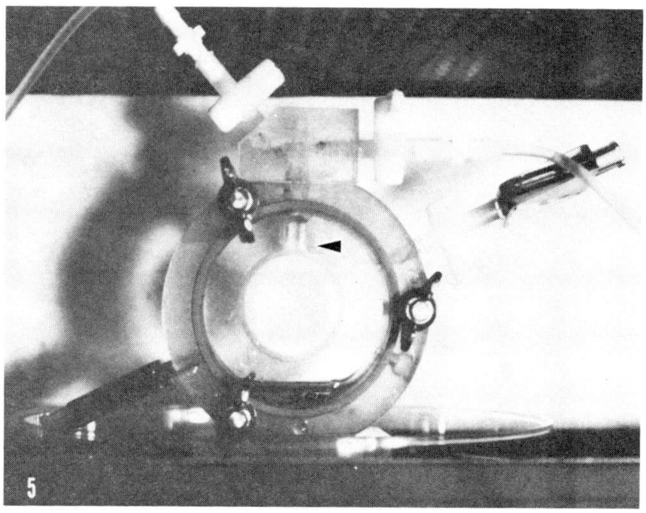

Fig. 5 -- The core of TESTSKIN (TM) is covered by the complete LSE on all sides. The LSE bonds to the neck of the TESTSKIN (TM) core. In the prototype shown, TESTSKIN (TM) is served by a closed circulatory loop.

The Histologic and Biosynthetic Likeness of the Living Skin Equivalent to Actual Skin: The LSE undergoes remarkably complete differentiation. The collagen concentration in the dermal equivalent approaches that of embryonic skin by the time the dermal equivalent reaches an equilibrium size. The fibroblasts of the dermal equivalent are surrounded by relatively well organized arrays of compacted collagen fibrils. This condition is brought about by an ongoing interaction between the cells and the originally random network of collagen fibrils. Throughout the period of maturation, the dermal fibroblasts are biosynthetically active. Collagen type I and small quantities of type III are synthesized, secreted, processed and added to the collagen matrix provided by the fabricators and organized by the cells [19]. These events are comparable to those which occur in vivo, and may be distinguished from what happens when cells are grown on a monolayer. On a monolayer, the same cells cannot process the collagen they synthesize [20,21,22], nor can the unprocessed collagen add to a preexisting substrate. In addition to collagen, we have shown that other molecules are added to the intercellular matrix of the dermal equivalent. These include fibronectin, hyaluronic acid, dermatan sulfate, and chondroitin sulfate. The latter glycosaminoglycan is usually present only in embryonic skin. The full range of molecular additions to the dermal equivalent by the resident cells has not yet been assayed, but it is likely to be much larger than the molecules already identified.

The coverage of the dermal equivalent by keratinocytes plated onto it is rapid. By four hours after plating, there is nearly a confluent monolayer of adherent cells. By four days, there are well-developed basal and suprabasal layers and as many as four to six strata of squamous cells in various stages of differentiation layered above the basal cells with numerous desmosomal attachments in the suprabasal layers (Fig. 6). In some areas, a horny layer can be seen.

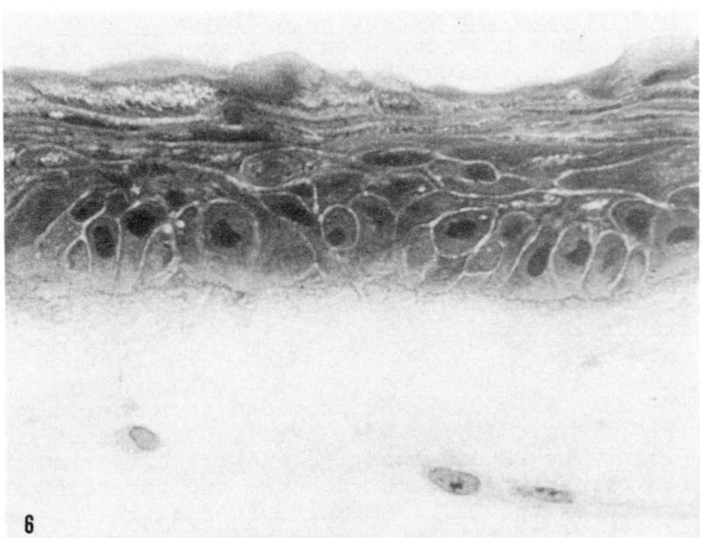

Fig. 6 -- The LSE four days after epidermalization is about 1.1mm thick. The dermis, shown in part, is 10x the thickness of the multilayered keratinizing epidermis. Basal, suprabasal and squamous layers are seen. The dermis has a well-organized mat of collagen fibrils.

A fully-differentiated stratum corneum is apparent by ten to twelve days [9,16] and by three to four weeks, a continuous basal lamina has developed between the dermis and epidermis [17]. The biosynthesis of keratins ranging between 55KD and 67KD by keratinocytes in the epidermis of the LSE has been demonstrated by PAGE [16,23] and by immunocytochemistry [24] staining of LSEs with monoclonal antibodies. Antibodies to filaggrin [24] stain the granules in the stratum granulosa and involucrin is present throughout the squamous layers.

The Graftability of the Living Skin Equivalent: Perhaps the ultimate test for judging the likeness of the LSE to actual skin is to ask whether it performs the functions of skin when it is grafted. These include being vascularized, blocking wound contraction, and being capable of self repair. it has been shown in grafts to experimental animal models that the LSE performs all of these functions [9-13]. It becomes so well integrated with adjacent host skin that it is difficult grossly to observe a suture line at the edge of the graft. The grafted skin does not become hypertrophic; it does develop a highly organized dermis in which the normal dense basket weave organization of the collagen matrix is observed. Most important, the grafted skin persists. Its persistence for the lifetime of the recipient animal, the rat, has been demonstrated by applying grafts fabricated with female cells to male hosts. Analysis by karyotyping of grafted skin at intervals after grafting provided rigorous proof that the female genotype characterized at least 50% of the graft cell population.

The Living Skin Equivalent as a Biotest System: The Dermal equivalent (DE) alone has been used as a wound healing model to access the effects of various hormonal substances such as cortisone and dexamethasone on the process of contraction brought about by the interaction of dermal fibroblasts with collagen fibrils [25]. In a study dealing with the biosynthesis of perinuclear peroxidases by fibroblasts in the dermal equivalent it was revealed that the permeability of dermal fibroblasts to various substances was determined by conditions of culturing. While cells in the DE, like cells in freshly biopsied tissue, were permeable to the reagent diaminobenzidine, cells grown on a plastic surface were relatively impermeable, suggesting that cells not incorporated into a tissue behave aberrantly.

The DE cast as a disk and provided with a skin punch biopsy in its center [14] (Fig. 7), has been used in studies of the disease psoriasis [15]. The DE was constituted with either normal or psoriatic fibroblasts from human donors, and the rate of outgrowth over the surface of the DE by normal epidermal cells, keratinocytes, was measured. Radial epibolic outgrowth of the epidermis was found to be proportional to the amount of newly made DNA synthesized by its cells. The significant finding was that psoriatic fibroblasts induced hyperproliferative outgrowth in normal epidermis, pointing for the first time to dermal cells as a possible cause of the disease.

CONCLUSION

The LSE has many properties of actual skin: it resembles skin morphologically, its biosynthetic repertoire is similar, it is

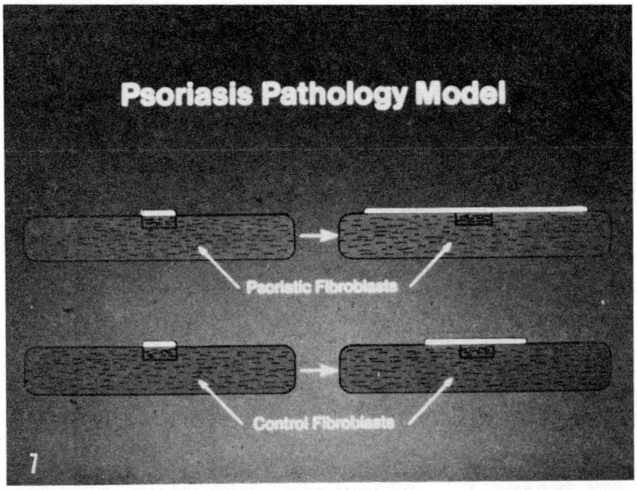

Fig. 7 -- Schematic of psoriasis model shows psoriatic or normal fibroblasts incorporated into dermal equivalents each provided with a punch containing normal keratinocytes. The cells grow out radially from the punch to cover the dermal equivalent. Hyperproliferation, induced by psoriatic fibroblasts, is characteristic of outgrowth of normal keratinocytes on the "diseased" dermal equivalent.

graftable, it can repair itself both in vitro and in vivo, but unlike excised human skin, it can be maintained in vitro as a living organ for many months, at least, and probably for much longer. In the form of TESTSKIN (TM), having a physically separated externum and internum equipped with a circulatory system, it mimics an organism and will hopefully be the first of many generations of hybrid organisms useful for a broad range of test applications.

REFERENCES

1. FRANZ, T.J., (1975), Percutaneous absorption. On the relevance of in vitro data. J. Invest. Derm., 61:190-195.

2. BRONAUGH, R.L., STEWART, R.F., CONGDON, E.R. and GILES, A.L. Jr., (1982), Methods for in vitro percutaneous absorption studies I. Comparison with in vivo results. Toxicol. Appl. Pharmacol., 62:474-480.

3. BRONAUGH, R.L., STEWART, R.F. and SIMON, M., (1986), Methods for in vitro percutaneous absorption studies. UII: USG of Excised Human Skin., J. Pharm. Sci., 75:1094-1097.

4. FELDMANN, R.J. and MAIBACH, H.I., (1970), Absorption of some organic compounds through the skin of man. J. Invest. Derm. 54:399-404.

5. BARTEK, M.J., LABUDDE, J.A. and MAIBACH, H.I., (1972), Skin permeability in vivo: comparison in rat, rabbit, pig and man. J. Invest. Derm., 58:114-123.

6. BRONAUGH, R.L. and MAIBACH, H.I., (1985), Percutaneous absorption of nitroaromatic compounds: in vivo and in vitro studies in human and monkey. J. Invest. Derm., 84:180-183.

7. MARZULLI, F.N. and MAIBACH, H.I., (1983), Contact Allergy: Predictive Testing in Humans in Dermatotoxicology, Second Edition, Marzulli, F. N. and Maibach, H. I. (eds.) Hemisphere Publishing Corp., N.Y., 279-296.

8. BELL, E., EHRLICH, H.P., BUTTLE, D.J., and NAKATSUJI, T., (1981), Living tissue formed in vitro and accepted as skin-equivalent tissue of full thickness. Science, Vol. 211:1052-1054.

9. BELL, E., SHER, S., HULL, B., MERRILL, C., ROSEN, S., CHAMSON, A., ASSELINEAU, D., DUBERTRET, L., COULOMB, B., LAPIERE, C., NUSGENS, B., and NEVEUX, Y., (1983), The reconstitution of living skin. The Journal of Investigative Dermatology, Vol. 81, No. 1, 2s-10s.

10. SHER, S.E., HULL, B.E., ROSEN, S., CHURCH, D., FRIEDMAN, L., BELL, E. (1983), Acceptance of allogeneic fibroblasts in skin equivalent transplants. Vol. 36, No. 5, 55.

11. HULL, B.E., SHER, S.E., ROSEN, S., CHURCH, D.A. and BELL, E., (1983), Structural integration of skin equivalents grafted to Lewis and Sprague-Dawley rats. The Journal of Investigative Dermatology, 81:429-436.

12. HULL, B.E., SHER, S.E., ROSEN, S., CHURCH, D. and BELL, E., (1983), Fibroblasts in isogeneic skin equivalents persist for long periods after grafting. The Journal of Investigative Dermatology. 81:436-438.

13. BELL, E., SHER, S. and HULL, B., (1984), The living skin equivalent as a structural and immunological model in skin grafting. Scanning Electron Microscopy.IV:1957-1962.

14. COULOMB, B., SAIAG, P., BELL, E., BREITBURD, F., LEBRETON, C., HESLAND, M. and DUBERTRET, L., (1986), A new method for studying epidermalization in vitro. British Journal of Dermatology. 114:91-101.

15. SAIAG, P., COULOMB, B., LEBRETON, C., BELL, E. and DUBERTRET, L., (1985), Psoriatic fibroblasts induce hyperproliferation of normal keratinocytes in a skin equivalent model in vitro. Science. 230:669-672.

16. COULOMB, B., DUBERTRET, L., BELL, E., MERRIL, C., FOSSE, M., BRETON-GORIUS, J., PROST, C. and TOURAINE, R., (1983), Endogenous peroxidases in normal human dermis: a marker of fibroblast differentiation. The Journal of Investigative Dermatology. 81:1:75-78.

17. TOPOL, B.M., HAIMES, H.B., DUBERTRET, L. and BELL, E., (1986), Transfer of melanosomes in a skin equivalent model in vitro. The Journal of Investigative Dermatology, 87:5:642-647.

18. BELL, E., IVARSSEN, B. and MERRILL, C. (1979), Production of a tissue-like structure by contraction of collagen lattices by human fibroblasts of different proliferative potential in vitro. PNAS, USA 76:3:1274-1278.

19. NUSGENS, B., MERRILL, C., LAPIERE, C. and BELL, E. (1984), Collagen biosynthesis by cells in a tissue equivalent matrix in vitro. Collagen Rel. Res. 4:351-364.

20. FREIBERGER, H., GROVE, D., SIVARAJAH, A. and PINNELL, S.R. (1980), Procollagen I synthesis in human skin fibroblasts: effect of culture conditions on biosynthesis. J. Invest. Dermatol. 75:425-430.

21. GOLDBERG, B., EPSTEIN, Jr., E.H. and SHEER, C.J. (1972), Precursors of collagen secreted by cultured human fibroblasts. Proc. Natl. Acad. Sci. USA. 69:3655-3659.

22. LAYMAN, D.L., MCGOODWIN, E.B. and MARTIN, G.R., (1971), The nature of collagen synthesized by cultured human fibroblasts. Proc. Natl. Acad. Sci. USA 68:454-458.

23. CHAMSON, A., FINLEY, J., HULL, B. and BELL, E., (1982), Differentiation and morphogenesis of keratinocytes grown on contracted collagen lattices. J. Cell Biol. 95:59a.

24. PARENTEAU, N., Unpublished results.

25. COULOMB, B., DUBERTRET, L., BELL, E. and TOURAINE, R., (1984), The Contractibility of fibroblasts in a collagen lattice is reduced by corticosteroids. Journal of Investigative Dermatol., 82:341-44.

A4

Cellular Responses of Cultured Human Epidermal Keratinocytes as Models of Toxicity to Human Skin

STEVEN T. BOYCE,[1] JOHN F. HANSBROUGH,[1]
and DAVID A. NORRIS[2]

[1]Department of Surgery
University of California
San Diego Medical Center
San Diego, CA
[2]Department of Dermatology
University of Colorado Health Sciences Center
Denver, CO

ABSTRACT

Major purposes for testing of local and systemic toxicity include evaluation for safety of externally applied consumer products, foods and drugs, occupational hazards, and environmental hazards. Conventional tests assess percutaneous absorption with cadaveric human skin, and irritation and corrosion with topical applications of compounds to the skin and eyes of animals. Studies with skin substitutes used for permanent skin replacement in surgery provide models for percutaneous absorption in vitro. Advances in dermatology and cell biology provide in vitro models of skin irritation and of skin corrosion with combinations of human epidermal keratinocytes (HK) and human leukocytes in culture. Cultured HK release inflammatory mediators (interleukins, arachadonic acid metabolites, leukocyte mitogen), express specific cellular antigens, and stimulate thymidine incorporation in lymphocytes which represent skin irritation. Cytotoxic lysis of cultured HK occurs by direct action of toxic agents, by leukocyte action (cell-mediated cytotoxicity; CMC), and by antibody plus leukocytes (antibody-dependent cellular cytotoxicity; ADCC) which represent skin corrosion. Adaptation and validation of these models for toxicology testing is anticipated to contribute to reduction in animal use, and to maintain rigorous standards of public safety.

INTRODUCTION

Public health and welfare are the objectives of safety testing of agents that are potentially toxic to humans. Human contact with toxic agents may occur by external application of consumer products, by intake of foods and drugs, or by exposure to occupational or environmental hazards. Animal subjects have served as models for human toxicity [1], but their use can be reduced or even eliminated with validation of alternative tests for human toxicity. Responses of cultured human epidermal keratinocytes (HK) provide alternative models for toxicity to human skin.

Conventional assays for testing of toxicity to skin include percutaneous absorption, acute dermal irritancy and corrosion, skin sensitization, and repeated dose dermal toxicity [2]. Human cadaveric skin has served as the preferred model for percutaneous absorption. Animal subjects have been utilized

Parts of this report supported by NIH grant GM 35068.

for safety testing because toxic responses produce the external manifestations of inflammation (erythema and edema) or of corrosion (ulceration). Semi-quantitative measurement of these responses in animal testing has provided the bases for the Draize dermal and ocular irritancy assays [3] and for assays of dermal and ocular corrosion. Irritation is defined in the Guidelines of the Organization for Economic Co-operation and Development (OECD) [2] as reversible inflammatory changes in the tissue to which a test substance is applied. Reversible changes of inflammation resolve and lead to recovery of the injured tissue. Corrosion is defined by the OECD as irreversible tissue damage after application of a test substance. Irreversible tissue necrosis resolves by regenerative mechanisms of wound healing. Although the manifestations of dermal irritation and of corrosion are relatively simple to perceive and score, they result from complex physiologic reactions that involve both parenchymal and immune cells present in the skin. Validation of cultured human epidermal keratinocytes as animal alternatives requires understanding and consideration of the cellular and molecular mechanisms of dermal inflammation and ulceration.

MECHANISMS OF SKIN TOXICITY

Skin toxicity may be manifested as inflammation (reversible changes) or as necrosis (irreversible damage). However, multiple mechanisms may contribute to these manifestations as represented diagrammatically in Figure 1.

Epidermal Penetration. Initiation of most toxic responses or of drug delivery requires transmission of a compound across the epidermis where it can interact with components of the vasculature. The barrier functions of skin can be attributed predominantly to the cornified layers of the epidermis and to the lipids that seal the spaces between individual cornified envelopes. After penetration, foreign antigens can interact with mast cells to cause degranulation, with T-lymphocytes or other immune effector cells to initiate cellular or humoral immune responses, or with sensitized T-lymphocytes or specific antibodies directed against the antigens.

Mast Cell Degranulation. Subcellular vesicles (granules) in mast cells contain histamine, seratonin, prostaglandins of the E series and leukotrienes, which are potent vasodilators. Release of these vesicles, or degranulation, affects vasodilation and capillary leakage to produce manifestations of erythema and edema. Mast cell degranulation can result from several inflammatory pathways: direct interaction of antigen with IgE on mast cells in acute inflammation; eosinophil induction in immediate hypersensitivity; T-lymphocyte induction in delayed hypersensitivity; or induction by plasma mediators, C3a and C5a in chronic inflammation. Mast cell degranulation is the predominant mechanism of skin inflammation, although kinins and neuroendocrine factors can also induce capillary leakage that result in erythema and edema.

Epidermal Cytokines. Leukocyte chemotaxis, activation and proliferation are central to inflammatory and immune processes. Cellular mediators, or cytokines, have been shown to be released directly from epidermal keratinocytes in culture [4-6]. Among the cytokines characterized in bioassays are: Epidermal Thymocyte Activating Factor (ETAF) [7], Interleukin 1 and 2-like activities [8], Interleukin 3 [6], Granulocyte-Macrophage Colony Stimulating Factor (GM-CSF) [9], and arachidonic acid metabolites including prostaglandins, leukotrienes, and eicosaniods [10]. Human epidermal keratinocytes participate in the immune functions of skin by synthesis and release of cytokines that constitute specific components of general mechanisms of cutaneous inflammation and ulceration.

Epidermal Antigens. Expression of cellular antigens by epidermal keratinocytes occurs in response to specific stimuli. Class II transplantation antigens (HLA-DR) are synthesized and expressed on the surfaces of cultured human keratinocytes in response to gamma-interferon [11, 12]. Antibodies against

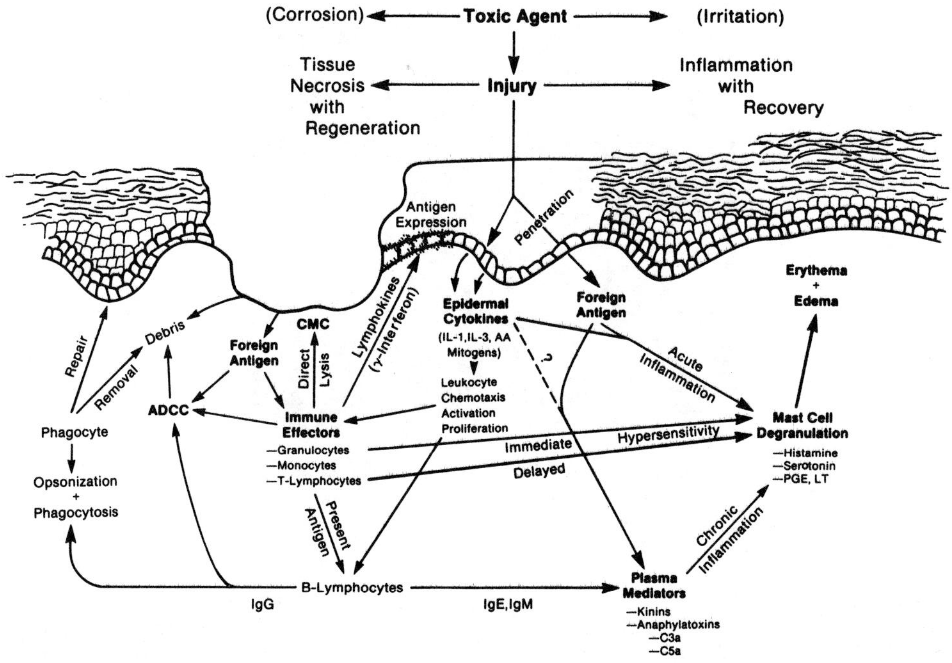

Figure 1. Diagrammatic illustration of cellular and humoral mechanisms of dermal irritation and corrosion. Abbreviations: IL-1, IL-3, interleukins 1 and 3; AA, arachidonic acid metabolites; PGE, prostaglandins of the E series; LT, leukotrienes; CMC, cell-mediated cytotoxicity; ADCC, antibody-dependent cellular cytotoxicity; Ig, immunoglobin.

antigens associated with lupus erythematosis (ribonuclear protein, Smith, Sjogren syndrome antigens) are bound by epidermal keratinocytes after exposure to UV light [13]. These antigens are associated with certain skin pathologies, and may represent responses to specific stimuli after cellular injury.

Epidermal Cytotoxicity. Corrosion of protective epidermis may occur by at least three general mechanisms. Direct keratinocyte lysis by action of the toxic compound causes immediate corrosion of the epidermis from the external surface. Cell-Mediated Cytotoxicity (CMC) results from lytic action of immune effector cells (lymphocytes, monocytes, neutrophils) on epidermal keratinocytes. Antibody-Dependent Cellular Cytotoxicity (ADCC) occurs by lysis of keratinocytes that have bound specific antibodies which make the epidermal cells susceptible to attack by immune effectors that bear Fc receptors [14].

CULTURED HUMAN EPIDERMAL KERATINOCYTES

Human epidermal keratinocytes (HK) participate in dermal inflammation and can be destroyed by cellular and humoral mechanisms, and therefore, constitute valid components of toxicity to human skin. HK cells can be readily cultured in serum-free media, stored in liquid nitrogen and recovered into culture for experimental testing [15,16]. Figure 2 shows an actively replicating culture of HK in serum-free medium. Serum-free and biochemically defined media [17,18] for HK are particularly sensitive for detection of very low (physiologic) concentrations of released cellular metabolites and for HK stimulation with low concentrations of toxic or physiologic compounds. Actively replicating HK

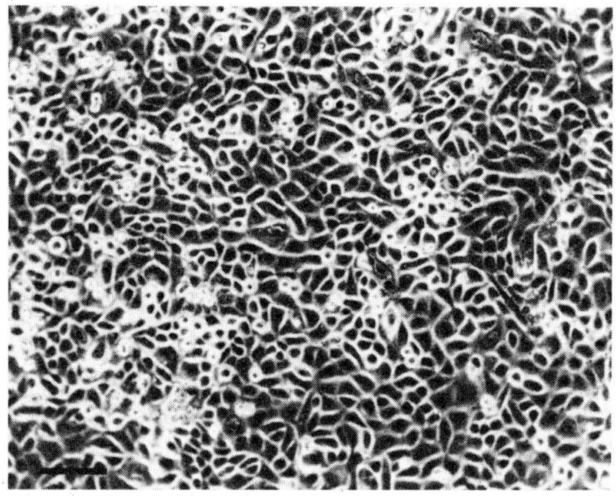

Figure 2. Phase contrast micrograph of HK culture showing confluent sheet of HK cells within a large colony. Note that many mitotic (refractile) cells are present. Scale bar = 0.1 mm.

cultures are suitable for studies of dermal irritation [19]. Epidermal differentiation can be regulated in vitro by adjustment of calcium concentration [18] or addition of fetal bovine serum (FBS) [20] to the culture medium to reform stratified, cornified human epithelia in vitro. Stratified HK cultures provide an in vitro model for percutaneous absorption.

PERCUTANEOUS ABSORPTION MODELS

Surgical need for treatment of burns and skin loss injuries has led to the development of permanent skin substitutes designed to restore the structure and function of human skin. All permanent skin substitutes contain an epidermal component [18, 21] and others contain both epidermal and dermal components [22, 23]. Skin substitutes contain only a subset of the complex cellular and biochemical compositions of native skin, and to describe skin substitutes as "equivalent" to native skin is a misnomer both of terminology and biology. For studies of percutaneous absorption in vitro, the dermal component of skin substitutes may prove to be relatively unimportant, except as a culture substrate. Dermal vasculature in vivo approximates the dermal-epidermal junction, and consequently, native dermis does not contribute significantly to barrier functions of the skin. Therefore, the dermal component of skin substitutes will more closely model native skin if it does not interfere greatly with the movement of compounds from the "external" surface of application to the "internal" surface of detection.

Stratified cultures of HK can be prepared on the surfaces of porous collagen-glycosaminoglycan (GAG) substrates [22, 24] to generate dermal-epidermal skin substitutes that are histologically comparable to native skin as shown in Figure 3. Development of a stratified, cornified epithelium is critical to the establishment in vitro of an epithelial barrier that restricts the transfer of applied compounds. Rat keratinocytes have also been shown to develop into stratified, cornified epithelia on synthetic membranes [25]. Although epidermal substitutes stratify and cornify in vitro, detailed analyses are lacking of synthesis, release and location of epidermal lipids in these tissue analogues, and whether epidermal lipids contribute to epithelial barrier function in vitro is not well described. Consequently, full utilization of cultured epithelium as an alternative to human cadaveric skin will probably require direct comparisons of transmission of standard compounds across the two materials. Comparative

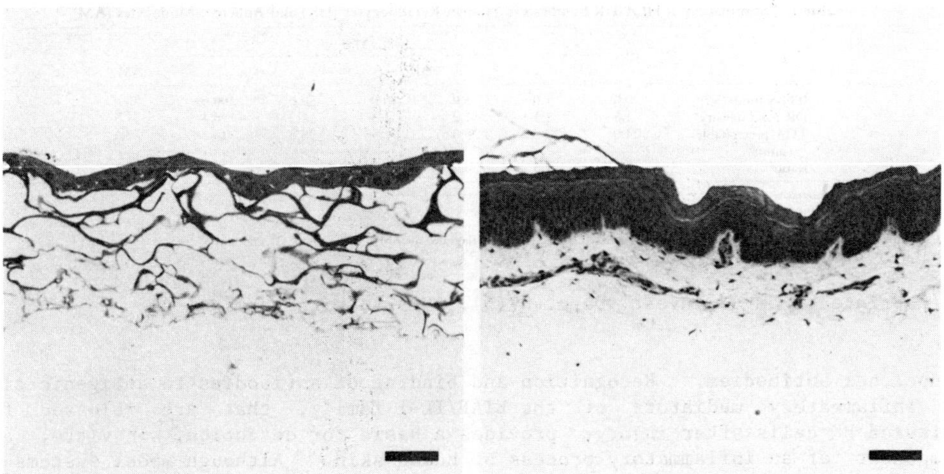

Figure 3. Light micrographs of a cultured skin substitute and of split-thickness human skin. Left panel, dermal-epidermal skin substitute consisting of a porous collagen-glycosaminoglycan dermal substitute covered on its surface with cultured human epidermal keratinocytes. Extension of culture period beyond 5 days and modification of culture conditions results in development of stratified, cornified epithelium in vitro [22]. Right panel, split-thickness human skin. Scale bars = 0.1 mm.

studies of cultured epithelium to native skin are not extensive at present, but will provide the basis for validation of cultured epithelium as a test subject for percutaneous absorption.

INFLAMMATION MODELS

Dermal inflammation results from highly integrated, regulated cellular and molecular processes in which components of skin epithelium, local leukocyte populations, vasculature and connective tissue participate. Production and release of epidermal cytokines contributes to leukocyte chemotaxis, activation and proliferation. Peptide cytokines reported to be produced by HK cells include Epidermal Thymocyte Activating Factor (ETAF) [7,26,27], Interleukin-1-like activity (IL-1) [28,29], Interleukin-2-like activity [8], Interleukin-3-like activity (IL-3) [6,8,30], Epidermal Cell Natural Killer Activating Factor (ENKAF) [4], Granulocyte Colony Stimulating Factor (G-CSF) [31], and Granulocyte-Macrophage Colony Stimulating Factor (GM-CSF) [32], also termed Keratinocyte Thymocyte Growth Factor (KTGF) [9]. Arachidonic acid metabolites known to be released from human keratinocytes are prostaglandins E_2 and $F_{2\alpha}$ [10], and leukotrienes B_4 and C_4 [33].

ETAF can be distinguished by DNA restriction mapping from two different forms of IL-1, IL-1α and IL-1β [34], but the biological functions of these compounds cannot be distinguished. ETAF/IL-1 is family of highly homologous molecules that has multipotent actions at the cellular, local tissue and systemic levels of inflammation. These actions include T-cell activation [7], chemotaxis of neutrophils [35] and of T-cells [36], systemic fever induction, production of acute phase plasma proteins, and muscle proteolysis [37]. These actions represent the early events of inflammatory reactions induced by apparently separate gene products that have been purified by high-performance liquid chromatography [5] and used to generate monoclonal antibodies [38]. ETAF/IL-1 molecules contain common antigenic determinants which cross-react with the

Table I. Stimulation of HLA-DR Synthesis in Human Keratinocytes (HK) and Adherent Monocytes (AM)

	Cell Type						
	HK						AM
IFN-γ (units/ml)[a]	0.0	1.0	5.0	10.0	50.0	100.0	50.0
DR band density[b]	1.5	1.1	1.2	1.3	11.2	18.4	17.5
TCA-precipitable counts[c]	24.0	12.8	20.6	11.5	28.6	16.0	2.6
Ratio[d]	0.9	1.3	0.9	1.7	5.8	17.1	100.0

[a] γ-Interferon concentration.
[b] Band density in arbitrary units.
[c] Expressed as millions of cpm.
[d] Ratio of band density to TCA-precipitable counts expressed as a percentage of the value for AM.

(Reprinted from J. Invest. Derm. 87(5):559-564, with permission)

monoclonal antibodies. Recognition and binding of antibodies to antigenic sites on inflammatory mediators of the ETAF/IL-1 family, that are released from cultured HK cells after injury, provides a basis for detection, in vitro, of a component of an inflammatory process of human skin. Although model systems of this kind are not yet described or validated for toxicology testing, it would be expected that results from this type of assay would correlate well with skin inflammation both in humans and in animals.

Other mediators of skin inflammation include IL-3, hemopoietic colony stimulating factors, and arachadonic acid metabolites. Keratinocyte IL-3 is reported to stimulate proliferation and chemotaxis of mast cells [4]. Several hemopoietic factors including G-CSF, GM-CSF and epidermal cell leukocyte stimulating activity (ELSA) [39,40] are produced by epidermal keratinocytes and result in leukocyte activation and proliferation. Arachadonic acid metabolites produced by cultured keratinocytes include prostaglandins E_2 and $F_{2\alpha}$ which are mediators of acute inflammation [10]. Leukotriene B_4 that causes leukocyte migration and adherence, and leukotriene C_4 that causes smooth muscle contraction have also been isolated from human epidermal keratinocytes in vitro [33]. Therefore, the participation of epidermal keratinocytes in the processes of skin inflammation is clear, but in vitro assays for detection of epidermal cytokines must be standardized before correlation of in vitro assays with animal models can be performed.

Expression of certain antigens by HK is associated with inflammatory skin conditions. Exposure of cultured HK to ultraviolet light (UV) stimulates binding of antibodies from sera of patients with lupus erythematosus (LE) [13]. The antibodies identify the ribonuclear protein, Smith, and Sjogren syndrome-A antigens that are associated with photosensitive lesions of LE. HK express the Class II transplantation antigen, HLA-DR, in a variety of inflammatory skin diseases, such as graft-vs-host disease, lichen planus, mycosis fungoides, and skin graft rejection. HK do not express HLA-DR after 7-14 days in culture, but will re-express HLA-DR in response to concentration-dependent administration of gamma-interferon [11,12]. Table I compares the relative induction of HLA-DR by gamma-interferon in HK and in human monocytes. After normalizing HLA-DR expression to total amount of protein synthesized, these studies showed that maximal HLA-DR expression by HK is approximately 17% of expression by monocytes. Although HLA-DR antigen is associated with inflammatory diseases of the skin, particularly in presentation of foreign antigen by Langerhans cells in sensitization of T-lymphocytes [41], the functional role of HLA-DR expression by HK in the inflammatory process is not fully clarified.

CYTOTOXICITY MODELS

Irreversible damage to skin tissue can result from exogenous or endogenous agents. Direct destruction of skin after contact with corrosive compounds, as in

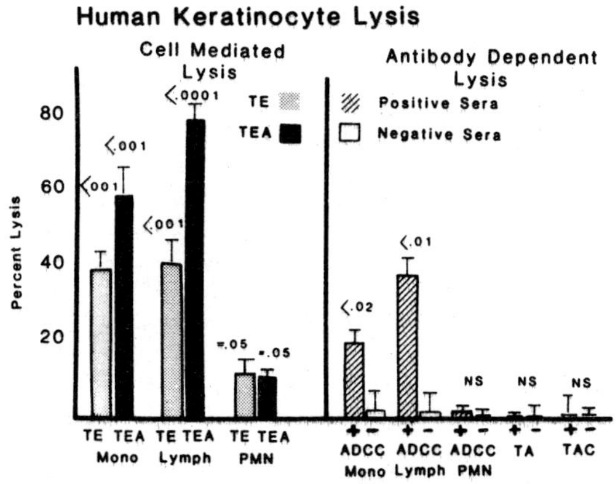

Figure 4. Percent lysis of TNP-coated human keratinocytes is shown as bars representing the mean ± SEM. Different combinations of targets (T), effectors (E), antibody (A), and complement (C) are summarized under the appropriate bars. Left, lysis by effectors alone (TE) or by effectors plus antibody (TEA) for monocytes (Mono), lymphocytes (Lymph), or neutrophil (PMN) fractions. Effector to target ratios: Mono 10:1, Lymph 100:1, PMN, 25:1. ADCC is defined as TEA-TE. Right, comparison of ADCC to lysis by antibody alone (TA) or by antibody plus complement (TAC) with either positive anti-TNP sera (+) or a negative control sera (-). Statistical significance is indicated by p values above bars or by NS (not significant). (Reprinted from J. Immunol. 135(2):1073-1079, with permission)

chemical burns, characterizes skin corrosion. These kinds of injuries produce ulcerations that resolve by coagulation of exudate from the wound followed ultimately by re-epithelialization or scar formation. Release of the dye, neutral red from cultured cells has provided an elegant and sensitive assay for evaluation of immediate cellular lysis by test compounds [42]. Assays for metabolic toxicity to cultured cells, including HK, after exposure to test compounds have measured uridine uptake and protein synthesis [19,43,44].

However, epidermal necrosis and ulcerations can also result over longer periods of time from cellular or humoral agents of the immune system. Lymphocytes, monocytes, and neutrophils are major subsets of leukocytes that are capable of acting as immune effector cells in vivo. Keratinocyte lysis occurs in various skin diseases including lupus erythematosis, lichen planus, graft-vs-host disease, erythema multiforme, and eczematous dermatitis. Keratinocyte destruction is often associated with epidermal antibody deposition. Cultured HK have been demonstrated to act as cytotoxic targets in vitro for combinations of immune effectors and specific antibody [14]. HK can be labelled with the radioisotope, ^{51}Cr, which is released into the culture medium after cell lysis. Experimental scintillation counts are compared to background as a baseline and to detergent lysed targets as 100% lysis value. Figure 4 compares lysis of labelled HK targets in vitro after coating the targets with trinitrophenol (TNP), an artificial antigen, and testing combinations of targets (T), effectors (E), specific antiserum (A) to TNP or non-immune serum, and complement (C). Cell-mediated cytotoxicity (CMC) results predominantly from HK lysis by lymphocytes and monocytes, and to a lesser extent, neutrophils. Addition of anti-TNP antiserum enhances target lysis by lymphocytes and by monocytes, but not by neutrophils. The additional target lysis in the presence of antiserum is antibody-dependent cellular cytotoxicity (ADCC). This type of assay system provides a model for evaluation of intermediate-term and long-term toxicity where cellular and humoral responses to specific agents occur.

VALIDATION

Animal models of dermal irritancy and corrosion are inherently valid because the complex processes of skin inflammation and ulceration are highly regulated in vivo. Ideally, in vitro tests would be equally well regulated, and wound identify and quantitate individual mechanisms of skin toxicity. However, because in vitro tests contain only a subset of the anatomical, cellular and humoral components of skin, only a subset of skin responses can be measured by any single endpoint. Consequently, greater numbers of endpoints will tend to increase test validity, assuming that the endpoints correlate with skin irritancy and corrosion in vivo. Because in vitro tests are analogous, but not homologous with animal assays, certain strengths and weaknesses will always distinguish the two test formats.

Advantages to validation for use of cultured HK in place of animals include: a) assay endpoints that produce quantitative rather than semi-quantitative data; b) greater mechanistic definition of the cellular and molecular processes of dermal irritation and corrosion; c) greatly decreased cost per test point; d) greater numbers of test points handled per person; e) greater ease of handling; and f) no taxonomic extrapolation from animal to human responses of skin toxicity.

Disadvantages to validation for cultured HK as an in vitro model of skin toxicity include: a) less biologic complexity and possible absence of regulatory factors in vitro; b) requirement for qualified interpretation of data due to less biologic complexity; c) requirement for multiple endpoints to define a sublethal toxic response in vitro.

Validation of in vitro toxicology tests is a multi-step process that involves test development, test standardization, correlation of in vitro results with animal results, and acceptance by regulatory agencies [45,46]. For assays with cultured HK, the process will involve: a) selection and standardization of endpoints relevant to dermal irritation and corrosion; b) independent correlation by multiple investigators of results from in vitro and animal tests; c) acceptance by regulatory agencies; and d) constant improvement of available tests and addition of new endpoints for measurement of skin toxicity.

CULTURED HUMAN KERATINOCYTES AS AN ALTERNATIVE TO ANIMALS

Normal human epidermal keratinocytes in culture provide a very promising model of toxicity to human skin as an alternative to animal toxicity testing. Stratified and cornified HK cultures may prove to be useful in studies of drug and chemical penetration of the skin. HK targets in cytotoxicity assays have been demonstrated to be useful as a screen for irreversible cellular damage. Sublethal concentrations of toxic agents will be anticipated to induce reversible cellular changes associated with synthesis and release of inflammatory mediators and expression of cellular antigens associated with inflammatory conditions. Adaptation of these existing models for the purpose of safety testing of consumer products, foods and drugs, and environmental and occupational hazards can result in the development and acceptance of guidelines for in vitro tests with cultured HK. Continued progress toward this objective can reduce or eliminate animal testing, and provide equivalent or superior standards of health and safety to the general public.

REFERENCES

1. WHO Publication (1978), Environmental Health Criteria 6, Principles and Methods for Evaluating the Toxicity of Chemicals, Part I; Geneva.

2. Organization for Economic Cooperation and Development Guidelines for Testing of Chemicals (1987), In, "Dermatotoxicology, third edition," F.N. Marzulli and H.I. Maibach, editors; Hemisphere Publishing, Washington, pp 713-761.

3. Draize, J.H., Woodard G. and Calvery, H.O. (1944), Methods for the study of irritation and toxicity of substances applied topically to the skin and mucous membranes. J Pharmacol Exp Ther 82:377-390.

4. Luger, T.A., Kock, A., Danner, M., Colot, M. and Micksche, M. (1985), Production of distinct cytokines by epidermal cells. Br J Derm 113, supplement 28:145-156.

5. Kock, A. and Luger, T.A. (1985), High-performance liquid chromatographic separation of distinct epidermal cell-derived cytokines. J Chromatography 326:129-136.

6. Luger, T.A., Wirth, U. and Kock, A. (1985), Epidermal cells synthesize a cytokine with interleukin 3-like properties. J Immunol 134(2):915-919.

7. Sauder, D.N., Carter, C.S., Katz, S.I. and Oppenheim, J.J. (1982), Epidermal cell production of thymocyte activating factor (ETAF). J Invest Derm 79(1):34-39.

8. Kupper, T.S. (1986), Interleukin 1, 2, and 3-like activity released by keratinocytes: a novel perspective on post burn immunosuppression. Program of the 18th Annual Mtg of Amer Burn Assoc, Abstract No. 154.

9. Kupper, T.S., Coleman, D.L., McGuire, J., Goldminz, D., and Horowitz, M.C. (1986), Keratinocyte-derived T-cell growth factor: a T-cell growth factor functionally distinct from interleukin 2. Proc Natl Acad Sci 83(12):4451-4455.

10. DeLeo, V.A., Midlarsky, L., Harber, L.C., Kong, B.M. and DeSalva, S. (1987), Surfactant-induced cutaneous primary irritancy: an in vitro model. Proc Soc for Exper Biol & Med 184:477-482.

11. Wikner, N.E., Huff, J.C., Norris, D.A., Boyce, S.T., Cary, M., Kissinger, M. and Weston, W.L. (1986), Study of HLA-DR synthesis in cultured human keratinocytes. J Invest Derm 87(5):559-564.

12. Basham, T.Y., Nickoloff, B.J., Merigan, T.C. and Morhenn, V.B. (1984), Recombinant gamma interferon induces HLA-DR expression on cultured human keratinocytes. J Invest Derm 83:88-92.

13. LeFeber, W.P., Norris, D.A., Ryan, S.R., Huff, J.C., Lee, L.A., Kubo, M., Boyce, S.T., Kotzin, B.L. and Weston, W.L. (1984), Ultraviolet light induces binding of antibodies to selected nuclear antigens on cultured human keratinocytes. J Clin Invest 74:1545-1551.

14. Norris, D.A., Ryan, S.B., Kissinger, R.M., Fritz, K.A. and Boyce, S.T. (1985), Systematic comparison of antibody-mediated mechanisms of keratinocyte lysis in vitro. J Immunol 135(2): 1073-1079.

15. Boyce, S.T. and Ham, R.G. (1985), Cultivation, frozen storage, and clonal growth of normal human epidermal keratinocytes in serum-free media. J Tiss Cult Meth 9(2):83-93.

16. Boyce, S.T. and Ham, R.G. (1986), Normal human epidermal keratinocytes, in, "In Vitro Models for Cancer Research"; Vol. 3, Carcinomas of the Mammary Gland, Uterus and Skin", Weber, M.M., and Sekely, L.I., eds.; CRC Press, Boca Raton, Florida, pp. 245-274.

17. Tsao, M.C., Walthall, B.J. and Ham, R.G. (1982), Clonal growth of normal human epidermal keratinocytes in a defined medium. J Cell Physiol 110:219-229.

18. Boyce, S.T. and Ham, R.G. (1983), Calcium-regulated differentiation of normal human epidermal keratinocytes in chemically defined clonal culture and free serial culture. J Invest Derm 81(1), supplement:33S-40S.

19. Shopsis, C. (1987), In vitro ocular irritancy prediction: comparison of cell systems and assay conditions. In Vitro Cell & Devel Biol 23(3):44A.

20. Pittelkow, M.R. and Scott, R.E. (1986), New techniques for the in vitro culture of human skin keratinocytes and perspectives on their use for grafting of patients with extensive burns. Mayo Clin Proc 61:771-777.

21. Gallico, G.G., O'Conner, N.E., Compton, C.C., Kehinde, O. and Green, H. (1984), Permanent coverage of large burn wounds with autologous cultured human epithelium. N Engl J Med 311:448-51.

22. Boyce, S.T. and Hansbrough, J.F. (1987), Biological attachment, growth and differentiation of cultured human epidermal keratinocytes on a graftable collagen and chondroitin-6-sulfate substrate. Surgery, in press.

23. Bell, E., Sher, S., Hull, B., Merrill, C., Rosen, S., Chamson, A., Asselineau, D., Dubertret, L., Coulomb, B., Lapiere, C., Nusgens, B. and Neveux, Y. (1983), The reconstitution of living skin. J Invest Derm 81(1), supplement:2s-10s.

24. Hansbrough, J.F. and Boyce, S.T. (1984), What criteria should be used for designing artificial skin replacements and how well do the current materials meet these criteria. J Trauma 24(9), supplement, S29-S35.

25. Vaughan, F.L., Gray, R.H. and Bernstein, I.A. (1986), Growth and differentiation of primary rat keratinocytes on synthetic membranes. In Vitro Cell & Devel Biol 22(3):141-149.

26. Goldminz, D., Kupper, T.S. and McGuire, J. (1987), Keratinocyte membrane-associated epidermal cell-derived thymocyte-activating factor (ETAF). J Invest Derm 88(1):97-100.

27. Luger, T.A., Stadler, B.M., Katz, S.I. and oppenheim, J.J. (1981), Epidermal cell (keratinocyte) derived thymocyte activating factor (ETAF). J Immunol 127:1493.

28. Bell, T.V., Harley, C.B., Stetsko, D. and Sauder, D.N. (1987), Expression of mRNA homologous to interleukin 1 in human epidermal cells. J Invest Derm 88(4):375-379.

29. Kupper, T.S., Ballard, D.W., Chua, A.O., McGuire, J.S., Flood, P.M., Horowitz, M.C., Langdon, R., Lightfoot, L. and Gubler, U. (1986), Human keratinocytes contain mRNA indistinguishable from monocyte interleukin 1α and β mRNA. Keratinocyte epidermal cell-derived thymocyte-activating factor is identical to interleukin 1. J Exp Med 164(6):2095-2100.

30. Danner, M. and Luger, T.A. (1987), Human keratinocytes and epidermoid

carcinoma cell lines produce a cytokine with interleukin 3-like activity. J Invest Derm 88(4):353-361.

31. Denburg, J.A. and Sauder, D.N. (1986), Granulocyte colony stimulating activity derived from human keratinocytes. Lymphokine Res 5(4):261-274.

32. Coleman, D.L., Kupper, T.S., Flood, P.M., Fultz, C.C. and Horowitz, M.C. (1987), Characterization of a keratinocyte-derived T cell growth factor distinct from interleukin 2 and B cell stimulatory factor 1. J Immunol 138(10):3314-3318.

33. Rosenbach, T., Grabbe, J., Moller, A., Schwanitz H.J. and Czarnetzki B.M. (1985), Generation of leukotrienes from normal epidermis and their demonstration in cutaneous disease. Br J Derm 113, supplement 28:157-167.

34. Sauder, D.N., Arsenault, T.V., Stetsko, D. and Harley, C.B. (1987), Isolation and partial characterization of a putative ETAF cDNA clone (kIL-1): ETAF is distinct from IL-1 or IL-1 . J Invest Derm 88(4):515.

35. Sauder, D.N., Mounessa, N.L., Katz, S.I., Dinarello, C.A. and Gallin, J.I. (1984), Chemotactic cytokines: the role of leukocytic pryogen and epidermal cell thymocyte-activating factor in neutrophil chemotaxis. J Immunol 132(2):828-832.

36. Sauder, D.N., Monick, M.M. and Hunninghake, G.W. (1985), Epidermal cell-derived thymocyte activating factor (ETAF) is a potent T-cell chemoattractant. J Invest Derm 85(5):431-433.

37. Sauder, D.N. (1985), Biologic properties of epidermal cell thymocyte-activating factor (ETAF). J Invest Derm 85:(1), supplement:176s-182s.

38. Luger, T.A., Danner, M. and Kock, A. (1986), Monoclonal anti-IL 1 is directed against a common site of human IL 1 alpha and IL 1 beta. Immunobiol 172(3-5):346-56.

39. Denburg, J.A. and Sauder, D.N. (1985), Hemopoietic colony stimulating activity derived from human keratinocytes. Clin Res 33(2):633A.

40. Luger, T.A., Kapp, A., Mickshe, M. and Danner, M. (1987) Characterization of distinct epidermal cytokine with multiple immunoregulatory properties. J Invest Derm 88(4):504.

41. Edelson, R.L. and Fink, J.M. (1985), The immunologic function of skin. Sci Amer 252(6):46-53.

42. Borenfreund, E. and Puerner, J.A. (1985), Toxicity determined in vitro by morphological alterations and neutral red absorption. Tox Lett 24:119-124.

43. Shopsis, C., Borenfreund, E., Walberg, J. and Stark, D.M. (1985), A battery of potential alternatives to the draize test: uridine uptake inhibition, morphological cytotoxicity, macrophage chemotaxis and exfoliative cytology. Fd Chem Tox 23(2):259-266.

44. Shopsis, C. and Eng, B. (1985), Rapid cytotoxicity testing using a semi-automated protein determination on cultured cells. Tox Lett 26:1-8.

45. Stark, D.M., and Shopsis, C. (1983), Developing alternative assay systems for toxicity testing. Annals New York Academy of Sciences 406:92-103.

46. Nardone, R.M. (1981), Ocular toxicity testing: An in vitro strategy. In, Proceedings of the Symposium on Trends in Bioassay Methodology: In Vivo, In Vitro, and Mathematical Approaches, pp. 163-173; NIH, Bethesda, Md.

A5

Surfactant-Induced Cutaneous Primary Irritancy: An *In Vitro* Model—Assay System Development

VINCENT DELEO,[1] JACQUELINE HONG,[1] SARA SCHEIDE,[1] BETTY KONG,[2] SALVATORE DESALVA,[2] and DANIEL BAGLEY[2]

[1]Department of Dermatology
Columbia University
New York, NY 10032
[2]Department of Pharmacology and Toxicology
Research and Development
Colgate-Palmolive Company
Piscataway, NJ 08854

ABSTRACT

Primary irritancy in human skin, when induced by surfactant contact, is mediated in part by molecules derived from cellular membrane lipids. Utilizing human epidermal keratinocytes in culture as an in vitro model system we have shown that the irritant process involves surfactant-induced stimulation of phospholpases. Studies were done in an effort to use this mechanism of phospholipase activation as an assay for irritancy. Cells in culture were prelabelled with either (^{3}H) arachidonic acid or (^{3}H) choline. The cells were treated with five different finished products (surfactant mixtures) of known irritancy in animal skin (Primary Dermal Irritancy Index-PDII). Release of radiolabel was assayed and the dilution of product necessary to induce release at 150% of control was calculated (ID 150%). The rank order of the PDII and ID 150% correlated fairly well for the five products. In addition, a commercially available human keratinocyte line (NHEK-Clonetics) was used in release assays and the response of these cells to that of primary keratinocyte cultures showed an excellent correlation.

INTRODUCTION

Primary cutaneous irritancy occurs when an agent induces direct toxicity in human skin. Such reactions occur frequently in societies like ours that use large quantities of soap and detergent containing personal care and household products. We have been involved with developing in vitro models for studying the mechanism of this response. We have grown mouse fibroblasts (C3H 10T1/2) and normal human epidermal keratinocytes (HK) in culture; prelabelled the cells with either (^{3}H) arachidonic acid (AA) or (^{3}H) choline (CH); treated the cells with surfactants; and assayed the effect of such treatment on cellular phospholipid metabolism. In previous communications (1-4) we have reported that anionic surfactant treatment stimulated release of both (^{3}H)AA and (^{3}H)CH from prelabelled cells. The response to surfactant treatment was dose dependent and the magnitude of release of label among different pure surfactants correlated with their in vivo irritancy in animal skin (1-4). In addition, surfactant treatment resulted in stimulation of production of inflammatory mediators of lipid origin by both cell types (1,3). Further data suggested that surfactants stimulate specific phospholipase activation in HK in culture (2,4).

In the present studies we extend our observations to a commercially available human epidermal keratinocyte line (NHEK-Clonetics) and examine the effect of complex surfactant mixtures (finished products) on release of label assays.

METHODS

Cell Culture Systems:

Human epidermal Keratinocytes. We utilized the system of Eisinger et al described in detail previously (5). A single cell suspension of epidermal cells was produced from surgical specimens and diluted with growth medium (5) and seeded at appropriate densities. Assay medium was of the same composition but without fetal calf serum.

NHEK. This is a commercially available normal human epidermal keratinocyte system. The cells are supplied with all media and reagents necessary for a propagation and maintenance of the system. Growth Medium for these cells is as supplied while assay medium is the same as for the HK system. The cells were a generous gift of the Clonetics Corporation, San Diego, CA.

Experimental Procedure: Release of Label Assay. Cells were seeded into dishes at a constant density in growth medium. Cells were allowed to attach and grow to 90% confluency. Cells were then labelled with either of the following in growth media:

(^{3}H)-Arachidonic Acid 1uCi/ml

(^{3}H)-Choline 1uCi/ml

After a 24 hour labelling period labelling media were removed and cells were washed three times with assay media.

Assay medium alone (control) or assay medium containing surfactant or finished product was added to triplicate dishes. Cells were incubated at 37°C.

At selected times, media were removed from dishes; centrifuged (10,000 rpm) to remove detached cells; and an aliquot was assayed for radioactivity by liquid scintillation counting.

Results are presented in terms of mean total release of label into media.

Finished Products. Six finished products were supplied by Colgate-Palmolive to our laboratory. The composition of these were unknown to us and these we labelled A-F. The products were diluted in distilled water to a stock solution of 1%. At the completion of the studies, the Primary Dermal Irritancy Index(PDII) score for the products was made available to us for analysis of data.

Analysis of Data. The release of label for each of the products at multiple dilutions was determined and calculated as percent control:

$$\text{Percent Control} = \frac{\text{Mean CPM Surfactant}}{\text{Mean CPM Control}} \times 100$$

The release of label for the dilutions were compared and subjected to linear regression analysis to plot a best fit line. The formula for this line was then used to compute the Irritant Dilution 150% (ID 150%). ID 150% was the dilution calculated to induce release at a level of 150% of control. The rank order of the ID 150% for the products was then determined and compaired to the rank order irritancy of the product in terms of PDII.

RESULTS

Six finished products were supplied in a blinded fashion. The agents were diluted to the 1% level in distilled water before dilutions into media. One of the products (F) was not completely soluble in this dilution and it was not utilized for further studies.

The other five agents were used in multiple assays at dilutions between 0.0001 and 0.1% to treat HK cells prelabelled with both (^3H)AA and (^3H)CH. As in previous reports these products induced release of label in a concentration dependent manner, except for product C, which did not induce release above control level at dilutions assayed (data not shown).

Data for each product were then examined statistically to compute dilution of product necessary to induce release of label at 150% of control release. This level was designated the Irritant Dilution 150% (ID 150%) for each product in both assays ((^3H)AA and (^3H)CH). The ID 150% for the five products are given in Table I. The ID 150% ranged from 0.0147 to >0.1% for the (^3H)AA assay and 0.012 to >0.05% for the (^3H)CH assay.

Table I also lists the Primary Dermal Irritancy Index (PDII) scores for the five products. These scores were furnished by Colgate-Palmolive. A product with PDII a score of 0 - 0.5 is considered a negligible irritant; 0.5 to 2 is considered a mild irritant; 2 to 5 is a moderate irritant; and greater than 5 is a severe irritant (6). Products A, B and D, therefore, would be classed as moderate irritants and C and E as negligible irritants.

In Table II, the rank order of the <u>in vivo</u> and <u>in vitro</u> for the five products are compared. In both assays the rank order for the 5 products was good (Spearman Rank Order Correlation = 0.9). The three moderate irritants (A, B, D) as determined by PDII were also the agents considered most irritating by the <u>in vitro</u> ID 150%. The two negligible irritants (C, E), were the least irritating by ID 150% scores. The rank order of these two agents were however reversed.

Preparation of primary human keratinocyte cultures is time consuming and requires access to fresh human skin from surgical specimens. Since this might be difficult for industrial groups interested in utilizing the release of label assays for pre-market testing , we have begun examining the feasability of using a commercially available normal human keratinocyte culture system in our assays. NHEK (Clonetics) were prelabelled with (^3H)AA or (^3H)CH and treated with the pure surfactant LAS (Linear Alkyl Benzene Sulfonate). HK cells were treated similarly in parallel studies. As shown in Table III, the two culture systems responded to LAS treatment with comparable release of label. In preliminary studies the NHEK cells also responded to treatment with finished products in a manner similar to HK cells (data not shown)

Table I. Finished Products - Primary Dermal Irritancy Index (PDII) and ID 150% in Release of label Assay - HK Cells.

Product	PDII	ID 150%*	
		(3H)AA	(3H)CH
A	4.0	0.0168	0.017
B	2.8	0.0195	0.024
C	0.4	>0.1	>0.05
D	4.8	0.0147	0.012
E	0	0.02	0.05

*ID 150% - dilution of product (in percent) necessary to induce release at 150% of control release.

Table II. Rank Order* Comparison of PDII and ID 150% in Release of Label Assay in HK Cells for Finished Products.

Product	RANK ORDER		
	PDII	ID 150%	
		(3H)AA	(3H)CH
A	4	4	4
B	3	3	3
C	2	1	1
D	5	5	5
E	1	2	2

*Rank order - on a 1 to 5 scale. 5 indicating highest irritancy rating; 1 indicating lowest rating.

Table III. The effect of LAS on Release of Label in two Different Keratinocyte Systems.

LAS Concentration (Linear Alkyl Benzene Sulfonate) (UM)	Release of Label (% control)			
	HK		NHEK	
	(3H)AA	(3H)CH	(3H)AA	(3H)CH
0	100	100	100	100
5	104	126	97	103
25	160	122	116	81
50	257	200	338	202

Data are based on means of triplicate observations.

SUMMARY

The data presented in this communication suggest that a system of human epidermal keratinocytes (HK) in culture, prelabelled with either (^{3}H)AA or (^{3}H)CH can be used as an in vitro assay system for irritancy of water soluble surfactant mixtures. In addition, a commercially available human keratinocyte culter system (NHEK-Clonetics) appears to be a viable source of cells for these assays. Future work to validate these systems is in progress.

REFERENCES

1. DeLeo V., Harber L., Kong B., DeSalva S. Alternative Methods in Toxicology 3: 466-481, 1985.

2. DeLeo V., Harber L., Kong B., DeSalva S. Proc. Soc. Exp. Bio. Med. 184: 477-482, 1987.

3. DeLeo V., Midlarsky L., Harber L., Kong B., DeSalva S., Alternative Methods in Toxicology 5: 129-138, 1987.

4. DeLeo V., Hanson D., Scheide S., Kong B., DeSalva S. Submitted to Tox Applied Pharmac, 1987.

5. Eisenger M., Lee J., Hepton J., Darsynkiewicz Z., Chaio J., DeHaven E. Proc. Nati. Acad. of Sci. USA 76: 5340-5343, 1979.

6. Gad S., Walsh R., Dunn B. J. Toxicol.- Cut. & Ocular Toxicol. 5(3): 195-213, 1986.

A6

Summary of Panel Discussion

YALE GRESSEL

Avon Products, Inc.
Division Street
Suffern, NY 10901

Lowell Goldsmith started the session off by pointing out the marvelous complexity of skin architecture and function by using the analogy with a shopping mall and its suborganization. It leads one to wonder, can we really expect to develop in vitro alternatives that can even come close to reflecting this complex organ that we call the skin? As if Dr. Goldsmith's excursion through the shopping mall was not enough to humble us, Dr. Gerald Lazarus discussed the very important roles of mast cell degranulation and the proteolytic enzymes in cutaneous toxicity. He noted their involvement in cell movement, cell adhesion and in the activation of the inflammatory cascade.

He described the 2 types of plasminogen activators, the tissue type and the urokinase type. The latter binding to the cell surface. He noted that we have now moved from the era of the Langerhans cell to the decade of the mast cell and described its involvement in the inflammatory process and in a number of disease states such as urticaria and eczema. Two types of mast cells were identified with different tissues differing in the preponderance of the type present.

Mast cell involvement in blistering or separation of the epidermis and dermis and in vascular tone was described. Finally Dr. Lazarus projected several mast cell models that might be used in the future for studying cutaneous toxicity such as an epithelial cell culture to which one would add the materials to be tested and then measure the release of proteinases.

Dr. Eugene Bell then described the preparation of the living skin equivalent, prepared by first plating human dermal fibroblasts and developing a dermal equivalent. Then after this, seeding human keratinocytes on its surface. The epidermal cells spread across the surface and differentiate. A multilayered epidermis with a well organized collagen skeleton forms. Stratum corneum is complete in 1 to 14 days. Various skin cells such as melanocytes can be added.

He then further went on to describe a chamber which would allow profusion of dermal media. This would allow removal of aliquots to measure materials diffusing through or materials that excreted into the bathing media. Obviously one could visualize and some of the discussion that took place further indicated, that there may well be a variety of applications for preparations of this type. There was some discussion on its utility for percutaneous penetration. It was pointed out that the intracellular lipids have still not been defined and of course they play a key role in skin permeability.

Dr. Stephen Boyce then discussed the cellular responses of cultured human epidermal keratinocytes as a model for toxicity assessment of human skin. He reviewed the current tests commonly employed in safety testing. He then noted that materials can produce inflammation by directly acting on mast cells or by release of epidermal cytokines that then lead to mast cell degranulation. He described the conditions necessary for optimal growth of human epidermal keratinocytes and the development of a multilayer epithelium similar to the split skin preparation. This differs in some respects from skin as for example in the lack of melanocytes and the various appendages. He discussed the epidermal cytokines and projected the use of cultured keratinocytes in irritancy assays by exposing the culture to various agents and measuring the release of interleukin-1. The use of cultured keratinocytes in cytotoxicity assays was further discussed.

Finally the importance of validation and the advantages and disadvantages of the use of keratinocyte cultures was elucidated.

Dr. Vincent De Leo described his very elegant model for assessing surfactant induced primary irritancy. He used several cell types i.e. primary human keratinocytes, a commercial source of human keratinocytes, and the C3H 10t 1/2 mouse embryo fibroblasts and he indirectly measured the release of arachidonic acid metabolites subsequent to cell exposure to irritants. He looked at a number of anionic, cationic and nonionic surfactants of known human irritancy. He found an excellent dose response relationship and good correlation with the in vivo situation.

I just finished sitting through a very tedious day with Alan Goldberg and his expert review committee looking at a variety of grant applications and one couldn't help but note that there were many, many proposals that focussed on a variety of different end points for dealing with skin irritation. One had to speculate on why we need so many different tests. I think as we walk through Dr. Goldsmith's shopping mall, we recognize that we have an extraordinarily complex situation. It is very doubtful, at least in my humble estimation that all irritants act by the same mechanism. Therefore how can one test be a catchall for everything? How could we have one test that's going to give us all of the answers? Our critics expect a panacea, the pot of gold at the end of the rainbow to occur any day now but the complexity of the in vivo situation works against this. I had a great deal of difficulty trying to summarize in a short period of time the very complex material that was thrown my way which leads me to believe that it is very naive for any of us to think that we are going to come up with a simple cure-all. I think we have to do something very much akin to what Dr. De Leo has done with the surfactants. We have to look at the mechanisms involved, class by class and determine which procedure, which end point of the many that have been elucidated and the many that I think we can see are available to us based on some of the information thrown our way today. It's a very, very complex situation and I'm not saying that it's insoluble, I think we will find ways of dealing with the situation, but it's not something that's going to happen tomorrow.

Thank you very much.

B. Recent Advances in Tissue Culture

B1

Introduction

PETER WARD

Department of Pathology
University of Michigan Medical School
Ann Arbor, MI 48109

The following two presentations will describe in vitro approaches for further defining basic cell biological principles as well as mechanisms leading to cell injury. The first presentation, by Dr. Una Ryan, describes in some detail how endothelial cell cultures can be adapted for the probing of their responses to various environmental factors, the production by endothelial cells of mediators such as endothelial cell derived relaxing factor, the susceptibility of endothelial cells to injury produced by stimulated phagocytic cells, to list only a few examples. Dr. Ryan together with her colleagues have over the years demonstrated how the careful application of tissue culture approaches can provide important insights into the behavior of vascular endothelial cells.

The second speaker, Dr. John Farber, has a distinguished record demonstrating how hepatocytes can be adapted in tissue culture to yield insight into the mechanism of hepatotoxicity induced by drugs and environmental toxins. Dr. Farber has mapped the oxidant generating pathways in hepatocytes and has been one of the first to suggest that metabolism of drugs and toxins within hepatocytes can be related ultimately to the intracellular generation of toxic oxygen species which in some cases also requires mobilization of intracellular iron, presumably to yield Fenton reactions such as the hydroxyl radical.

The two speakers should establish the point that cell culture systems, when used appropriately and with certain constraints, can yield important new insight into cell biology. Their presentations will demonstrate beyond doubt the utility of tissue culture approaches in the field of toxicology.

B2

Cultured Endothelial Cells as Probes for *In Vivo* Biology

UNA S. RYAN and JAMES M. VANN

Department of Medicine
University of Miami School of Medicine
Miami, FL 33101

ABSTRACT

Methods for maintaining pulmonary endothelial cells in culture have been available for approximately 12 years and are constantly developing. Using current techniques, endothelial cells in culture have been shown to maintain a wide variety of functions, including processing of vasoactive substances, generation of growth factors, angiogenic factors, hemostatic factors, immunologic and complement components, and (despite loss of receptors for some agonists) synthesis of a wide variety of active molecules. As a consequence of their important location within the vasculature, and their ability to replicate in culture while retaining many characteristic functions, cultured endothelial cells are ideal probes of vascular functions and dysfunctions. This paper describes model systems for studies of endothelial cell interactions with bacteria.

INTRODUCTION

The use of endothelial cells in culture developed, in the first instance, as a means of validating in vivo or in situ preparations. For example, pulmonary endothelial cells were first isolated to show that the degradation of bradykinin and conversion of angiotensin I to angiotensin II, processing functions that appeared to be conducted on the vessel wall, were accomplished solely by endothelial cells (1,2). Once isolated the cells had to be characterized and the original research aim (localization of angiotensin converting enzyme) now became a tool for the characterization of endothelial cells (3,4). As success with culture grew, so that pulmonary endothelial cells could be maintained in long-term, large-scale culture (5,6), the continuing presence of ACE activity provided the means for validating cultures for preservation of differentiated properties characteristic of the cell in vivo or in early passages in vitro. The need for simple assays for ACE lead to the development of ^{3}H acylated peptides that could be used for assessing ACE of cells in culture (3,4). These proved useful in clinical assays and could be used for testing ACE levels of patients on the orally effective ACE inhibitors (Captopril, Enalapril) and estimating patient compliance. Now they can be used for assessing vascular surface area.

Now that the culture of endothelial cells is a routine procedure, studies using these cells have shown a vast array of endothelial properties. For example endothelial cells are now known to play a role in the control of blood pressure, hemostasis, gas exchange, inflammation and immune reactions (7) and interact with blood-borne and tissue-derived molecules to engage in cell-matrix interactions and cell-cell interactions with blood cells and the underlying layers of the vascular wall (8). The strategic position of the endothelium at the interface between the blood and tissues makes it ideally suited both as a regulator of vascular events and as a target for vascular injury. The wealth of activities shown to be maintained in cultured endothelial cells makes them an ideal model for studies of the metabolism of bioactive molecules, the release of endothelium-derived products, and for interactions with cells or microorganisms.

Recently, the ability of endothelial cells to phagocytize particulate material has been recognized. We have used endothelial cells in culture to study phagocytosis of bacteria. Our model allows us to measure the recognition, binding and ingestion of bacteria and the consequences of phagocytosis on endothelial cell immunologic properties, respiratory burst response and behavioral kinetics. In addition we have begun to study the bactericidal ability of endothelial cells and the effects of endothelial ingestion on the susceptibility of bacteria to antibiotic action.

These studies have yielded information on the basic mechanisms of phagocytosis in endothelial cells and may throw light on the pathogenesis and treatment of a number of disease states without incurring the need for large numbers of experimental animals.

PHAGOCYTOSIS OF PARTICULATES BY ENDOTHELIAL CELLS

Endothelial cells are not normally considered to be "professional" phagocytes. However, both in vivo and in vitro endothelial cells are capable of ingesting particulates (9) including bacteria (9-13). Endothelial cells in culture phagocytize unopsonized polystyrene spheres, uptake is rapid (minutes) and after several hours of exposure individual cells could contain as many as 15 or more beads. The range of sizes of ingested spheres is from 0.2 μm to 15 μm. Spheres of 20-25 μm are partially surrounded by endothelial cells, while spheres of more than 30 μm are treated as microcarriers and can be used for the isolation (14,15) and large scale culture of endothelial cells (5,6,17). Fluorescent staining using monoclonal antibodies to vimentin suggest that the endothelial cytoskeleton forms a meshwork retaining ingested microbeads and appears to be involved in drawing outlying beads "captured" by cell extensions to the interior of the cell (18).

Cells that have undergone phagocytosis of many spheres express receptors for the Fc portion of IgG on their surface (10), these receptors may be unmasked in a manner similar to that of endothelial cells injured by viral infection, white cell lysates or endotoxin (10,19).

PHAGOCYTOSIS OF SAMMONELLA MINNESOTA

Endothelial cells are capable of phagocytizing both living and dead Salmonella minnesota. We have studied different strains of S. minnesota to determine the effects of the bacteria on the endothelial cells and, conversely, the effects of the endothelial cells on the bacteria.

Endothelial cells bind and ingest the mutant (Re) form of S. minnesota while the wild (S) type is not phagocytized to any great extent (Fig 1) (18).

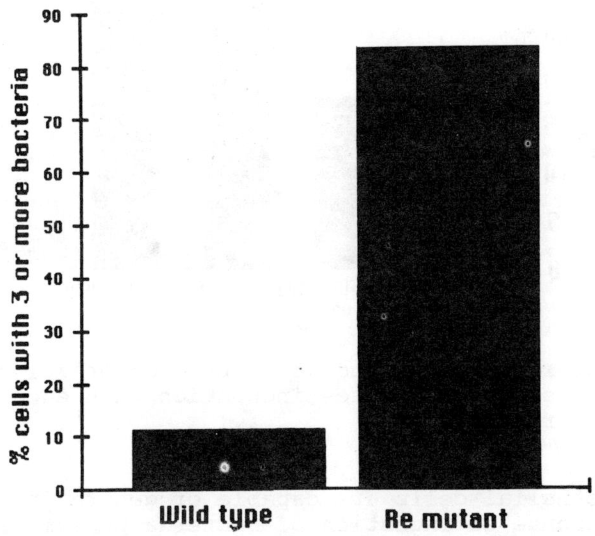

Figure 1. Phagocytosis of S. minnesota by pulmonary endothelial cells. The wild type (S form) is not phagocytized to any great extent, while the Re mutant binds and undergoes phagocytosis (from ref 18).

The binding of the Re type is mediated by C1q; a subunit of the first component of complement, that binds to the Re mutant but not to the S-type (20). Endothelial cells possess receptors for C1q (21) and these receptors bind the collagen-like tail region of C1q leaving the Fc binding heads to interact with the S. minnesota Re bacteria. Experimental evidence indicates that incubation of endothelial cells and Re type bacteria with C1q-depleted serum inhibits binding. Preincubation of either endothelial cells or S. minnesota Re with C1q enhances binding, but incubation of both endothelial cells and Re mutant with C1q prior to co-incubation of cells and bacteria reduces binding presumably due to lack of unoccupied C1q binding sites available for interaction (20).

Ingestion of S. minnesota Re type induces a respiratory burst in endothelial cells. Measurement of superoxide anion generation in endothelial cells in response to the Re mutant in comparison with the effects of calcium ionophore (A23187) and an activator of protein kinase C (phorbol myristate acetate) acting independently and synergistically are shown in Fig 2.

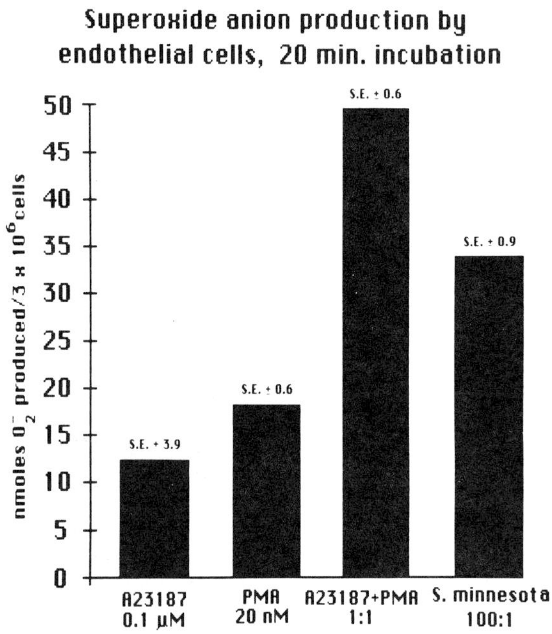

Figure 2. Superoxide anion production by endothelial cells in response to 20 minutes incubation with each reactant (from ref 22).

Thus, endothelial cells are capable of generating oxygen radicals in response to ingestion of bacteria presumably as a bactericidal mechanism. However, the ability of endothelial cells to kill S. minnesota Re is not highly effective (9,18). The bactericidal effectiveness of endothelial cells appears to vary with the toxin producing characteristics and anti-oxidant activities of the bacteria and is regulated by exogenous substances (see below). Nevertheless, endothelial cells must be regarded as a source of oxidant damage with the potential for deleterious effects on the vasculature (22).

PHAGOCYTOSIS OF STAPHYLOCOCCUS AUREUS

S. aureus is a leading cause of infectious endocarditis and there have been reports that endothelial phagocytosis occurs in vivo (9,16). Recently we have shown that endothelial cells in culture phagocytize both living and dead S. aureus (10-13). Intracellular S. aureus do not proliferate but can be cytotoxic to endothelial cells as estimated by the release of ^{3}H-adenine from endothelial cells, depending on the size of the inoculum, strain and time (13). The degree of cytotoxicity of S. aureus seems to be heavily determined by whether or not α-hemolysin is produced, since

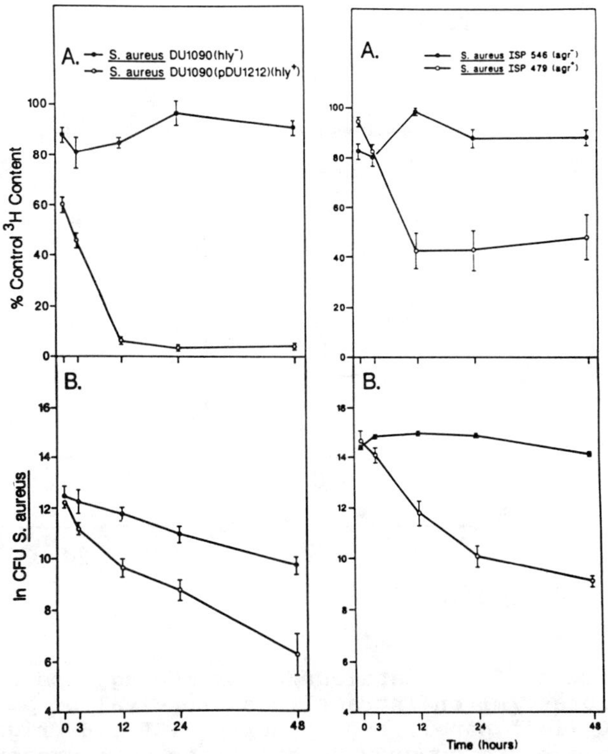

Figure 3. Effect of intracellular S. aureus DU 1090 and DU 1090 (pDU 1212) (left panels) and ISP 546 and ISP 479 (right panels) on endothelial cell monolayers. Endothelial cell cultures $\pm{}^3$H-adenine label were exposed to S. aureus for 3.5 hours, then lysostaphin was placed in the culture to destroy extracellular S. aureus. At subsequent times, content of ^{3}H-adenine (panel A) or intracellular S. aureus CFU (panel B) were assayed (from ref 13).

α-hemolysin-producing DU 1090 and ISP 546 were not found to be cytotoxic whereas α-hemolysin-producing DU 1090 (pDU 1212) was cytotoxic (Fig 3) (13).

However, in addition to the effects of bacteria on the endothelial cells, the latter clearly are not passive victims. Viable intracellular S. aureus decrease in number without damage to the endothelial cell monolayer suggesting bactericidal activity. As indicated above endothelial cells are capable of generating superoxide anion (O_2^-). We investigated the effects of catalase, SOD (Fig 4) and adenosine (Fig 5) and found that each of these substances decreases the bactericidal activity of endothelial cells, indicating the importance of reactive oxygen metabolites in bactericidal activity (22,24,25).

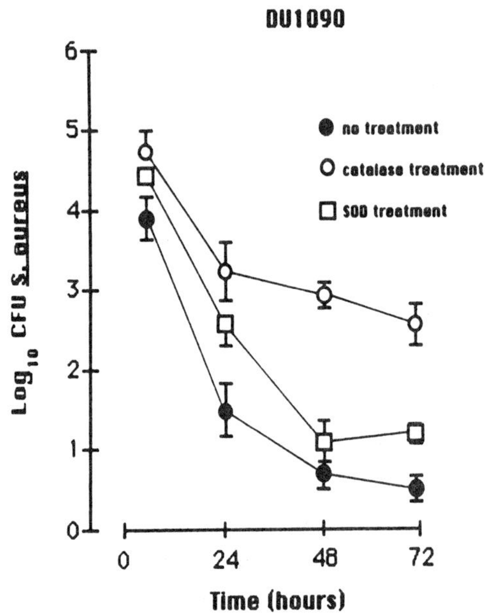

Figure 4. Effect of 50 μg catalase/ml or 100 μg superoxide dismutase/ml on intracellular survival of S. aureus DU 1090 (left panel) and S. aureus ISP 546 (right panel). Catalase and superoxide dismutase were present in the medium when S. aureus were added.

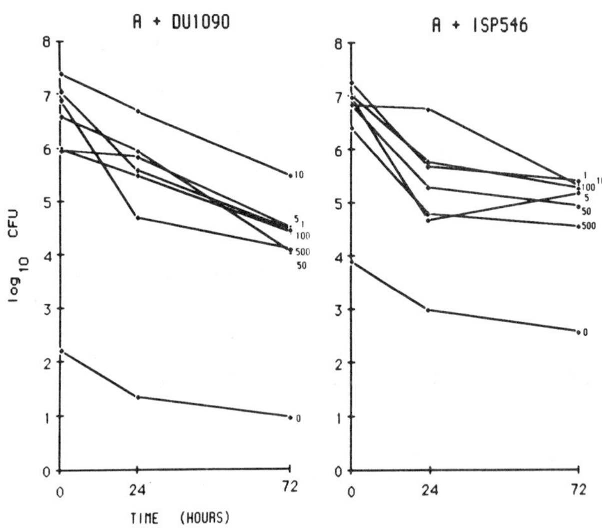

Figure 5. Effect of varying concentrations of adenosine on endothelial cell bactericidal activity. The concentrations indicated, in μg/ml, were present in the medium when S. aureus DU 1090 (left panel) or S. aureus ISP 546 (right panel) were added to the cultures.

The effect of hypoxanthine on bactericidal activity is similar to that of adenosine , and studies using dipyridamole, an inhibitor of adenosine uptake but not binding, indicate that binding of adenosine to its receptors rather than metabolism of adenosine, is important in reducing bactericidal activity. It is interesting that in order for adenosine to produce its effect on bacterial killing it must be incubated with endothelial cells at the time of ingestion of bacteria not after ingestion has occurred (Fig 6) suggesting an effect on receptors in the phagosome membrane rather than on the external plasma membrane (25).

Pre- and Post-phagocytosis Addition of Adenosine

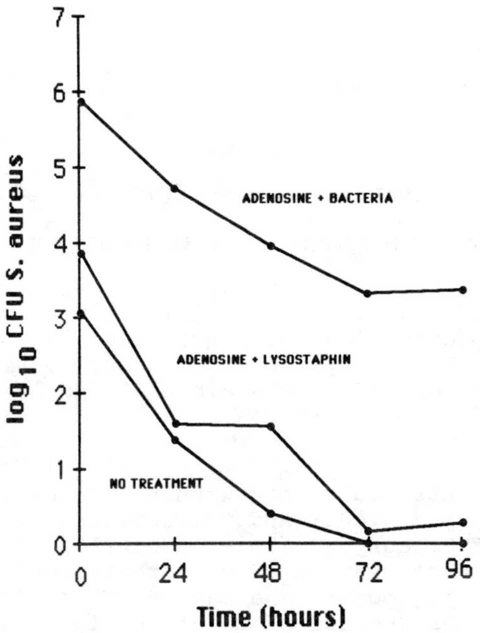

Figure 6. When adenosine was added to endothelial cultures at the same time as the bacteria, killing was inhibited. However, adenosine was not effective if added after phagocytosis (at the time lysostaphin was added to remove extracellular bacteria).

We next tested various antibiotics for their effects on S. aureus (ATCC 25923) within endothelial cells. Clindamycin, penicillin G, rifampin and tetracycline were used at concentrations well in excess of their MIC or MBC. Their effects on intracellular survival (colony forming units) by endothelial cells that had been incubated (1:100) with S. aureus are shown in Fig 7.

The data suggest that the antibiotics tested do not decrease survival of S. aureus within endothelial cells. Clindamycin and

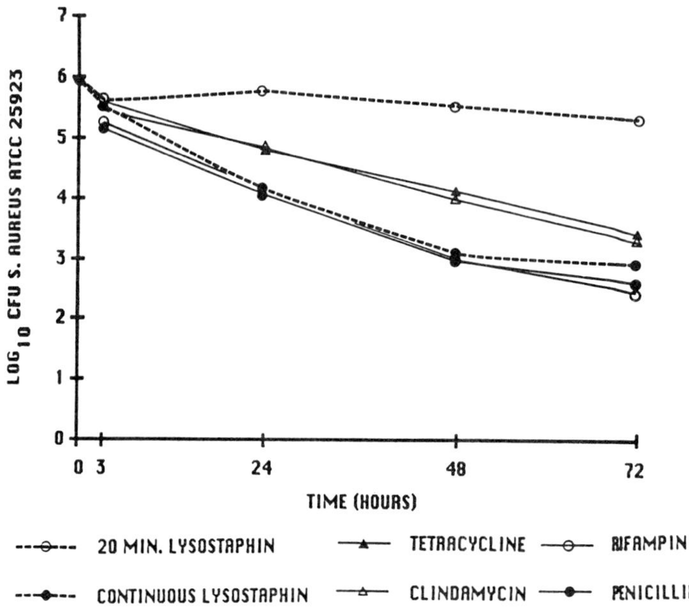

Figure 7. Effect of antibiotics on intracellular survival of S. aureus ATCC 25923. Endothelial cells were allowed to ingest S. aureus for 3.5 hours, then medium containing 2.5×10^{-5} M tetracycline, clindamycin, rifampin, or penicillin, or medium containing 10 μg lysostaphin / ml was placed in the cultures.

tetracycline are concentrated 3-fold within endothelial cells. At 24 hours clindamycin ($p > 0.005$) and tetracycline ($p > 0.01$) increased survival of S. aureus within endothelial cells (26).

Taken together these results suggest that endothelial cell phagocytosis of S. aureus occurs and may result in damage to the endothelial layer. Consequences of damage or lysis of endothelial cells would include the exposure of subendothelial collagen allowing platelet adhesion and aggregation leading to the development of a thrombotic vegetation at the infected site. In addition, bacteria harbored within endothelial cells are protected from host defenses (such as macrophages) and from antibiotics. However, endothelial cells respond to phagocytosis by releasing toxic oxygen species which could further damage surrounding vascular tissues as do reactive oxygen metabolites derived from neutrophils. Lysis of endothelial cells would have the effect of releasing bacteria into the circulation which could produce cycles of bacteremia and further phagocytosis by endothelial cells. Thus, these effects could explain the prolonged antibiotic therapy required for the treatment of subacute bacterial endocarditis and how sepsis leads to pulmonary diseases such as the adult respiratory distress syndrome.

EFFECTS OF PHAGOCYTOSIS ON ENDOTHELIAL CELL BEHAVIORAL KINETICS

Phagocytosis is an example of the several properties shared by endothelial cells and macrophages (27). Recently, we have been able to show that endothelial cells can be activated by phagocytosis of 5-10 μ polystyrene beads (18). Using a wounded monolayer assay (28) endothelial cells of a stationary confluent monolayer are exposed to beads for 15 mins, the monolayer is then wounded by removal of two-thirds of the cells with a rubber policeman. The cells migrate out from the wound line to fill the space. The cells are tracked by Quiktrak, a computer program specifically developed for (29) analysis of endothelial cell behavioral parameters. Phagocytosis causes a dramatic increase in the rates of migration (22 μm/hr v 9 μm/hr), division (interdivision interval - hv 90 h) and further phagocytosis (9,18,30).

CONCLUDING COMMENTS

We have studied phagocytosis of bacteria and particulates using endothelial cells in culture. The studies have thrown light on the basic mechanisms of interaction between endothelial cells and pathogens and of the mechanisms of regulation and inhibition of bactericidal activity. It is hoped that, in addition, the research described has demonstrated that endothelial cells in culture can provide powerful tools for improving understanding of fundamental biological mechanisms and clinical implications while avoiding the use of large quantities of experimental animals.

ACKNOWLEDGEMENTS

Supported by grants from the National Heart Lung and Blood Institute (HL 21568, HL 33064) and the Council for Tobacco Research (814).

REFERENCES

1. RYAN, U.S., RYAN, J.W., WHITAKER, C. and CHIU, A. (1976), Localization of angiotensin converting enzyme (kininase II). II. Immunocyto-chemistry and immunofluorescence. Tissue & Cell, 8:125-146.
2. RYAN, U.S. (1985), Processing of angiotensin and other peptides by the lungs. In Handbook of Physiology - The Respiratory System 1 (eds. A.P. Fishman and A.B. Fisher), Amer. Physiol. Soc., Bethesda, MD, Chapter 10, pp. 351-364.
3. RYAN, U.S., CLEMENTS, E., HABLISTON, D. and RYAN, J.W. (1978) Isolation and culture of pulmonary artery endothelial cells. Tissue & Cell, 10:535-554.
4. RYAN, U.S. and MAYFIELD, L.J. (1986), Assay and computation of angiotensin converting enzyme activity of endothelial cells. J. Tissue Cult. Methods, 10:15-25.
5. RYAN, U.S., MORTARA, M. and WHITAKER, C. (1980), Methods for microcarrier culture of bovine pulmonary artery endothelial cells avoiding the use of enzymes. Tissue & Cell, 12:619-635.
6. RYAN, U.S. (1984), Culture of pulmonary endothelial cells on microcarrier beads. In Biology of the Endothelial Cell (ed. E.A. Jaffe), Martinus Nijhoff, The Netherlands, Chapter 4, pp. 34-50.
7. RYAN, U.S. (1986), Metabolic activity of pulmonary endothelium: Modulation of structure and function. Ann. Rev. Physiol., 48:263-277.

8. JOHNS, A., KHALIL, R.A., RYAN, U.S. and VAN BREEMEN, C. (1987), Endothelium-Derived Relaxing Factor. In Endothelial Cells. (ed. U.S. Ryan) CRC Press, Boca Raton, Florida, in press.
9. RYAN, U.S. (1987), Phagocytic properties of endothelial cells. In Endothelial Cells. (ed. U.S. Ryan) CRC Press, Boca Raton, Florida, in press.
10. RYAN U.S. (1986), The endothelial surface and responses to injury. Fed. Proc., 45:101-108.
11. HAMILL, R.J., VANN, J.M. and PROCTOR, R.A. (1986), Phagocytosis of Staphylococcus aureus by Cultured Bovine Aortic Endothelial Cells: A Model for Post-Adherence Events in Endovascular Infections. Infect. Immun. 54: 833-836.
12. VANN, J.M. and PROCTOR, R.A. (1987), Ingestion of Staphylococcus aureus by Bovine Endothelial Cells Results in Time and Inoculum-Dependent Damage to Endothelial Cell Monolayers. Infect. Immun. 55:2155-2163.
13. VANN, J.M. and PROCTOR, R.A. (1987), Cytotoxic Effects of Ingested Staphylococcus aureus on Bovine Endothelial Cells: Role of S. aureus Alpha-Hemolysin (Submitted to Microbial pathogenesis).
14. RYAN, U.S. and WHITE, L. (1986), Microvascular endothelium, isolation with microcarriers: Arterial, venous. J. Tissue Cult. Methods, 10:9-13.
15. RYAN, U.S., WHITE, L., LOPEZ, M. and RYAN, J.W. (1982), Use of microcarriers to isolate and culture pulmonary microvascular endothelium. Tissue & Cell 14:597-606.
16. DOMAGK, G. (1924), Über die Bedeutung der Endothelien für die Abwehr von Infektionserrengern und die Entstehung des Amyloids. Klin. Wchnschr, 3:1338-1339.
17. RYAN, U.S. and MAXWELL, G (1986), Microcarrier cultures of endothelial cells. J. Tissue Cult. Methods, 10:7-8.
18. RYAN, U.S. (1987), Endothelial cell activation responses. In Pulmonary Endothelium in Health and Disease. (ed. U.S. Ryan), Marcel Dekker, Inc., N.Y., 32:3-33.
19. RYAN, U.S., SCHULTZ, D.R. and RYAN, J.W. (1981), Fc and C3b receptors on pulmonary endothelial cells: Induction by injury. Science, 214:557-559.
20. RYAN, U.S., SCHULTZ, D.R., GOODWIN, J.D., VANN, J.M. and HART, M.A. (1987), Role of C1q in phagocytosis of S. minnesota by pulmonary endothelial cells. submitted.
21. ZHANG, S.C., SCHULTZ, D.R. and RYAN, U.S. (1986), Receptor - mediated binding of C1q on pulmonary endothelial cells. Tissue & Cell, 18:13-18.
22. RYAN, U.S. and VANN, J.M. (1987), Endothelial cells: A source and target of oxidant damage. In Proceedings of the 4th International Congress on Oxygen Radicals. (ed. M.G. Simic, K.A. Taylor and A.F. Ward), in press.
23. RYAN, U.S., GOODWIN, J.D., CURLESS, B.L. and SCHULTZ, D.R. (1987), Endothelial cell responses to bacterial ingestion. Fed. Proc. 46:971, (Abstr. 3813).
24. VANN, J.M. and RYAN, U.S. (1987), Engagement of adenosine receptors results in decrease of endothelial cell bactericidal activity. submitted.
25. VANN, J.M. and RYAN, U.S. (1987), Adenosine decreases the bactericidal activity of endothelial cells. J. Cell Biol. 105:326a, (Abstr. 1840).
26. VANN, J.M. and RYAN, U.S. (1987), Bactericidal activity of endothelial cells for ingested S. aureus. 27th ICAAC, New York, N.Y. (Abstract 508).

27. RYAN, U.S. (1987), The macrophage-like properties of endothelial cells. NIPS, submitted.
28. RYAN, U.S., ABSHER, M., OLAZABAL, B.M., BROWN, L.M. and RYAN, J.W. (1982), Proliferation of pulmonary endothelial cells: Time-lapse cinematography of growth to confluence and restitution of monolayer after wounding. Tissue & Cell, 14:637-649.
29. RYAN, U.S. and MAYFIELD, L.J. (1986), Video analysis of endothelial cell genealogy, migration and division. J. Tissue Cult. Methods, 10:55-60.
30. RYAN, U.S. and MAYFIELD, L.J. (1987), Computer tracking of endothelial activation responses. In Vascular Endothelium in Health and Disease. (ed. S. Chien), in press.

B3

Cultured Rat Hepatocytes in the Study of the Hepatotoxicity of Acetaminophen

JOHN L. FARBER

Department of Pathology
Thomas Jefferson University
Philadelphia, PA 19107

ABSTRACT

The results of the author's studies of the killing of cultured hepatocytes by acetaminophen are reviewed and compared with the hepatotoxicity of acetaminophen in the intact rat. The data allow the tentative conclusion that the mechanisms of the killing of cultured hepatocytes by acetaminophen are not necessarily different from those that obtain in the intact animal.

Isolated rat hepatocytes are increasingly used to study the mechanisms of toxic liver cell injury. An essential assumption that the use of such an in vitro system implies is that the mechanisms determining the lethal injury of isolated hepatocytes are essentially the same as those that determine liver cell necrosis in the intact animal. However, in only a very few cases has this assumption been specifically verified.

Acetaminophen is a commonly sued analgesic-antipyretic. While generally devoid of toxicity at therapeutic doses, overdosage can result in a severe centrilobular hepatic necrosis that depends upon metabolism of the toxin by the mixed function oxidases (1,2). However, the mechanism coupling such metabolism to the necrosis of hepatocytes is a matter of continuing study. Previous studies related the extent of the covalent binding of acetaminophen metabolites to cellular macromolecules with the production of liver necrosis (2-5).

We have been using cultured rat hepatocytes to study the hepatotoxicity of acetaminophen (6,7). We have obtained evidence for the participation of activated oxygen species in the genesis of lethal cell injury by acetaminophen. In addition, we have begun to compare the results of these in vitro studies with the features of the hepatotoxicity of acetaminophen in the intact animal. The present report summarizes the results of these initial studies.

Hepatocytes isolated from male rats were insensitive to as much as 10 mM acetaminophen. Sensitivity of the cultured hepatocytes to acetaminophen was induced by pretreatment of the rats with 3-methylcholanthrene or phenobarbital (6). Hepatocytes prepared from the livers of rats pretreated with methylcholanthrene were more sensitive to acetaminophen than hepatocytes from rats induced with phenobarbital. Napthoflavone, a specific inhabiter of mixed function oxidase activity, prevented the killing of hepatocytes from methylcholanthrene-induced rats (6). By contrast, SKF-515A, another specific inhabiter of mixed function oxidase activity, prevented the killing of hepatocytes from phenobarbital-induced rats but not from those pretreated with methylcholanthrene. The effects of these inhibitors document that the toxicity of acetaminophen for cultured hepatocytes depends on the metabolism of the drug, a situation similar to that occurring with intact animal (1,2).

Inhibition of glutathione reductase by bis-chloro-nitrosourea (BCNU) with the resultant inhibition of the GSH-GSSG cycle potentiates the toxicity of an acute oxidative stress that results from the generation of hydrogen peroxide in the culture medium by the bacterial enzyme glucose oxidase (8) or by the intracellular generation hydrogen peroxide formed as a result of the metabolism of quinonoid compounds, particularly menadione (8) and adriamycin (9). In a liver cell, quinones undergo a one-electron reduction to yield the corresponding semiquinone radical. Oxidation of such semiquinone radicals by molecular oxygen produces superoxide anions with regeneration of the parent compound. In turn, the enzymatic or spontaneous dismutation of the superoxide anions gives hydrogen peroxide. Inhibition of glutathione reductase by treatment of methylcholanthrene induced hepatocytes with BCNU very strikingly potentiates the toxicity of acetaminophen (6). After a 4 hour exposure to either 750 or 1000 uM acetaminophen there was essentially no loss of viability of the cultured cells. By contrast, with BCNU present these same doses killed virtually all of the hepatocytes. Importantly, this increased killing was achieved without any increase in the extent of the covalent binding of [^{3}H]acetaminophen to total hepatocyte proteins. In other words, the use of BCNU allowed the definition of situations in which either essentially all or none of the cultured hepatocytes are killed by acetaminophen without any difference in the extent of covalent binding.

The killing of cultured hepatocytes by hydrogen peroxide is dependent on an endogenous source of ferric iron (10). Cultured hepatocytes pretreated with the ferric iron chelator deferoxamine are resistant to the toxicity of hydrogen peroxide generated either by glucose oxidase or by the metabolism of menadione. Pretreatment with deferoxamine similar prevents the cell killing by acetaminophen (6). Pretreatment of the hepatocytes with 20 mM deferoxamine prior to the exposure to BCNU and acetaminophen prevented the cell killing. Again, protection against the liver cell injury was achieved without any reduction in the extent of the covalent binding of [^{3}H]acetaminophen (6). The addition of ferric iron to the culture medium restored the sensitivity of hepatocytes that were pretreated with deferoxamine to acetaminophen without change in covalent binding (6). These data indicate that it is possible to manipulate the iron content of the hepatocytes to vary in either direction the toxicity of acetaminophen without any effect on the extent of the covalent binding of metabolites of [^{3}H]acetaminophen to total hepatocyte proteins.

The data reviewed above demonstrate that the toxicity of acetaminophen for cultured rat hepatocytes can be dissociated from the covalent binding of its metabolites and support the alternative hypothesis that lethal cell injury is the consequence of an acute oxidative stress. The ability of both superoxide dismutase and catalase to prevent the metabolism-dependent cytotoxicity of acetaminophen directly implicates oxygen radicals in this process (7).

Superoxide dismutase or catalase added to the culture medium prevented the killing of cultured hepatocytes by acetaminophen (7). While almost all the hepatocytes can be killed following exposure to acetaminophen and BCNU, less than 10% were irreversible injured in the presence of superoxide dismutase or catalase, respectively. Heat-inactivated (boiled) superoxide dismutase or catalase have no effect on the extent of cell killing. The hydroxyl radical scavenger mannitol also protected hepatocytes from the cytotoxicity of acetaminophen (7).

As noted above, the killing of cultured hepatocytes by acetaminophen depends upon a cellular source of ferric iron. Addition of superoxide dismutase to the culture medium prevents the restoration of sensitivity to acetaminophen by ferric iron in deferoxamine-pretreated cells but not that produced by ferrous iron. By contrast, catalase is effective in preventing the killing of cells in the presence of either ferric or ferrous iron (7).

The main conclusion to be drawn from the above data is that both ferric iron and superoxide ions are required for the killing by acetaminophen of cultured hepatocytes from methylcholanthrene-induced rats. Furthermore, the data argue that this iron acts to generate hydroxyl radicals by the Fenton reaction. It is suggested that intracellular ferric iron derived from ferritin is reduced to ferrous iron by superoxide anions. The ferrous iron then reacts with hydrogen peroxide formed as a result of the oxidative metabolism of acetaminophen to form hydroxyl radicals.

By what mechanisms do hydroxyl radicals lethally injure hepatocytes that are intoxicated with acetaminophen? We have defined two distinct mechanisms by which acetaminophen kills cultured hepatocytes prepared from 3-methylcholanthrene-pretreated male rats (11). With 0.5 to 5 mM acetaminophen cell killing within 4 hours depended on the inhibition of glutathione reductase with BCNU and was accompanied by the peroxidation of cellular lipids as assessed by the accumulation of malondialdehyde (MDA) in the culture medium (11). The antioxidant diphenyl phenylenediamine (DPPD prevented both the peroxidation of lipids and the death of the cells. By contrast, DPPD had no effect on the metabolism of acetaminophen as assessed by the extent of the covalent binding of [^{3}H]acetaminophen, by the rate and extent of the depletion of glutathione, and by the accumulation of acetaminophen metabolites in the culture medium. It is concluded that the peroxidation of the phospholipids of cellular membranes is most likely the first mechanism whereby acetaminophen lethally injures cultured hepatocytes.

With 10-20 mM acetaminophen, there was no evidence of lipid peroxidation, and DPPD had no effect on the number of dead cells (11). Thus, the second mechanisms of lethal cell injury is independent of lipid peroxidation and insensitive to antioxidants. Its chemical nature remains to be determined. Damage to the inner mitochondrial membrane with loss of mitochondrial function is suspected to play a role in the cell killing by the second mechanism.

The essential features of the killing of cultured hepatocytes by acetaminophen reviewed above can be reproduced in the intact animal (12). Male rats had no evidence of liver necrosis 24 hours after administration of up to 1000 mg/kg acetaminophen. Inducers of mixed function oxidase activity increased the hepatotoxicity of acetaminophen. In particular, the livers of rats treated with methylcholanthrene are more sensitive to acetaminophen than are those that are induced with phenobarbital. Inhibition of glutathione reductase with BCNU increased markedly the liver cell necrosis produced by 500 mg/kg acetaminophen in methylcholanthrene-induced rats (12). There was no evidence of liver necrosis in rats treated with BCNU alone for up to 48 hours. BCNU reduced the GSH content of the liver by 40%, but the potentiation of liver necrosis cannot be attributed to this depletion of GSH. Reduction of the GSH content by 40% with diethylmaleate did not potentiate the toxicity of 500 mg/kg acetaminophen in methylcholanthrene-induced rats (12).

The antioxidant DPPD and the ferric iron chelator deferoxamine prevented the liver necrosis produced by 500 mg\kg acetaminophen in rats pretreated with BCNU (12). By contrast, neither protective agent prevented the fall in GSH induced by acetaminophen (12). Preliminary studies indicate that superoxide dismutase administered in liposomes similarly prevents the hepatotoxicity of acetaminophen in methylcholanthrene-induced rats (13).

These features of the hepatotoxicity of acetaminophen closely reproduce the conditions of the killing of hepatocytes cultured from the livers of similar rats. Thus, these data allow the tentative conclusion that the mechanisms of the killing of cultured hepatocytes by acetaminophen are not necessarily different from those that obtain in the intact animal.

REFERENCES

1. Mitchell, J.R., Jollow, D.J., Potter, W.Z., Davis, D.C., Gillette,. J.R., and Brodie, B.B. (1973) J. Pharmacol. Exp. Ther. 187, 185.

2. Jollow, D.J., Thorgeirsson, S.S., Potter, W.Z.,

Hashimoto, M., and Mitchell, J.R. (1974) Pharmacology 12. 171.

3. Jollow, D.J., Mitchell, J.R., Potter, W.Z., Davis, D.C., Gillette, J.R., and Brodie, B.B. (1973) J. Pharmacol. Exp. Ther. 187, 195.

4. Potter, W.Z., Davis, D.C., Mitchell, J.R., Jollow, D.J., Gillette, J.R., and Brodie. B.B. (1973) J. Pharmacol. Exp. Ther. 187, 203.

5. Mitchell, J.R., Thorgeirsson, S.S., Potter, W.Z., Jollow, D.J., and Keiser, H. (1974) Clin. Pharmacol. Ther. 16, 676.

6. Gerson, R.J., Casini, A., Gilfor, d., Serroni, A., and Farber, J.L. (1985) Biochem. Biophys. Res. Commun. 126, 1129.

7. Kyle, M.E., Miccadei, S., Nakae, D., and Farber, J.L. (1987) Biochem. Biophys. Res. Commun. 149, 889, 1987.

8. Starke, P.E., and Farber, J.L. (1985) J. Biol. Chem. 260, 86.

9. Babson, J.R., Abell, N.S., and Reed, D.S. (1981) Biochem. Pharmacol. 30, 2299.

10. Starke, P.E., and Farber, J.L. (1985) J. Biol. Chem. 260, 10099.

11. Farber, J.L., Serroni, A., Leonard, T.B., and Rogers, S.A. Unpublished data.

12. Nakae, D., Oakes, J.W., and Farber, J.L. Unpublished data.

13. Nakae, D., and Farber, J.L. Unpublished data.

C

Update: A Critical Evaluation of Alternatives to Acute Ocular Irritancy Testing

JOHN M. FRAZIER

Department of Environmental Health Sciences
The Johns Hopkins University
School of Hygiene and Public Health
615 North Wolfe Street
Baltimore, MD 21205

ABSTRACT

Alternatives to in vivo acute ocular irritation testing have been developing over the past 10 years. The status of these approaches was reviewed in the Bausch & Lomb sponsored workshop in the Spring of 1986 and the report published as Volume 4 of the Alternative Methods in Toxicology book series in early 1987. Since that time, progress has been made to implement these tests in a strategy for toxicological risk assessment. These developments are reviewed in this report.

INTRODUCTION

The purpose of this discussion is to update progress related to the development of alternatives to in vivo ocular irritation testing which has taken place since the last CAAT symposium. As many of you will recall, in conjunction with that symposium (Progress in In Vitro Toxicology) CAAT conducted a workshop on this particular subject which was sponsored by Bausch & Lomb. The outcome of this workshop was the publication of Volume 4 of the series Alternative Methods in Toxicology - A Critical Evaluation of Alternatives to Acute Ocular Irritation Testing (Frazier, Gad, Goldberg and McCulley - 1987). At the symposium and in Volume 4, I described a methodological approach to validation of alternative test systems (Chapter 7 - Volume 4). It was hoped at that time, nearly one and a half years ago, that this validation procedure would be applied to the existing test systems in order to establish a battery of accepted in vitro tests which could be utilized by regulatory agencies as an alternative for in vivo acute ocular irritation testing. Progress toward that goal is discussed below as well as recent developments in some of the previously identified tests. In addition, several new test systems are described.

Before addressing the specific issue at hand, a few comments about the overall objective and strategy of in vitro testings are in order. The objective of toxicity testing is to develop a scientific database which can be used to evaluate the potential toxicological risk of a chemical to man, be it a commercial household product, a drug or an industrial chemical. The traditional approach to this problem is based on in vivo testing methodologies using animals as model systems to generate the database employed by regulatory agencies to make risk assessments (Table 1). The basic set of in vivo tests includes acute, subchronic and chronic tests which provide data ranging from LD50's to carcinogenic potential of the test chemical. In addition, specific tests are conducted to evaluate reproductive toxicity, including teratogenicity, skin and ocular risks as well as immunological responses such as hypersensitivity. In any particular situation, all of these tests or some subset will be conducted depending on the characteristics of the chemical and its potential utilization. The database provided by this basic set of animal tests is evaluated in terms of scientific quality, interpreted in terms of consistency (are rat and mice data consistent - if not what additional studies, such as metabolic studies, can resolve discrepancies) and integrated into the human risk assessment process. The specific tests to generate the database and the procedures to utilize this data have evolved over the past 50 to 60 years to provide regulatory agencies with the necessary information to make safety evaluations and regulatory decisions.

TABLE 1: Specific Toxicity Tests Employed for Risk Assessment Analysis

CLASSICAL ANIMAL TESTING	IN VITRO TESTING
Acute	Cytotoxicity (Target Organ)
Subchronic	Cell Specific Function
Chronic (Carcinogenicity)	Genotoxicity
Toxicokinetics	Metabolism
Reproductive	Teratogenicity
Ocular/Skin	Ocular/Skin Inflammation
Hypersensitivity	

The question we are asking today is whether a totally new database provided by in vitro test systems can in fact replace the traditional approach utilizing whole animal data. Obviously, twenty years ago the question would not even have been asked. The biotechnology, both cell culture techniques and bioanalytical methodologies, were not sufficiently developed to make in vitro test systems a viable option to whole animal test systems at that time. This situation is rapidly changing with both technological developments as well as our growing understanding of toxicological principles. In vitro toxicity test systems which have developed specifically for toxicity testing purposes over the past decade can be classified as in Table 1. Listing both in vivo and in vitro tests in the same table is designed to illustrate that there is parallelism between the two approaches. For example, in vitro cytotoxicity tests provide data which are relevant to acute toxicity questions. In vitro xenobiotic metabolism studies have correlates with in vivo toxicokinetic studies. For more specific toxicity questions - teratogenicity, ocular irritation, skin irritation, etc. - there are strong parallelisms between in vitro and in vivo test systems. However, it should be apparent that there is not a one-to-one parallelism. Clearly in vitro cytotoxicity tests do not provide in and of themselves a direct replacement for an in vivo acute toxicity study. Hence, the data generated by any one in vitro test does not provide an equivalent set of data which can be incorporated into the existing risk assessment process in place of in vivo data. The new spectrum of data generated by a battery of in vitro tests must be integrated into a new approach, in a sense a new formula, to conduct a scientifically valid safety evaluation.

Bringing this discussion to focus on the issue of acute ocular irritation testing, an in vitro approach must employ a battery of tests which provide a spectrum of data which encompasses the range of toxicological processes which contribute to ocular irritation. No single test system will provide both a necessary and sufficient database for a complete evaluation of potential risk for human ocular irritation. When researchers claim in scientific publications and presentations that their test system is a replacement for the Draize test it reduces the credibility of not only their specific test but of the in vitro approach to toxicity testing in general. There is no credible scientific evidence that any single in vitro test will directly replace any in vivo toxicological test. As a result of over enthusiastic claims, potentially useful test systems, as components of test batteries, may be discredited because of unattainable expectations.

The previous discussion was intended to point out the basic difference in the type of data generated by in vivo versus in vitro test systems. The second major component of the risk assessment process is to extrapolate those data from the model system to man. The mere generation of reproducible numbers is not enough; the meaning of the numbers in the context of potential human toxicity is what is important. The traditional whole animal approach to toxicity testing involves various extrapolation processes (Table 2). The procedures to extrapolate animal data have been studied over the years and in spite of well recognized problems, the perception is that the methods work. Furthermore, with the inclusion of safety factors, safe conditions for human exposure to chemicals can be established. To switch to in vitro approaches for toxicity testing, the fundamentally different database generated requires a new formulation of the extrapolation process. Some of the types of extrapolation required are given in Table 2 and again have similarities to whole animal methodologies. One advantage of in vitro systems is the potential to utilize human cells in the test system. This allows one to eliminate a large set of difficult problems related to interspecies extrapolation. However, the advantage gained in this respect is offset by the problems of in vitro to in vivo extrapolation. Because the concept of using in vitro toxicity data as a basis for prediction of human risk is really quite new (less than 10 years old), the problem of in vitro to in vivo extrapolation is a new and challenging area of toxicology.

TABLE 2: Specific Extrapolation Processes Employed to Make the Transition from Model to Man

WHOLE ANIMAL	IN VITRO
High Dose to Low Dose	In Vitro to In Vivo
Species	Toxicokinetics
Toxicokinetics	Interactions
Sensitivities	(Species)
Route to Route	Acute to Chronic
Acute to Chronic	High Risk Groups
High Risk Population	

In the particular case of acute ocular irritation testing, the extrapolation process is somewhat simplified since many of the factors involved in the more general toxicological process (absorption, distribution, excretion, metabolism, etc.) are not operative. Thus, it is possible to calibrate in vitro test systems with known toxic substances (ocular irritants) and present results as relative classifications rather than having to explicitly define absolute exposure concentrations and conditions which are safe.

With this overall conceptualization of the purpose of toxicity testing, i.e. database generation for inclusion in the risk assessment process and the extrapolation to the human, in vivo situation, we can proceed to some observations on the validation process. Validation of an in vitro testing strategy means establishment of the credibility of process such that predictions based on this approach are accepted at the regulatory /legal/ethical levels as adequately protecting human health and welfare. Thus, validation involves establishing the credibility of the whole procedure, both data generation and risk prediction. In the case of acute ocular irritation testing the basic protocol for the validation process has been presented previously (Frazier, 1986). The various phases of the validation process are summarized in Table 3. The purpose here is not to go over the details of the validation process, but to comment on developments to date or the lack thereof in implementing this process to validate alternatives to acute ocular irritation testing. With respect to potential tests, the Bausch & Lomb project basically summarized the identifiable tests as of the Spring, 1986. Several of the specific tests identified in that report have been further developed, and some of these are discussed below. In addition several new approaches have been proposed and are also discussed below.

TABLE 3: The Validation Process

PHASE 1: PRELIMINARIES

A. Definition of test objective
B. Identification of potential alternative tests
C. Selection of test chemicals
D. Establishment of "Gold Standard"

PHASE 2: MICROVALIDATION - PRIMARY LABORATORY

A. Protocol standardization
B. Blind feasibility study (20 test chemicals)

PHASE 3: MACROVALIDATION - SECONDARY LABORATORY

A. Test implementation - QC samples
B. Blind study (50-100 test chemicals)
C. Statistical evaluation

PHASE 4: TEST BATTERY OPTIMIZATION

The situation concerning selection of a set of test chemicals for the validation process can be summarized simply as "still to be resolved". Following the Bausch & Lomb workshop, CAAT attempted to establish a mechanism to address the issue but support for such a project was not available. It is extremely important to convene a panel of experts to select a set of test chemicals to be used to validate individual test systems. Some of the criteria for selection have been previously discussed (Frazier, 1987). The establishment of a "chemical bank" to provide these chemicals "blind" to researchers developing new tests also has high priority. Such a resource must be established to act as an impartial intermediary to break the code and evaluate the test results.

When critical evaluations of test results are performed, the "gold standard" for the toxicity classification of the test chemicals is needed. The problem is that the major source of scientifically documented test data is derived from the Draize test in rabbits. It would clearly be better to have a human database for validation studies rather than the de facto default to animal data. However, in the absence of such human data the selection of test chemicals should not include any chemicals about which there is controversy over the correlation between the Draize classification and available human data. Neither of these two activities, selection of a set of test chemicals and documentation of the toxicology database for these test chemicals, has been completed for acute ocular irritation testing

UPDATE OF IN VITRO TESTS

At the time of the acute ocular irritation workshop sponsored by Bausch & Lomb a total of 34 test systems was identified. These tests were classified according to the component of the ocular irritation response to which they applied as determined by the end point measurements performed. Progress has continued on several of these tests and some observations on recent developments follow:

1. Test Number: B.1.e. and B.3.d.

   Principal Researcher: Charles Shopsis - Rockefeller University and Adelphi University

   In studies described in more detail in the Poster Presentations (See Part 2, #20 of this volume), it was determined using several cell types and endpoint assays (uridine uptake inhibition and protein accumulation) that correlations between *in vitro* test data and *in vivo* Draize irritation scores were significantly better when serum was excluded from the medium. These studies involved a series of surfactants. Whether this relationship will hold true for other classes of chemicals must be established.

2. Test Number: D.2.

   Principal Researcher: Salwa Elgebaly - University of Connecticut

   This methodology is continuing to be developed (see Poster Presentations, #10). The test aims at developing an assay for release of inflammatory mediators (leucocyte chemotactic factors) from cultured bovine cornea. The chemotactic factors are currently being isolated for development of an ELISA assay which will allow the method to be automated.

3. Test Number B.3.d.

   Principal Researcher: Ellen Borenfreund/Harvey Babich - Rockefeller University

   The Neutral Red Assay has been used to evaluate additional classes of test chemicals and incorporation of a metabolizing (S-9) component has been investigated (Poster Presentations - #2). This assay system has been implemented in several laboratories indicating it has good properties for technology transfer.

4. Test Number: D.5.

   Principal Researcher: Norman Dubin - Johns Hopkins University

   The rat vaginal segment/prostaglandin release assay has been extended to additional test chemicals with promising results (see Poster Presentations - #9). This test may be useful since it evaluates the response of a mucous membrane.

5. Test Number: F.1.

Principal Researcher: Virginia Gordon - National Testing Corporation

The EYTEX test has undergone extensive evaluation including both micro- and macro-validation (Commercial Poster Presentations #1). The test has been quite successful in evaluating toxicity of a wide range of chemicals. The test protocol has been extended to accommodate non-soluble test chemicals.

6. Test Number: F.2.

Principal Researcher: Kurt Enslein, et al - Health Designs, Inc.

The rabbit eye irritation correlation model is continuing to be developed. These are purely statistical correlative methods and have the greatest application in product development rather than regulatory evaluation.

Over the last year and a half several new approaches to acute ocular irritation testing have developed. In some cases the test system is not necessarily new but represents a new application of an older test system. Some comments on these developments follow:

1. Drs. Hainsworth and Mowrey-McKee - Bausch & Lomb, Inc.

Endpoint: Cytotoxicity

Microwell Liquid Assay - Mouse L929 fibroblast are plated in 96 well microtiter plates. Cells are cultured for 18 h in the presence of the test chemical. At the end of the incubation period cells are stained with Erythrocin B and the LD_{50} determined. This test was used to evaluate optimal formulations for product development.

2. Dr. Dale Meyer - University of Texas - Dallas

Endpoint: Multiple

Using both rabbit corneal epithelial and endothelial cell cultures, the test evaluates acute and delayed effects following a short term exposure to a test chemical (see Poster Presentations - #17). Acute effects are measured 4 h after exposure and evaluate membrane leakage/lysis and morphology. Delayed effects are evaluated at 24 h by morphology, exfoliation and protein synthesis. Initial data suggest that different parameters can differentiate between different types of damage as well as the associated severity.

3. Dr. Ruy Tchao - Medical College of Pennsylvania

Endpoint: Physiology

Monolayers of Madin-Darby Canine Kidney (MDCK) cells are grown on Millipore - Millicell chambers. Confluent monolayers are impermeable to Na-Fluorescein, however chemical damage will result in diffusion of the fluorescent dye across the epithelium. This test system is described in Poster Presentations (Part 2, #24). Preliminary data indicate the test system may discriminate toxicity of chemicals which have previously been difficult to test - Tween compounds.

4. Dr. Edward Jackson - Noxell Corporation

Endpoint: Cytotoxicity

The Noxell Corporation and North American Science Associates (NAmSA) of Northwood, Ohio developed the agarose diffusion test method previously used to test medical devices, as a potential replacement for the Draize eye irritancy test on cosmetic products. Details about this work were recently presented at the Cosmetic, Toiletry and Fragrance Association's Scientific Conference in Boston, Massachusetts October 27, 1987. A manuscript on the application of this method for testing cosmetic products has been accepted by the Journal of Toxicology: CUTANEOUS AND OCULAR TOXICOLOGY (Volume 6, Number 4:239-250). The agar overlay assay is based on monolayer cultures of mouse L929 cells. The cells are overlayed with agar and the toxicant placed on the agar surface. The extent of cytotoxicity is evaluated and graded for the ranking of chemical toxicity. Extensive studies of various chemical classes have been undertaken.

5. John Shadduck - University of Illinois

Endpoint: Exfoliation

In studies which compared ultrastructural changes *in vitro* with *in vivo* responses to a test chemical it was observed *in vivo* that early detachment of corneal epithelial cells occurs without lysis. It may be possible to develop an *in vitro* assay using rapid cell detachment as the assay endpoint.

One additional development which is relevant to the validation discussion is the availability of new *in vivo* data for evaluation of *in vitro* test systems. The Procter and Gamble Company research group under the direction of Dr. Jack Griffith has compared the human experience with ocular irritants to the low volume Draize test (Freeberg, et al., 1986). The data indicate that this procedure (using 0.01 ml of test chemical) gives better correlation than the standard test (which uses 0.1 ml). The most striking effect is the improved correlation with time-to-recovery which was seriously overestimated in the standard volume test.

Although these comments have been brief, they illustrate the continuing research activities directed toward the development of alternatives to *in vivo* acute ocular irritation testing.

VALIDATION PROGRAMS

In a general sense the application of the validation process to *in vitro* methods for toxicology testing really began with the long process of validating the Ames assay for carcinogenicity testing. This assay is based on the hypothesis that mutagenicity, i.e. alteration in DNA, is an initial step in the carcinogenic process. As we now know this is only part of the carcinogenicity story, however the studies over the past 15 years to develop the Ames assay as an acceptable *in vitro* toxicity test (i.e. a system to generate data which are relevant to evaluating the carcinogenic potential of a test chemical) have provided useful insights into the mechanics of validation.

A second step towards the current situation for validation of acute ocular irritation test systems was the work performed by FRAME (Fund for the Replacement of Animals in Medical Experimentation) in England under the guidance of Dr. Michael Balls. The validation program of FRAME focused on a specific *in vitro* cytotoxicity test using total protein content of BCL-D1 cell cultures as a replacement for the LD50. Again, this project was extremely beneficial in identifying the factors which are important in transferring *in vitro* toxicity test technology from one laboratory to another. Many of the problems encountered in the Ames assay experience and the FRAME activity are directly reflected in the strategy for validation presented in Table 3.

More specifically for acute ocular irritation testing, the preliminary validation project undertaken by the Soap and Detergent Association through the Arthur D. Little Corporation has been the only direct attempt to validate these alternative test systems. The original project, which has been termed a pilot study, has been completed and publication of the results will occur in the near future. The project has been extended to a second phase which focuses on fewer test systems and more test chemicals to provide better statistics for evaluation purposes. The design of these studies appears to conform to the microvalidation phase in Table 3.

At the present time, the Soap and Detergent Association study is the only validation program specifically addressing the issue of *in vitro* alternatives to acute ocular irritation testing. The main limitation to the implementation of a more comprehensive validation program which would take the tests through all necessary phases of validation has been funding. There have been significant difficulties in identifying support mechanisms which utilize the interested parties: industry, government and social activist groups. Without adequate funding, the validation process will progress in an unorganized, and hence inefficient, fashion and will take 10-20 years as did the acceptance of the Ames assay.

To end on a positive note, there have been important advances in several specific tests. In fact, four tests have been submitted to the United States Pharmacopeial Convention as stimuli for consideration as standardized tests for ocular irritation testing (Table 4). Acceptance of these tests will lend credibility to the *in vitro* approach to toxicity testing and thus facilitate its introduction and acceptance.

TABLE 4: Test Submitted for Consideration by The United States Pharmacopeial Convention, Inc.

1. Chorioallantoic Membrane (CAM) Assay
2. Neutral Red Uptake Assay
3. Total Cell Protein Assay
4. Rabbit Corneal Epithelial Cell Wound Healing Assay

(Goldberg and Stark, 1987)

In summary, the progress towards validation of *in vitro* alternatives to acute ocular irritation testing has been slow. However, significant progress has been made. Scientifically we have a much better idea of what components are needed for a battery of *in vitro* tests to replace whole animal testing for acute ocular irritation. In addition, many specific tests continue to develop, both established tests as well as new approaches. In terms of validation some small steps have been taken but there is still a long way to go. Moreover, the basic hypothesis of *in vitro* toxicity testing as a methodology to provide the database for toxicity risk assessment has been accepted as worthy of further evaluation. Acceptance of the basic concept has been a difficult barrier to progress in the field and this barrier has been overcome. Scientists now talk about how and where *in vitro* approaches will be used in toxicity testing, as opposed to several years ago when the question was if *in vitro* approaches would be used.

REFERENCES

1. FRAZIER, J.M. (1987), The validation approach of The Johns Hopkins Center for Alternatives to Animal Testing, *Alternative Methods in Toxicology*, Mary Ann Liebert, Inc., 4:87-90.

2. FRAZIER, J.M., Gad, S.C., Goldberg, A.M. and McCulley, J.P. (1987), A critical evaluation of alternatives to acute ocular irritation testing. Alternative Methods in Toxicology, Vol. 4, Mary Ann Liebert, Inc., New York.

3. FREEBERG, F.F., Nixon, G.A., Reer, P.J., Weaver, J.E., Bruce, R.D., Griffith, J.F. and Sanders, L.W. (1986), Human and rabbit eye responses to chemical insult. Fund. Appl. Toxicol. 7:626-634.

4. GOLDBERG, A.M. and Stark, D. (1987), Eye irritancy testing. Pharmacopeial Forum, Nov.-Dec., pp.3235-3239.

D. Biotechnology and *In Vitro* Toxicology

D1

Issues in the Safety Assessment of Products of Biotechnology

GERHARD ZBINDEN

Institute of Toxicology
Swiss Federal Institute of Technology and University of Zurich
Schwerzenbach, Switzerland

ABSTRACT

Because of their unique chemical structures and biological actions, biotechnology products cannot be subjected to the routine safety tests developed for small molecular drugs. Current experience shows that experiment with live laboratory animals provide little useful information on the adverse properties of these substances. However, a number of biological characteristics that are relevant for the toxicity of the agents can be investigated in in vitro models. For the study of certain effects, cell culture and tissue explant methods are the only means to obtain relevant information. This is particularly the case for the investigation of the cross-reactivity phenomenon of monoclonal antibodies, the binding to cell receptors specific for humans, and the proliferative or cytotoxic responses resulting from such interactions. Cell culture techniques are also of use for monitoring contamination of biotechnology products with live microorganisms.

GENERAL CONCEPTS

When the biotechnology products of the first generation, e.g. antisera, vaccines and immunostimulants such as live or inactivated BCG were introduced in human therapy, some thoughts were given to the potential toxicity of these agents (7,8). The major concerns with vaccines were contamination with pyrogens and other reactive substances, e.g. dermonecrotic factor and histamine-sensitizing toxin, and the sensitizing effects of components of the culture medium. However, only minimal formal preclinical safety studies were required by drug regulatory agencies.

The arrival of the biotechnology products of the second generation, e.g. monoclonal antibodies, proteins and peptides manufactured by recombinant DNA technology, their synthetic and semisynthetic analogs, and various tissue fractions and extracts, was greeted with a different attitude. Safety of these substances soon became an important issue, and testing guidelines were prepared by several public health agencies. This response is understandable if one considers the high biological activity and extreme specificity of many of these substances, and the fact that some of them, e.g. recombinant human insulin, are administered for a prolonged period of time. Moreover, the unexpected multiplicity and severity of side-effects encountered with interferons (IFN) and interleukins (IL) in man (3) were a clear indication that biologically active proteins, even those occurring naturally in the human organism, could not a priori be assumed to be harmless at any dose.

The chemical nature of biotechnology products precludes the indiscriminate application of conventional safety testing protocols, mainly because the repeated administration often induces neutralizing antibodies. Moreover, in some cases, e.g. the interferons and interleukins, laboratory animals lack specific receptors for the human proteins, and thus do not show the pharmacological and toxicological responses observed in man (10). These facts are acknowledged by drug regulatory agencies world-wide, as shown in the recent draft guidelines of the Japanese Ministry of Health (March 31, 1987). The section on toxicology starts with the following statement:

> "Toxicity studies on drug products obtained by cell culture should generally be performed based on views and by methods different from those for conventional pharmaceuticals because of their unique properties. As we have limited findings and experiences in the subject area, and as we expect increased diversity in types and properties of drug products obtained by cell culture and in the applicable methods to their clinical use, we believe that it is not reasonable to establish uniform standards and methods of studies at this time point".

This view is in line with the concepts of the US Food and Drug Administration (4) and the drug regulatory agency of the Federal Republic of Germany (1) which have also advocated a "case-by case approach" to safety testing of biotechnology products.

TESTING PRIORITIES

The possibility to evaluate biotechnology products on an individual basis should please the toxicologists who often complain about the rigid check-list approach to drug safety testing. But before protocols can be developed, the potential toxicological targets and the adverse responses resulting from interactions with these targets must be considered. The main areas of toxicological concern with these substances have been discussed previously (12). In many cases, the most important adverse responses are directly related to the pharmacodynamic properties of the drugs. If they are clearly identified, as in the case of human insulin and tissue plasminogen activator, the hazards for man can readily be predicted by rational extrapolation. With other compounds acting on complex or poorly defined targets, e.g. IFN, IL, tumor necrosis factor etc., the "pharmacodynamic activities" are less well understood, and for this reason, adverse responses associated with the pharmacodynamic effects are difficult to predict. Instead, the knowledge of the toxicological targets is essentially based on a narrow, but rapidly broadening pool of data obtained by clinical and epidemiological observations.

Next in importance are the adverse effects related to certain biological characteristics of the biotechnology products ("biological toxicity"). Of major concern is the immunogenicity of the substances that may lead to development of neutralizing antibodies and, less frequently, other manifestation such as local and generalized skin erythemas, anaphylactic reactions and immune-complex disease. In experiments on guinea pigs, we have demonstrated that the antigen-antibody reaction in animals exposed to rIFN-alpha may be associated with the appearance of reversible and irreversible, circulating platelet aggregates and pulmonary microembolism (Zbinden, unpublished observation). There is also much experimental evidence that certain biotechnology products are cytotoxic to cells having the appropriate receptors, or are stimulating lymphocytes or monocytes to secrete cytotoxic substances.

With monoclonal antibodies, an important concern is the possibility of cross-reactivity with cellular determinants other than those intended for the diagnostic or therapeutic application. This is particularly serious with monoclonal antibodies coupled to cytotoxic or radioactive components.

The third area of concern relates to "intrinsic toxicity". This is an ill-defined complex of adverse properties that are due to the molecule per se, and not clearly related to the pharmacodynamic and biological qualities described above. Liver and kidney toxicity and cardiac arrhythmias observed in some patients treated with IFN may, for want of a better explanation, be considered as expression of intrinsic toxicity.

A separate problem of toxicological relevance are adverse effects caused by contaminants. Among them, hypersensitivity reactions to culture medium components and toxic effects of small molecular impurities, e.g. heavy metals and antibiotics, are of greatest practical importance. Rigorous purification and quality control procedures are necessary to avoid undesirable and even dangerous adverse reactions caused by these contaminants. For biotechnology products manufactured with the help of bacteria, yeasts and mammalian cells, contamination with live microorganisms and oncogenic DNA is a possibility that must also be monitored by appropriate quality control measures.

DEVELOPMENT OF TOXICOLOGICAL PROTOCOLS

In this paper no attempt is made to review all possible approaches to safety testing of biotechnology products. The currently available procedures have been discussed at a recent international symposium and the proceedings are published (6). In keeping with the subject of this congress, possible applications of *in vitro* techniques for the safety evaluation of biotechnology products will be mentioned.

A great advantage of cell culture methods over the *in vivo* toxicity tests is the possibility to use human material. This is particularly important for the study of agents that act by binding to specific receptors or cell surface determinants. For example, the potential for cross reactivity of monoclonal antibodies directed against specific human cells with cells of other tissues cannot be investigated in animal models. It is, however, possible to study the affinity of specific monoclonal antibodies to various human cell lines and to aceton-fixed fresh biopsy material. Some antibodies may also bind to formalin-fixed and paraffin-embedded tissue, but if such preparations are used to check for cross-reactivity, the ability of the antibody to bind to equally preserved cells against which it is directed must be ascertained.

Compounds that bind to receptors at the cell surface may show marked species and tissue specificity. For example, thyrotropin stimulated growth of a rat thyroid follicle cell line FRTL and cultured dog thyroid cells, but has no effect on cultures of porcine and ovine thyroid cells. In monolayer cultures of human thyroid cells the hormone even caused growth inhibition (11). A similar observation was made with rIFN-gamma and recombinant tumor necrosis factor-alpha (r-TNF-alpha). These agents either inhibited growth and caused cell lysis, or had no effect on a variety of human and murine tumor cell lines in culture, but growth of several normal human cell types was stimulated (9). Biotechnology products can also alter other properties of cells. An example is stimulation of adherence of human peripheral neutrophile leukocytes to human endothelial cell monolayers by rTNF (5). In combination with receptor binding studies, such investigations can provide important information on potential, tissue-specific targets of toxicity.

In vitro techniques can also be used to investigate potentially toxic effects that are not related to an interaction with specific receptors. Due to electrical surface charges and other properties the large molecules of biotechnology products can affect membranes and might be expected to alter cell-cell contacts (e.g. platelet aggregation), cell motility or membrane permeability. In blood and tissues the biomolecules have the potential for interfering with enzymatic processes. For example, the IFN-inducer polyinosinic-polycytidylic acid (poly-IC) caused hypercoagulability probably due to activation of Hageman factor (13), and this effect resulted in hepatic vein thrombosis demonstrated in experiments with mice (Zbinden, unpublished observation). When incubated with rabbit hypothalamic minces, rTNF and IL-1 induced synthesis of prostaglandin E2, an effect that also occurs *in vivo* and that is responsible for the pyrogenic effects of these drugs (2).

Finally, cell culture techniques can also be used for the detection of contamination of the biotechnology products by microorganisms. An example is the reverse transcriptase assay in cell cultures for the detection of retroviruses. The possibility to detect relevant contamination of biotechnology products by oncogenic DNA using cultures of NIH 3T3 cells is presently under review.

REFERENCES

1. BASS, R., SCHEIBNER, E. and SCHNIEDERS, B. (1987), Preclinical safety of biotechnology products intended for human use: government regulatory position in the Federal Republic of Germany. In: *Preclinical Safety of Biotechnology Products Intended for Human Use*. C.E. Graham, ed. Alan R. Liss, Inc., New York pp. 31-48.

2. DINARELLO, C.A., CONNOR, J.G., WOLFF, S.M., BERNHEIM, H.A., BEUTLER, B., CERAMI, A., FIGARI, I.S., PALLADINO, M.A., Jr. and O'CONNOR, J.V. (1986), Tumor necrosis factor (cachetin) is an endogenous pyrogen and induces production of interleukin 1. J. Exp. Med. 163:1433-1450.

3. FENT, K. and ZBINDEN, G. (1987), Toxicity of interferon and interleukin. TIPS 8:100-105.

4. GALBRAITH, W.M. (1987), Safety evaluation of biotechnology derived products. In: *Preclinical Safety of Biotechnology Products Intended for Human Use*. C.E. Graham, ed. Alan R.Liss,Inc., New York pp. 3-14.

5. GAMBLE, J.R., HARLAN, J.M., KLEBANOFF, S.J. and VADAS, M.A. (1985), Stimulation of adherence of neutrophiles to umbilical vein endothelium by human recombinant tumor necrosis factor. Proc. Natl. Acad. Sci. 82:8667-8671.

6. GRAHAM, C.E. (1987), *Preclinical Safety of Biotechnology Products Intended For Human Use*. Alan R.Liss, Inc., New York

7. MARTIN, M., KHALIL, A., JURCZYK-PROCYK, S., DUBOUCHE, P., GHERORGHIU M., ORBACH-ARBOUYS, S. and RAPPAPORT, H. (1976), Experimental toxicity studies of fresh live BCG in mice and monkeys. Proc. European Soc. Toxicol. 17: 83-87.

8. RONNEBERGER, H. (1976), Toxicity testing of vaccines. Proc. European Soc. Toxicol. 17:88-94.

9. SUGARMAN, B.J., AGGARWAL, B.B., HASS, P.E., FIGARI, I.S., PALLADINO, M.A, Jr. and SHEPARD, H.M. (1985), Recombinant human tumor necrosis factor-alpha:effects on proliferation of normal and transformed cells in vitro. Science 230:943-945.

10. TEELMANN, K., HOHBACH, C., LEHMANN, H. and INTERNATIONAL WORKING GROUP (1986), Preclinical safety testing of species-specific proteins produced with recombinant DNA-techniques. An attempt to transfer current experience into future testing strategies. Arch. Toxicol. 59:195-200.

11. WESTERMARK, K., KARLSSON, F.A. and WESTERMARK, B. (1985), Thyrotropin modulates EGF receptor function in porcine thyroid follicle cells. Molec. Cell. Endocrin. 40:17-23.

12. ZBINDEN, G. (1973), Arzneimittelwirkungen als Thromboseursachen. Bull. Schweiz. Akad. Med. Wiss. 29:191-200.

13. ZBINDEN, G. (1987), Biotechnology products for human use, toxicological targets and research strategies. In: Preclinical Safety of Biotechnology Products Intended for Human Use. C.E. Graham, ed. Alan R. Liss,Inc., New York pp. 143-159.

D2

Recombinant DNA and Monoclonal Antibody Products

RAYMOND E. STOLL

Sandoz Research Institute
East Hanover, NJ 07936

ABSTRACT

Present day toxicologic assessment of rDNA-derived proteins and monoclonal antibodies entails in vivo models being utilized, in which the pharmacologic activity has previously been demonstrated. Complexity of a toxicologic study involves obtaining pharmacologic, toxicologic, immunologic and pharmacokinetic data within the duration of the study planned. An example of a rDNA-derived protein, GM-CSF derived from CHO cells is to be discussed. The paper concludes that use of in vitro test systems is minimal in today's toxicologic assessment of rDNA-derived proteins, in particular due in part to too few numbers of rDNA-derived products tested, as well as lack of proper validation of such in vitro methodologies correlated to in vivo findings.

INTRODUCTION

The task assigned me, was to provide some general perspective as to the approach taken today in regard to the toxicologic assessment of rDNA-derived proteins in animals, in anticipation of testing such proteins in man for both safety and efficacy.

In the 16 to 17 years that I have been involved in the safety assessment of drugs in animals and man, the approach advocated by many in both industry and regulatory agencies is one of the few occasions I can recall in which both industry and regulatory are in basic agreement, as how one should initially investigate the potential toxicity of a rDNA-derived protein. The common approach advocated by both parties is the major point I will make in today's discussion. As Dr. Zvinden had previously alluded to within his presentation, the approach to testing the potential toxicity of rDNA-derived proteins is by a case-by-case approach. The routine toxicologic approach for xenobiotics has been, and is, making sure two species (one rodent and one non-rodent), three dose levels per study, and the duration of study ranging routinely from 4 weeks up to 26 weeks is performed per compound, and an IND (Investigative New Drug Application) is submitted to the FDA (Food Drug Administration). Thus the case-by-case approach for rDNA-derived proteins has moved away from the xenobiotic approach as outlined above, into what I believe to be a more stimulating and challenging approach, and sometimes a much more complicated toxicologic study investigation.

Up until the last couple of years, most of the experience involving preclinical toxicologic testing has been comprised of literature on the rDNA-derived protein, interferon. When interferon was tested in mice, rats, rabbits and ferrets, no major side effects were observed. However, the monkey did exhibit some anti-viral effects. Upon testing of interferon in man, transient pyretic effects were observed and this effect was not initially observed in the monkey. Retrospectively, the chimpanzee did respond to interferon in that mild fever and a decrease in leukocyte counts were observed.

To provide a case-by-case approach in the toxicologic assessment of a rDNA-derived protein, I will present data on a recombinant DNA-derived protein we at the Sandoz Research Institute have been investigating, GM-CSF (Granulocyte Macrophage - Colony Stimulating Factor). The first point to be made in regard to a case-by-case approach concerns the identification of a species which one can demonstrate the pharmacologic efficacy of the protein, before the protein is tested toxicologically. Within our laboratories, neither the rat, dog nor rabbit exhibited a pharmacologic effect induced by GM-CSF. However, the monkey did exhibit a pharmacologic effect, an increase in total leukocyte count. Thus, the monkey was the model of choice for the toxicologic assessment of this particular rDNA-derived protein. One should not conclude that all rDNA-derived proteins would necessarily follow the same species profile scenario as GM-CSF (derived from chinese hamster ovary cells, CHO). Our laboratories have also tested GM-CSF derived from E. coli, and from our experience with CHO versus E. coli derived GM-CSF, there appears to be differences in degree of toxicity in the monkey. However, the case-by-case approach to be discussed herein will be limited to CHO derived GM-CSF.

GM-CSF was anticipated to be utilized in treatment within life-threatening situations in man, not prophylactically over the life-time of a patient. The compound was also anticipated to be administered to man via the intravenous route, and not in a bolus injection, but in an i.v. drip. A pre-IND meeting with the FDA is also advised, which is not usually the case in evaluating a potential xenobiotic drug. Having met with the FDA, we performed a two-week intravenous drip study in the Rhesus monkey (bred in captivity). Since we were to be administering GM-CSF in a life-threatening situation we have not performed any teratology studies to date.

If one is to perform mutagenicity testing, it is recommended by the FDA, that only mammalian cells be used in the various tests you may decide to perform. I would not routinely envision having to perform a carcinogenicity study on a rDNA-derived protein used in a life-threatening situation.

Thus, in toxicologic testing of a rDNA-derived protein, the following should be addressed:

- o use a relative animal model demonstrating a pharmacologic response to the rDNA-derived protein.
- o one species tested <u>in vivo</u> should be included in the IND.

The route of administration should be similar as the route in man. This point, particularly in regards to the intravenous route, starts to deviate from the normal xenobiotic approach in that if the rDNA-derived protein is to be administered as an intravenous drip, then an i.v. drip in the monkey should be considered. With the herein GM-CSF case, one hour daily i.v. drips were administered to 24 animals equally divided into four groups as follows:

Group	μg/kg/day of GM-CSF*	No. of Animals Males	Females
I (Control)	0	3	3
II (Low)	15	3	3
III (Mid)	75	3	3
IV (High)	300	3	3

*All animals were infused at a rate of 0.5 to 1.0 ml/min. for 50 to 60 minutes, 7 days per week for 15 to 16 consecutive days.

A major point of discussion within our laboratories concerned the issue of what test material should be administered to the animals for inclusion in an IND. We have routinely chosen to use test material from the same Lot/Batch of material anticipated to be administered to man in the initial clinical trial. There are known cases whereby the bioengineer did not achieve making the end product he or she believed they were making, or that the specific activity of the rDNA-derived protein significantly differed from a previous Lot/Batch used in the very early development of the drug.

Since test material during early development of a rDNA-derived protein is usually limited in quantity, an attempt to maximize obtaining as much pertinent data from one study adds complexity to a preclinical toxicologic study. For those of you not familiar with the time sequence of performing a two-week study in the monkey, the following timing sequence would routinely occur. In the case of GM-CSF, a six-week quarantine of animals was incorporated, plus a four-week Pretest Phase whereby baseline observations were taken, in order to assess normal variability in the various parameters, which were also evaluated in the Drug Phase of the study. Therefore, a total of 12 weeks was involved in this two-week study, not just two weeks in total. Once we necropsied animals, another 10 to 12 weeks were necessary before issuance of a final report, which provided the safety assessment of the rDNA-derived protein.

Dose level selection incorporated into the design of the study also should be a major point. Some scientists believe a 5 to 10 fold safety factor of the anticipated human dose is satisfactory. We chose to go with multiples of 5, 25 and 100 fold of the anticipated human dose on an equivalent µg/kg basis. Whereby some scientists may believe this to be an overkill, our experience would argue to the contrary. For the GM-CSF case herein, the study entailed the use of approximately 325 mg of test substance at a cost of approximately $1,000 per mg. Thus, the test material costs alone for this one study totaled $325,000.

To additionally demonstrate the complexity of such a two-week study, the pharmacologic effect as a function of time was evaluated per animal, and below the mean total leukocyte counts (thousand/µl) per group as a function of time are presented:

Group	Drug Week Drug Day	-5	-1	1 3	2 8	2 11	3 15
I (Control)		9.2	8.7	8.8	9.1	8.8	12.1
II (Low)		7.9	8.0	8.8	9.9	7.6	13.5
III (Mid)		7.6	8.0	10.3	16.4	12.7	20.0
IV (High)		8.4	8.0	15.7	36.0	35.3	54.2

These data demonstrated a dramatic increase in total leukocyte counts even by Drug Day 3 of the study, and by termination of the study a four to five fold increase was observed at the High dose level, as well as a pharmacologic effect being observed at the Mid dose level.

The pharmacokinetics of GM-CSF in this monkey study was also determined by evaluating the plasma concentration as a function of time on Drug Days 1 and 15. The results are expressed as mean CML dilution units/ml:

	During Infusion (45 min. post initiation)	Minutes Post Infusion				
		5	12	25	40	60
Drug Day 1						
Group						
Control	0	0	0	0	0	0
Low	101	66	37	4	0	0
Mid	176	361	280	116	75	35
High	792	2722	988	-	365	76
Drug Day 15						
Control	0	0	0	0	0	0
Low	69	152	74	65	65	19
Mid	939	1182	800	414	241	99
High	6660	10011	7359	8895	1800	2669

These data were derived by use of a bioassay which was based on the proliferation of a human leukemia cell line in response to GM-CSF. Proliferation was based on measured incorporations of ^{3}H-thymidine into DNA. One CML dilution unit equaled the concentration of GM-CSF, which gave a half-maximal response on the dilution curve. The calculated half-life for the Low, Mid and High dose levels was 10, 16 and 13 minutes on Drug Day 1 and 20, 16 and 24 minutes respectively on Drug Day 15. The differences in half-life were not considered to be biologically significant. Thus, instead of using modern day methodologies such as HPLC, a bioassay was the most accurate and reproducible methodology available to date for measuring GM-CSF plasma concentrations.

Testing recombinant DNA-derived proteins has also forced one to evaluate the antigenicity of the protein in the preclinical toxicologic assessment. Use of an ELISA (enzyme-linked immunosorbent assay) to monitor IgG, IgE, IgA and IgM was performed in Pretest and in Drug Days 3, 8, 11 and 15. In this study, GM-CSF was slightly immunoreactive based on a moderate increase of IgM and IgG in a few High dose animals. Besides monitoring for serum immunoglobulins, a delayed hypersensitivity skin test was also performed on Drug Days 13 and 14 on all animals, using the method of Stites[1]. These latter results were negative.

Therefore, in the two-week study discussed, the protein was shown to be pharmacologically active, weakly immunogenic, and the pharmacokinetics demonstrated GM-CSF to have a short half-life in the monkey when administered intravenously. Histopathologic examination of approximately 50 tissues per animal did not reveal any target organ toxicity.

In review of this case, the point to be made is that no *in vitro* testing was employed in evaluating the potential toxicity of this particular protein.

One area in biotechnology we, as a company, are pursuing whereby an *in vitro* evaluation may potentially suggest problems in man, regards the toxicologic assessment of monoclonal antibodies developed for therapeutic administration to man. We have performed an *in vivo* monkey study similar to what I outlined for GM-CSF, but we are also evaluating the potential cross-reactivity of the monoclonal antibody to human tissues. We are having this type of *in vitro* testing performed for us by Dr. Hector Battifora at the City of Hope National Medical Center, in Duarte, California. Although I am not aware of any select number of tissues being recommended to evaluate potential cross-reactivity, within a workshop in early 1987 held at CIIT, in North Carolina, a Commission of European Communities document[2] was presented with the following tissues being recommended:

Tonsil, thymus, lymph nodes, bone marrow,
Peripheral blood, lung, liver, kidney, spleen,
Stomach, intestine
Pancreas, parotid, thyroid, parathyroid, adrenal,
Pituitary
Brain, peripheral nerve, heart, striated muscle,
Ovary, testes, skin

The technique being investigated with use of frozen tissues is that reported by Dr. Battifora[3].

The case examples of GM-CSF and the cross-reactivity approach we are taking on human monoclonal antibodies, indicate the perspective one company at least is taking on the toxicologic assessment of biotechnology products, a case-by-case approach. In reference to in vitro testing being substituted for in vivo testing regarding toxicologic assessment, I do not believe in vitro testing holds much promise as a substitute for in vivo testing. The role of in vitro testing will be emphasized perhaps in regard to investigating toxicities previously having been demonstrated in vivo, and follow-up investigations to be performed in order to establish a mechanism of action for the observed in vivo toxicity noted. The major deficiency I have observed with in vitro tests, is in the lack of validation of such in vitro tests and lack of establishing good correlative predicitiveness with what was observed in vivo. Review of the impact of in vitro testing in routine toxicologic testing of xenobiotics is minimal at best, in regard to replacing in vivo test models. Putting in perspective the 'infancy' of where we find ourselves as scientists investigating rDNA-derived proteins, even less influence of in vitro testing will be commonplace in rDNA-derived toxicology versus that observed in testing xenobiotics, at least for the near future.

References:

[1] Stites, D.P., Clinical Laboratory Methods for Detection of Cellular Immune Function, Chapters, 20-26, in Basic and Clinical Immunology, 5th edition, editors Stites, Fudenburg and Wells, Large Publication, Los Altos, Calif., 1984, pp. 353-502.

[2] Commission of the European Communities on Requirements for the Production and Quality Control of Monoclonal Antibodies of Murine Origin Intended for Use in Man, June 9-10, 1986.

[3] Battifora, H., Methods in Laboratory Investigation - The Multitumor (sausage) Tissue Block: Novel Method for Immunohistochemical Antibody Testing, Lab. Investigation 55(2): 244-248, 1986.

D3

Tests for Worker Exposure to Products of Biotechnology

DENNIS K. FLAHERTY, PEGGY A. WINZENBURGER, and PAUL L. SHERMAN

Environmental Health Laboratory
Monsanto Agricultural Company and the Environmental Science Center
Environmental Sciences and Health Department
Monsanto Company, St. Louis, MO

ABSTRACT

Workers in fixed biotechnology production facilities may be exposed to airborne organic materials which affect human health. In the presentation, methods used to collect and quantitate potentially harmful organic material in the workplace are discussed. In addition, the utility of immunological methods used to measure the workers' responses to workplace antigens are described. The presentation concludes that rapid, inexpensive methods can be used to detect workplace exposure and the biological response to workplace antigens.

INTRODUCTION

Recombinant DNA technology is being used to produce various commercial products. The products may be: genetically altered microorganisms which prevent environmental stress or microbial degradation of cash crops; products of genetically altered microorganisms used as human or veterinary therapeutic agents, food additives or supplements; and monoclonal antibodies.

For purposes of this discussion workers in biotechnology facilities producing monoclonal antibodies are excluded from consideration. Usually, these products are produced under maximum biocontainment and sterility conditions. Hence, it is unlikely that the workers will be exposed to agents which could affect health.

The workers in other biotechnology facilities may be exposed to a variety of organic materials which include: growth medium components; intact microbes and microbial components; and the commercial product.

The growth medium is a complex mixture of proteins, carbohydrates and fatty acids. Often the components of the media are not well defined. Some of the components may be extracts of yeast or mammalian organs. Protein material in the extracts has the propensity to elicit an immune response in humans.

Normal soil microorganisms have been genetically modified for field application as commercial products. The bacteria may be Gram Stain positive (Bacillus) or negative (Pseudomonas) species. Conversely, modified Gram negative Escherichia coli and yeast (Sacchromycetes cerevisiae) are used as vehicles to synthesize commercial products in fixed biotechnology facilities.

In the design of a protocol to monitor workers for exposure to products of recombinant technology, several questions should be addressed:

1. What are the workplace agents which could affect human health?

2. What methods may be used to determine human exposure to these agents?

3. Is there evidence that suggests workers have been exposed to agents in the workplace?

4. What is the minimum concentration of material necessary to give evidence of exposure in the workplace?

5. What is the relationship between exposure and adverse health effects?

WORKPLACE AGENTS WHICH MAY AFFECT HUMAN HEALTH

The intact microorganisms used in biotechnology pose no health problems in normal, healthy subjects. These organisms are widely distributed in nature and subjects are exposed normally to the microbes. Normal wild type or genetically altered microbes can occasionally cause opportunistic infections in compromised hosts. The host can be compromised as a consequence of: age, immune defects, treatment with antibiotics, immunosuppressive drug therapy and certain disease states (1).

Exposure to high concentrations of certain bacterial components can induce adverse health effects in humans. Two components of the cell wall that are of medical interest are the endotoxins and the peptidoglycans.

Bacterial endotoxins are normal lipopolysaccharide constituents of the gram negative cell wall. The serologically reactive (O-specific) antigen consists of distinctive repeating units of simple sugars. Antibody responses are directed toward the O-antigen. The O-antigen is linked to a Core region containing L-glycero-D-mannoheptose or ketodeoxyoctonate. In turn, the Core region is linked to the Lipid A moiety. Lipid A is comprised of hexosamines linked by phosphodiester bonds. The amino groups on the hexosamines are substituted with even numbered saturated and unsaturated fatty acids (2).

The Lipid A molecule is the biologically active endotoxin component. If the Lipid A is inhaled in sufficient quantities the molecule causes pulmonary function changes. The Lipid A also causes the release of Interleukin 1 (IL-1) from macrophages (3). The IL-1 acts on the temperature regulating centers of the brain to cause chills and fever. Endotoxin shock is possible if the Lipid A enters the circulating blood (4). The immune system is also activated by Lipid A. The molecule is a potent macrophage activator (5) and induces the non-specific proliferation of antibody producing B cells (6). There is also evidence which suggests that the Lipid A can activate the complement cascade (7).

The backbone of both the gram positive and the negative cell wall is the peptidoglycan layer. The peptidoglycan consists of repeating units of N-acetylglucosamine and N-acetylmuramic acid with a B-1,4 linkage. The carboxyl unit of the lactic acid is linked to a tetrapeptide. In E. coli, the tetrapeptide consists of L-ala-D-glut-(L) meso diaminopimelic acid-(L)-D-ala. Tetrapeptides are linked together by peptide bridges of D-ala-D-meso-diaminopimelic acid (8).

Studies have demonstrated that the E. coli peptidoglycan induces the proliferation of B cells and the production of antibodies (9). The stimulatory effect of the peptidoglycan is equal to or greater than the homologous endotoxin. The molecular structure necessary for the production of antibodies is N-acetylmuramyl-L-ala-D-glut (10).

Peptidoglycans can also substitute for Mycobacteria in Freunds Complete Adjuvant and elicit delayed hypersensitivity reactions (11-12). This observation is not unexpected. The structure of the E. coli adjuvant molecule is similar to the molecular form of the Mycobacteria immunostimulant (N-acetylmuramyl-L-ala-D-isoglut).

The adjuvant properties of the peptidoglycans and endotoxin are of medical importance. Exposure to the adjuvant in conjunction with other material could elicit an immune response to molecules which would not normally evoke a response. In addition, the adjuvant effect may accelerate or increase an on going immunological response. In most cases, the augmented immune response would be beneficial to the host. However, augmentation of the immune response in subjects with allergic and autoimmune diseases would be detrimental to the host.

Assuming that the commercial commodity is a product of the microorganism, exposure may have an effect on human health. Some of the products are human therapeutic agents and, hence, would have biological activity in humans. Other products may be foreign proteins. These molecules may evoke an immune response. As a consequence of the immunological response to the protein, adverse effects may be observed. These effects include allergic and delayed hypersensitivity reactions (13), hypersensitivity pneumonitis, and immune complex vasculitis (14).

DETERMINATION OF WORKPLACE EXPOSURE

Inhalation is the most likely route of exposure in biotechnology processes. It has been documented that particles with a size between 4.7 and 10 micrometer diameter can be inhaled. These particles usually impact in the nose and upper airways. Smaller particles (0.5 to 2.0 micrometer) can reach the alveoli in the lung (15). It is possible that the small particles can cross the lung blood barrier and enter the circulation.

The Industrial Hygienist can determine whether respirable aerosols are present at each step of the manufacturing process. The Andersen Ambient Sampler can be used to collect and aerodynamically size all airborne solid or liquid particulate matter (16). Particulate matter can be separated into eight fractions from 10 to 0.4 micrometer diameter. The concentration of organic material in each fraction can be determined by gravimetric analysis. When respirable aerosols are demonstrated in the workplace, the area can be monitored by High Volume Air Sampling or air sampling using the Andersen Microbial Sampler.

If the volume of air passing through the sampler is determined, the Andersen Microbial Sampler can be used to quantitate airborne bacteria (17). The airborne bacteria are drawn into the sampler and deposited on Petri plates containing an agar medium. To identify bacteria, one can use a selective medium. The selective medium favors the growth of the bacteria used in the manufacturing process and retards the growth of other microorganisms. After deposition of the bacteria on the agar plates, the plates are incubated and the colonies quantified.

High Volume Air Sampling can be used concentrate airborne organic material in the workplace prior to quantitation of molecules of interest. In order to validate the sampling method, several preliminary studies must be conducted. A filter medium with a high collection efficiency for the molecules of interest must be selected. The filter efficiency must be demonstrable in recovery studies. In theory, quantitative elution of specific molecules from the filter medium would seem to be a simple procedure. Experience has shown that some materials are difficult to elute and that preliminary studies must be conducted to determine the proper filter composition to be used in the high volume air sampling.

Airborne organic material may be present in high concentrations for short periods or present in low concentrations for extended time periods. In order to impinge sufficient material for quantitative studies, it is essential that the work place be continuously monitored by high volume air sampling. The filter should be changed at eight hours (shift studies) or 24 hour intervals.

Several methods can be used to quantitate specific molecules present in solutions of organic material eluted from the filters used in High Volume Air Sampling. These methods include: chemical, immunological and enzymatic assays.

High pressure liquid chromatography can be used to quantitate simple molecules. Hence, HPLC can be used to quantitate the small molecular weight commercial products or media components found in high volume air samples. The disadvantages of the HPLC methodology are a lack of sensitivity (1.0 mg) and an inability to identify the more complex endotoxins and peptidoglycans.

If properly validated in terms of accuracy, precision and parallelism (18), antibody mediated immunoassays can also be used to quantitate specific endotoxins, peptidoglycans or a commercial product in a matrix of organic material eluted from the high volume air sampling. Antibodies are highly specific and react only with the molecule which elicited their production. Immunoassays are sensitive, rapid and inexpensive.

A basic tenet of immunology is that the immune system will respond to a molecule (antigen) if the molecule is foreign to the host. This tenet allows the production of antibodies to molecules from one species by immunization of another, non-related species. The nature of the response depends on the manner in which the molecule is presented to the immune system. Large molecular weight compounds (>3000 M.W.) can be directly presented to the immune system to induce the production of antibodies. Small molecular weight compounds or haptens (<3000 M.W.) can evoke an immune response when covalently bound to protein. The small molecular weight compounds will not evoke an immune response when they are presented to the immune system in the free form. Hence, it is often necessary to synthesize hapten-protein conjugates for the generation of antibodies.

Immunoassays may not be feasible for all small molecular weight compounds even when bound to protein. The haptenic molecule must have some specific stereo chemistry which can be recognized by the immune system. The presence of aromatic groups, carbon-carbon double bonds or sulfhydryl linkages confer molecular rigidity which allow recognition by the immune system.

Antibodies can be produced by two methods. Rabbits, goats, or horses can be immunized with the large molecular weight compounds or hapten-protein conjugates. Polyclonal antibodies will be generated to the high molecular weight compound or to the hapten. Each population of antibodies will have different affinities or binding constants for the antigen or hapten. Monoclonal antibodies are produced by tissue culture adapted cell lines (19). In this procedure, mice are immunized and resultant splenic immunocompetent cells are fused with tissue culture adapted antibody producing cell lines. After selection and cloning of hybrid cells, cell lines are established. Each cell line will produce antibodies which have a homogeneous binding constant and reactivity toward a single determinant.

There are advantages and disadvantages in using polyclonal and monoclonal antibodies in immunoassays. Because the polyclonal preparations contain antibodies with different affinities, the sensitivity of the assay system is increased. When polyclonal antibodies are used in immunoassays it is not uncommon to detect as little as 1-2 ng of antigen. The disadvantage of polyclonal antibodies is that the serum pool represents a finite source of antibody. When the pool is expended, a new antibody pool must be generated and used in the assay. This requires restandardization of the assay. In addition, the use of different antibody preparations creates problems in the interpretation of data from longitudinal studies.

Monoclonal antibodies have weak binding constants when compared to polyclonal antibody preparations (20). Hence, the monoclonal mediated immunoassays are usually less sensitive (50 ng). The advantage of the monoclonal antibodies is that the cell line produces an infinite amount of antibody. Cell lines can be frozen and reconstituted over decades with no change in antibody affinity.

It is important to carefully consider the form of the antigenic material used to produce antibodies used in immunoassays. If the structure or molecular sequence is known, the antigenic determinants can be predicted. The immune system will recognize only hydrophillic sequences. Some molecules produced by bacteria or yeast are modified during the manufacturing process. Enzyme treatment, protein folding, dimer or trimer formation, or polymerization may delete or alter antigenic sites. Hence, antibodies should be directed toward hydrophillic antigenic sites which are unaffected by the manufacturing process.

The serological reactivity of endotoxins may also change with the method of extraction and purification. When isolated from the bacteria, the endotoxin is usually in a salt form complexed with other amines and nucleic acids. Due to the presence of carboxyl groups and phosphates, the endotoxins are negatively charged macromolecules. Removal of the contaminating molecules causes conformational changes in the O specific carbohydrate sequence, which results in distinct differences in physiological and serological reactivity (21).

An immunological assay used to test for reactivity to peptidoglycan or the commercial product is the Enzyme Linked Immunospecific Assay (22). In the ELISA assay, the organic material is adsorbed to microtiter plate wells. After washing to remove the unbound material, rabbit or mouse antibody directed toward the peptidoglycan or product is added to the wells. Following incubation, the plates are washed. A second antibody (anti-rabbit or mouse immunoglobulin) labeled with alkaline phosphatase is added to the wells. After incubation and washing to remove unbound antibody, the substrate (P-nitrophenyl phosphate) is added. If the test is positive, the substrate will be converted to p-nitrophenol which can be quantitated as a simple color change from colorless to yellow.

Endotoxins do not bind strongly to the microtiter plate wells. Hence, it is difficult to quantitate endotoxins by direct binding (23). It is, however, possible to modify the system to detect endotoxin. Rabbits immunized with endotoxin will produce endotoxin specific antibodies. Monoclonal antibodies can also be generated by somatic cell hybridization as discussed previously. The mouse monoclonal antibodies can be attached to the wells in microtiter plates. Endotoxin is then bound to the mouse antibodies in the wells. In essence, the endotoxin is bound to the plates via the mouse antibody. Polyclonal antibodies directed toward the endotoxin are added to the plate. After addition of anti-rabbit immunoglobulin labeled with alkaline phosphatase, the substrate conversion is quantified as described above.

Because of the difficulties in the immunological determination of endotoxin in air borne samples, it may be advantageous to use alternative assays. The Limulus assay can also be used to ascertain the biological activity of endotoxins. In the presence of endotoxin, the blood of the Horse Shoe Crab (Limulus polyphemus) will undergo enzymatic changes which result in increased turbidity (24). Commercially available kits are available which can quantify endotoxin in high volume air samples. The disadvantage of the Limulus assay is that it requires pyrogen free reagents and glassware. It also requires a series of dilutions to reach the optimum test concentration.

WORKER EXPOSURE

The basic premise used in testing workers is that exposure to foreign material induces the formation of antibodies in human serum directed toward workplace antigens. The presence of antibodies directed toward workplace antigens is an index of exposure.

Blood samples should be obtained from workers prior to exposure or beginning work in the biotechnology facility. These blood samples serve as the baseline control for the study. Additional blood samples should be obtained at six month or yearly intervals. Similar samples should be obtained from a normal, non-exposed control population. Serum samples recovered from the blood can be frozen for use in determining worker exposure.

Blood samples from a non-exposed population are critical to the interpretation of immunological reactivity. It is conceivable that normal subjects have antibodies which are cross reactive with the endotoxin or the commercial product. The presence of antibodies in the control population may be due to the fact that some antigenic determinants occur on completely unrelated molecular structures. If a baseline level for antigen specific antibodies in the control assay is established, the noise factor for the assay is reduced.

In the design of the study, paired serum samples from the same subject are required. The paired sera should be the baseline sample and the sample drawn at the next time period. It is also possible that the paired sera could be samples from two successive time periods. This approach reduces the technical problems associated with testing samples with different sets of reagents.

It is necessary to determine whether the antibody levels observed in the workers are statistically different when compared to non-exposed controls. If the antibody levels in the control population are normally distributed, standard statistical analyses can be used to determine the normal limits in terms of the 95% confidence level. If the data are not normally distributed, non-parametric statistical analyses can be used to establish similar confidence levels. Antibody levels greater than the normal limits in the control population would be considered significant (25).

Immunofluorescent assays can be used to detect antibodies directed toward intact bacteria or yeasts. The microbial agent can be fixed on a microscope slide. The test serum is placed on the slide. After incubation and washing, anti-human IGG labeled with fluorescein isothiocyanate (FITC) can be added to the slide. After removal of unbound antibody, the slide is examined using a fluorescent microscope. When excited by the proper light source, the FITC will absorb light at 485 NM and emit the light at a different wave length (515 NM) which gives a blue green color to the microorganism (26).

The indirect immunofluorescent assay has several disadvantages. The assay is tedious and time consuming to perform. Moreover, it is not possible to test large numbers of samples in the assay.

Particle Concentration Fluorescent Immunoassays (PCFIA) are a reasonable alternative to indirect immunofluorescent assays. In this assay fixed microorganisms and human test sera are added to 96 well microtiter plates and allowed to react. The plates are placed in a Pandex screen machine which automates the assay. Liquid is removed, the cells washed, and anti-human IGG conjugated with FITC is added to the wells. After washing, the filtered plate is read by front surface fluorimetry (27). The PCFIA assay has several advantages. The assay is rapid. Assay determinations (N=96) are completed within 15 minutes. The assay rapidity allows one to test large numbers of samples in a short period of time. Moreover, the assay is as sensitive as immunofluorescent or ELISA determinations (28).

The ELISA can also be used to test for human exposure to workplace antigens. The commercial product, linked to protein or peptidoglycans, can bind directly to microtiter plate wells. The purified endotoxins can be immobilized on the plates via mouse anti-endotoxin antibodies. Human sera is added to the wells and incubated. After washing, anti-human IGG labeled with alkaline phosphatase is added to the plates. After washing, the conversion of substrate is quantified. Longitudinal studies of the antibody levels in workers are also useful in measuring the success of improved Industrial Hygiene or biological containment practices. In the presence of continued exposure, the antibody levels would be expected to increase or remain at the same level. If the exposure ceases, the antibody levels would decrease over time.

MINIMUM AIRBORNE EXPOSURE AND WORKER EXPOSURE

If the immunological and bacterial isolation studies are conducted in a manner which demonstrates acceptable levels of accuracy, precision and the quantitative relationship between airborne bacterial levels and plate counts, the workplace air monitoring will determine the concentrations of respirable air borne antigenic material in the workplace. The human studies measure the biological response to the same compounds. When workers convert from a negative to a positive antibody status or demonstrate a significant increase in antibody levels, the exposure level can be determined. Hence, the minimum level of each antigen evoking a response can be determined.

RELATIONSHIP BETWEEN EXPOSURE AND HEALTH EFFECTS

The presence of antibodies only documents a response to antigen in sufficient quantities to elicit an immune response. No pathological significance can or should be ascribed to the presence in serum of IGG antibodies directed toward antigens present in the workplace. The documentation of all adverse health effects induced by exposure to products of biotechnology is the responsibility of the Occupational Health Physician. Based on symptoms, clinical and work exposure history, the physician can make a tentative diagnosis as to whether exposure to the work place antigen played a role in the development of adverse health effects.

REFERENCES

1. PINCHING, A.J., (1985), Laboratory investigation of secondary immunodeficiency. Clin. Immunol. and Allergy. 5: 469-480.

2. KABIR, S., ROSENSTREICH, D.L., and MERGENHAGEN, S.E. (1978), Bacterial Endotoxins and Cell Membranes, Bacterial Endotoxins and Cell Membranes, J. Jeljaszwicz and T. Waldman (eds.) Academic Press, N.Y., 59-86.

3. OPPENHEIM, J.J and GREY, I., (1982), Interleukin 1 is more than an interleukin. Immunology Today. 3: 113-119.

4. RIBI., E.E., CANTRELL, J.L., Von ESCHEN, K.B., and SWARTZMAN, S. (1979), Enhancement of endotoxic shock by N-acetyl Muramyl-L-analyl- (L- Seryl)- D - Isoglutamine. Cancer Research. 39: 4756-4759.

5. WEINBERG, J.B., CHAPMAN, H.A. and HIBBS, J.B. (1978), Characterization of the effects of endotoxin on macrophage tumor killing. J. Immunol. 121: 72-80.

6. CHILLER, J.M., SKIDMORE, B.J., MORRISON, D.C. and WEIGLE, W.O. (1973), Relationship of the structure of bacterial lipopolysaccharides to its function in mitogenicity and adjuvanticity. Proc. Natl. Acad. Sci. USA. 70: 2129-2133.

7. MERGENHAGEN, S.E., SYNDERMAN, R. and PHILLIPS, J.K. (1973), Activation of the complement system by endotoxin. J. Inf. Dis. 128: (suppl.) S86-S90.

8. SCHLIEFER, K.H. and KANDLER, O. (1972), Peptidoglycan types of bacterial cell walls and their taxonomic relationship. Bacteriol. Rev. 36: 407-477.

9. CHEDID, L., AUDIBERT, F., LEFRANCIER, P., CHOAY, J. and LEDERER, E. (1976), Modulation of the immune response by a synthetic adjuvant and analogs. Proc. Natl. Acad. Sci. USA. 73: 2472-2475.

10. DAMIAS, C., BONA, C., CHEDID, L., FLECK, J., NAUCEIL, C. and MARTIN, J.P. (1975), Mitogenic effect of bacterial peptidoglycans possessing adjuvant activity. J. of Immunol. 115: 268-271.

11. NAUCEIL, C., FLECK, J., MARTIN, J.P., MOCK, M. and NGUYEN-HUY, H. (1974), Adjuvant activity of bacterial peptidoglycans on the production of delayed hypersensitivity and on antibody response. Eur. J. Immunol. 14: 352-354.

12. DAVID, J.R., (1966), Delayed hypersensitivity in vitro: Its mediation by cell free substances formed by lymphoid antigen interaction. Proc. Nat. Acad. Sci. USA. 56: 72-77.

13. GASPARI, A.A., LOTZ, M.T., ROSENBERG, S.A., STERN, J.B. and KATZ, S.I. (1987), Dermatological changes associated with Interleukin 2 administration. JAMA. 258: 1624-1629.

14. ROBERTS, R.C. and MOORE, V.L., (1977), Immunopathogenesis of hypersensitivity pneumonitis. Am. Rev. Respirat. Dis. 116: 1075-1090.

15. BROWN, J.H., COOKE, K.M., NEY, F.G., and HATCH, T.F. (1950), Influence of particle size upon the retention of particulate matter in the human lung. J. Am. Pub. Health Assoc. 40: 450-458.

16. ANDERSEN, A.A., (1966), Sampler for respiratory health hazard assessment. A.I.H.A. Journal. March/April: 27.

17. SAYER, W.J., MAC KNIGHT, N.M and WILSON, H.W. (1972), Hospital airborne bacteria as estimated by the Andersen Sampler versus gravity settling culture plate. Amer. J. Clin. Pathol. 58: 557-568.

18. ROBARDS, D., (1967), Statistical quality control and routine data processing for radioimmunoassays (RIA) and radioimmuno-metric (IRMA). Clin. Chem. 20: 1255-1270.

19. DIAMOND, B.A., YELTON, D.E. and SCHARFF, M.O. (1981) Monoclonal antibodies. New Engl. J. Med. 304: 1344-1349.

20. VAN HEYNINGEN, V., BROCK, D.J.H. and VAN HEYNINGEN, S. (1983), A simple method for ranking affinities of monoclonal antibodies. J. Immunol. Methods. 62: 147-153.

21. GALANUS, C., (1975), Physical state and biological activity of lipopolysaccharides. Toxicity and immunogenicity of the Lipid A component. Z. Immuno. Forsch. Bd. 149: 214-279.

22. VOLLER, A.,(1978), The enzyme linked immunosorbent assay (ELISA). La Ricerca Clin. Lab. 8: 289-298.

23. GAFFIN, S.L., BADSHA, N., BROCK UTNE, J.G., VORSTER, B.J. and CONRADIE, J.D. (1982), An ELISA procedure for detecting human anti-endotoxin antibodies in serum. Ann. Clin. Biochem. 19: 191-194.

24. LEVIN, J. and BANG, F.B. (1964), The role of endotoxin in the extracellular coagulation of Limulus blood. Bull. Johns Hopkins Hospital. 115: 265-274.

25. De SAVIGNEN, D. and VOLLER, A. (1980), Communication of ELISA data from the laboratory to the clinician. J. of Immunoassay. 1: 105-128.

26. KAWAMURA, A., (1977), Fluorescent antibody techniques University Park Press, Baltimore, Md., 86-94.

27. JOLLEY, M.E., WANG, C.H.I., EKENBERG, S.J., ZUELKE, M.S. and KELSO, D.M. (1984), Particle concentration fluorescence immunoassay (PFCIA): a new rapid immunoassay technique with high sensitivity. J. of Immunol. Methods. 67: 21-35.

28. DAWSON, M., JOLLEY, M.E., and BETHELL, D.R. (1984), The use of particle concentration fluorescence immunoassay for the detection of bacterial surface antigens. Hybridoma. 13: 80-86.

D4

Summary

ROBERT A. SCALA

Exxon Biomedical Sciences, Inc.
Mettlers Road
East Millstone, NJ 08875-2350

I'll spend just a minute summarizing what we heard in the last four papers and then turn over to Dr. Goldberg to introduce the Hildegard Doerenkamp-Gerhard Zbinden Foundation Scientific Award.

The first speaker of this afternoon was Dr. Gerhard Zbinden and at the end of his talk he said that unique chemical structures present in biotechnology materials preclude the use of conventional animal toxicology assays. From that he developed the concept of the importance of the case-by-case approach. A number of the interesting keys which he looked at included toxicology related to pharmacodynamic effects, toxicology related to biological effects such as hypersensitivity, and studies related to intrinsic toxicity.

Zbinden then talked about the development of protocols, what can be tested in animals and what can be tested on human cell lines. He included for the latter receptor reaction, surface charge phenomenon and activation of enzymatic processes. I think the take home message was that with these biotechnology products, you are concerned about both the product itself and its contaminants. Perhaps you can control the contaminant question by following standard quality control methods in manufacture but you have to deal with both of those and you should deal with them on a case-by-case approach because of the uniqueness of those materials.

The second speaker was Dr. Raymond Stoll who discussed recombinant DNA and monoclonal antibody products. He too turned to this case-by-case approach and described their experience with preclinical testing of GMCSF, granulocyte macrophage colony stimulating factor. He took us through the standard approaches that a toxicologist uses including species selection (in his case they felt that the species in which a pharmacologic effect was produced was the most appropriate one for toxicity testing), route and duration, both of which mimic the human situation.

How do you come by the test material? I was surprised by $323,000 test material costs to do a two week study. I think that I would have been shot back home if I had tried it. I am impressed by his persuasiveness.

He compared and contrasted the testing goals using xenobiotic materials and species-specific proteins. Next Stoll outlined the design and conduct of a two week monkey study including a bioassay of the plasma GMCSF levels and the evaluation of immunogenicity. He spent just a few moments on monoclonal antibodies. Again the take home message was the importance of the in vitro work done for the IND; the cost of test species (primates) and the reinforcement of the case-by-case approach.

The third speaker was Dr. Jack Dean who talked about in vitro techniques for identifying immunomodulating chemicals and use of these methods to improve risk assessment. He examined immune dysfunction induced by chemical exposure and the important learning for me was his use of this parallelogram. The adverse effect was described in rodents in vivo. They then tried to produce this event first in vitro in rats and then in a parallel human system in vitro. At the very end he extrapolated to what is the probable risk for humans in vivo.

The materials he used were DMBA, dioxins and some related material. He compared the ED 50's and ID 50's (median immunosuppressive dose) and showed us where the margin of safety fell. He also mentioned in passing what CDC and ATSDR were doing in terms of a recommended screening set for immunotoxicology and finally their work in their own employees.

The last speaker was Dr. Dennis Flaherty who really represented a change of pace from the previous speakers. He talked about what his company is doing to evaluate worker exposure to products. They are concerned about worker exposures in large scale fermentation operations, and in a sense he asked us three questions, What are the agents? What's the evidence for exposure? And how do we control exposure and attendant risk?

The agents were the media, intact organisms, components of organisms including peptidoglycans and endotoxins and the commercial product. Exposure was assessed by a variety of techniques but largely monoclonal antibodies or polyclonal antibodies with ELISA assays. They also have sampling methods for worker's sera to determine what their exposures were. The final step is a team approach with toxicologists, immunologists, industrial physicians and industrial hygienists to provide a final health assessment.

That in a capsule is what I carried away from what was said over the last hour and a half or so. I appreciate four very fine speakers putting on a stimulating program.

I turn now to Dr. Goldberg for the final event of the afternoon.

Part 2

Poster Presentations

A. Poster Presentations

Poster A1

Functional Characteristics of Proximal Tubule Cells in Primary Culture: A New *In Vitro* Model for Studying Nephrotoxicity

MICHAEL D. ALEO and PAUL J. KOSTYNIAK

State University of New York at Buffalo
Department of Pharmacology and Therapeutics
and Toxicology Research Center
127 Farber Hall
Buffalo, NY 14214

ABSTRACT

Cell culture systems offer unique advantages for the study of chemical-induced toxicity on a cellular level within the cell type in question. These advantages are underscored by the lack of knowledge about the characteristics of explanted cells that have adapted to culture conditions. The primary goal of these studies was to document the growth and biochemical properties of rabbit renal proximal tubule cells in primary culture grown in antibiotic-free medium. Renal epithelial cells grown in antibiotic-free medium reached confluence twice as fast as cells grown in antibiotic-supplemented medium. The renal brush border enzymes alkaline phosphatase and gamma-glutamyltranspeptidase decreased in culture while the cytosolic and lysosomal enzymes lactate dehydrogenase and N-acetyl-glucosaminidase increased. Other enzyme systems responsible for xenobiotic metabolism like cytochrome P-450 associated mixed-function oxidase and glutathione S-transferase activity decreased in culture while cellular glutathione levels and redox state were well maintained in culture. Cellular protein content was stable throughout most of the culture period. Release of

---

1. Portions of this work were presented at the 25th Meeting of the Society of Toxicology and the 1987 Gordon Research Conference Mechanisms of Toxicity subsection.
2. Keywords: primary tissue culture, proximal tubule cells, and *in vitro* renal toxicology.
3. Abbreviations: AP, alkaline phosphatase; BND, benzphetamine N-demethylase; CDNB, 1-chloro-2,4-dinitrobenzene; ECOD, ethoxycoumarin O-deethylase; EDTA, ethylenediamine tetraacetate; EROD, ethoxyresorufin O-deethylase; FIPT, freshly isolated proximal tubules; GSH, reduced glutathione; GSSG, oxidized glutathione; GST, glutathione S-transferase; γ-GTP, gamma-glutamyltranspeptidase; HEPES, (N-2-Hydroxyethylpiperazine-N'-2-ethanesulfonic acid); LDH, lactate dehydrogenase; MFO, mixed-function oxidase; NAG, N-acetyl-glucosaminidase; TGS, total glutathione (oxidized + reduced).

potentially useful enzyme markers into the culture medium stabilized after the cells reached confluence. These data showed that a number of specific proximal tubule characteristics were retained in culture, albeit not at their *in vivo* levels, while other characteristics like protein, glutathione content, and cellular redox state were maintained at physiologically relevant levels. The results of these studies support the utility of this culture system as an *in vitro* model for studying chemical-induced nephrotoxicity.

INTRODUCTION

Although mammalian cells have been grown in culture for years, their applicability to studying mechanisms of xenobiotic metabolism and toxicity are only recently being realized and developed. *In vitro* models are extremely advantageous to use since they offer rapidity of response, freedom from hormonal and nervous system influence, and the ability to replicate observations with cells maintained in a highly controlled environment [1]. Some tissue culture systems have been characterized and developed to the point of being promoted as *in vitro* alternatives to live animal testing as is the case with alternatives to the Draize eye irritancy test [2-4]. These promising developments have created a greater interest and demand in the development and characterization of other tissue culture systems as *in vitro* models for toxicity studies. However, the progressive development of tissue culture models for toxicology depends upon either an appreciation for their overall limitations and applicability or their ability to mimic the *in vivo* situation as closely as possible.

Use of primary culture systems has its own intrinsic advantages and disadvantages over using established cell lines. One advantage is that since primary cultures are derived from tissue obtained directly from animals they should *ideally* express transport and hormonal properties like those found *in vivo*. This is in contrast to using established cell lines which have transformed in culture resulting in the expression of differentiated functions dissimilar from those of the cells from which they were derived [5-9]. The typical disadvantages of cells in primary culture are their limited life span in culture, the presence of multiple cell types, even when prepared from defined nephron segments [10] and phenotypic instability in culture [11-12]. These inherent disadvantages can limit their usefulness, and therefore proper characterization of the cells in culture is required before they are used as *in vitro* models for studying chemical-induced toxicity.

Advances have been made in developing rabbit renal proximal tubule cells in primary culture using antibiotic-supplemented hormonally-defined medium [13]. These cells in culture grow into confluent monolayers 14 days after plating and retain numerous differentiated functions typical of proximal tubule cells *in vivo* including transepithelial solute transport (as evidenced by multicellular dome formation), a Na^+/H^+ antiporter, Na^+-dependent inorganic phosphate uptake, Na^+-dependent alpha-methylglucoside transport, a functional hexose monophosphate shunt, parathyroid hormone sensitive cyclic AMP production, plus the presence of the brush border enzymes leucine aminopeptidase, alkaline phosphatase, and gamma-glutamyltranspeptidase [13-16]. This culture system offers significant improvements over previously developed primary kidney cell culture systems which utilized serum in the medium, resulting in either fibroblast overgrowth or extensive loss of highly differentiated functions [13,17].

As originally developed, the primary renal proximal tubule culture system utilized antibiotics in the culture medium. Since antibiotics inhibit organic anion transport [18] and protein synthesis *in vivo* [19], and since these cellular processes are potential indicators of nephrotoxin exposure; the growth of renal proximal tubule cells in antibiotic-free medium would offer distinct advantages for studying chemical-induced nephrotoxicity. Additionally, since the various segments of the proximal tubule are differentially sensitive to different chemicals it would also be of interest to identify the segment of the proximal tubule which is isolated during preparation. The purpose of this study was to characterize the growth pattern of rabbit renal proximal tubule cells grown in antibiotic-free medium, and to characterize the time dependent changes in biochemical markers, including Phase I and Phase II drug metabolizing systems.

MATERIALS AND METHODS

Materials:

Dulbecco's Modified Eagle Medium, Ham's F-12 Nutrient Mix, Penicillin "G", Trypsin·EDTA, Horse Serum, Soybean Trypsin Inhibitor, and Trypan Blue were obtained from Gibco Laboratories (Grand Island, NY). Streptomycin sulfate, HEPES, Trizma·acetate-(Tris[hydroxymethyl]aminomethane acetate), tissue culture hormones, transferrin, γ-GTP, GST, GSSG, other biochemicals, and standards were obtained from Sigma Chemical Co. (St. Louis, MO). Collagenase (Type IV) was obtained from Cooper-Biomedical (Malvern, PA). Calf thymus DNA was purchased from Calbiochem (La Jolla, CA) and potassium flame standards were purchased from Radiometer (Copenhagen). GSH, CDNB, and resorufin were obtained from Eastman Kodak Co. (Rochester, NY). Ethoxyresorufin and the bicinchoninic acid protein assay reagent were purchased from Pierce Chemical Co. (Rockford, IL). Bio-Rad protein assay kit was obtained from Bio-Rad Chemical Division (Richmond, CA). Benzphetamine·HCl was a gift from the Upjohn Company. The nylon sieves were obtained through Tetko Inc. (Elmsford, NY). Iron Oxide was prepared by the method of Cook and Pickering [20] and stock solutions of 50 mg/ml iron oxide in normal saline were sterilized and diluted with phosphate-buffered saline before use. All other reagents were of the highest purity commercially available.

Methods:

Isolation and Culture Conditions:

Proximal tubules were isolated by a modification of the method described by Brendel and Meezan [21] and prepared for culture as described by Chung *et al.* [13] with further modifications described by Aleo *et al.* [22]. Purified proximal tubules were incubated for 3 min at 25 °C in medium containing 0.2 mg/ml Collagenase (Type IV) and 0.002% (wt/vol) soybean trypsin inhibitor, centrifuged for 5 min at 50 x g, then resuspended in antibiotic-free medium supplemented with hormones and plated on 35 mm Falcon plastic tissue culture dishes at a plating density of 0.1-0.3 mg protein/dish. The cultures were maintained in a humidified 95% air/ 5% CO_2 incubator at 37 °C. The medium was changed every 1-2 days.

The basal culture medium was a 50:50 mixture of Dulbecco's Modified Eagle Medium and Ham's F-12 Nutrient Mix supplemented with 15 mM HEPES buffer and 14.3 mM sodium bicarbonate. The water used for medium preparation was first house distilled then deionized using a Millipore Reagent Grade Water System. The pH of the culture medium was adjusted to 7.35 before filter sterilization and the osmolarity routinely checked with a Micro Osmometer from Precision Systems (Natick, MA). This antibiotic-free medium was hormonally supplemented with bovine insulin (5 μg/ml), human transferrin (5 μg/ml), and hydrocortisone (5×10^{-8} M) immediately before use. The antibiotic-supplemented medium used during the isolation procedure also contained 192 IU/ml penicillin "G" and 200 μg/ml streptomycin.

Experimental Design:

Renal proximal tubule cells were cultured as described above and maintained for periods of up to 15 days in culture unless otherwise noted. In order to minimize variations due to hormonal and nutrient consumption, culture medium was changed 24 hours before each experiment in which growth and biochemical measurements were performed. A minimum of 2 rabbits were used as a source of cells for each parameter measured. All parameters measured including cell counts, enzyme assays, protein, and DNA determinations were performed on 3 culture plates from each of at least 2 separate proximal tubule cell isolations. Assay samples which were not sensitive to low temperature storage were frozen at -75 °C until analysis. Results are uniformly expressed as Mean ± S.E.M. unless noted otherwise.

Cell Growth, Protein, and DNA Determinations:

Cell growth was monitored throughout a 2 week period in culture. Cell counts were determined from triplicate culture plates using a Coulter Counter Model ZM and Channelyzer 256. The cells were dislodged by incubation with Trypsin·EDTA, the proteolytic action was then inhibited by soybean trypsin inhibitor, and the cell suspension diluted with counter diluent. Protein and DNA determinations were performed from parallel plates using modifications of the methods of Bradford [23], using bovine serum albumin as standard, and Labarca and Paigen [24], using calf thymus DNA as standard, respectively. The samples were solubilized with 0.1 *N* NaOH.

Marker Enzyme Activities:

Cellular enzymes LDH, AP, and NAG were determined by modifications of the methods of Mitchell *et al.* [25], Linhardt and Walter [26], and Maruhn [27], respectively. Cellular enzyme activities were determined from Triton solubilized FIPT and cells in culture. FIPT and proximal tubule cells in culture were washed with ice-cold phosphate buffered saline and lysed with 0.1% (v/v) Triton X-100 buffer containing 100 mM Tris-base and 150 mM NaCl (pH 7.5 at 25 °C) followed by sonication before enzyme measurements. Determination of cellular enzymes and protein released into culture medium has been described in further detail by Aleo and Kostyniak [28].

Cytochrome P-450 Content and Associated MFO Activities:

Confluent cultures of proximal tubule cells, grown in antibiotic-supplemented medium, were harvested 14 days after plating by dislodging the cells with Trypsin·EDTA. After the cells were freed from the plates, the proteolytic action of Trypsin was minimized with 10% Horse serum. The cells were collected and centrifuged at 50 x g for 5 min, rinsed with 10 mM Tris-acetate buffer (pH 7.4 at 4 °C) containing 1 mM EDTA and 20% glycerol, and recentrifuged at 50 x g for 5 min. The cellular pellet was homogenized in the same buffer with a tight pestle dounce homogenizer, and the homogenate was spun at 10,000 x g for 30 min. The resulting 10,000 x g supernatant was assayed immediately. Cytochrome P-450 content and associated MFO activities were also measured in microsomes from kidney cortex prepared by the method of Guengerich [29].

Cytochrome P-450 content was determined by measuring the carbon-monoxide difference spectrum of dithionite-reduced protein by the method of Omura and Sato [30] as modified by Guengerich [29]. Benzphetamine N-demethylase (BND) activity was determined by measuring the formation of formaldehyde essentially as described by Guengerich [29]. The incubation mixture consisted of 1.5 ml of a 50 mM potassium phosphate buffer (pH 7.4) with 5 mM $MgCl_2$, 0.5 mM $NADP^+$, 3 IU of glucose-6-phosphate dehydrogenase, 10 mM glucose-6-phosphate, and 1 mM Benzphetamine·HCl. The total incubation period was 50 min. 7-Ethoxycoumarin O-deethylase (ECOD) and 7-ethoxyresorufin O-deethylase (EROD) activities were measured by the fluorescent methods described by Prough *et al.* [31] with minor modifications. The stock solutions consisted of 0.01 mM 7-Hydroxycoumarin, 2 μM Resorufin, and 2.74 mM NADPH. The excitation/emission wavelengths were 380/460 nm and 530/585 nm for ECOD and EROD assays respectively. All MFO activities were linear over time and protein concentrations.

Glutathione Content, Redox State, and Related Enzyme Activities:

TGS concentrations, reduced and oxidized, were measured by a modification of the enzymatic method of Tietze [32] as described by Mulder and Kostyniak [33]. Cultures were washed with ice-cold PBS and then deproteinized with ice-cold sulfosalicylic acid (4% wt/vol) for 20 minutes. The culture plates were scraped and transferred to microfuge tubes. The tubes were spun in a Beckman microfuge for 5 min and the supernatant used for TGS determinations. TGS and GSSG determinations were performed in triplicate using the standard addition technique of Mulder and Kostyniak [33].

GST measurements were performed by a modification of the method of Habig *et al.* [34] using CDNB as substrate and authentic standard derived from rabbit liver. Substrate concentration in the assay was 1 mM for CDNB and reduced glutathione. Spectrophotometric enzyme determinations were performed at 340 nm in 100 mM phosphate buffer (pH 6.5) at 25 °C. Freshly isolated proximal tubules and proximal tubule cells in culture were washed with ice-cold phosphate buffered saline and homogenized in 200 mM potassium phosphate buffer (pH 6.5) using an ice-cold bath sonicator.

γ-GTP activity was determined by the method of Orlowski and Meister [35], as described by Meister *et al.* [36], using gamma-glutamyl-p-nitroanilide as substrate and glycylglycine as the amino acid acceptor. Enzyme activities were compared against authentic standard obtained from bovine kidney. Samples of FIPT and cells in culture were washed in ice-cold phosphate buffered saline and then permeabilized by a 50 mM Imidazole-HCl buffer (pH 7.2 at 25 °C) containing 1% (v/v) Triton X-100. Protein measurements on these samples were determined by the bicinchoninic acid protein assay as described by Smith *et al.* [37].

RESULTS

The time course for growth of renal proximal tubule cells in culture is illustrated in Figure 1. The amount of protein per plate was stable over 3 days then increased until a plateau was reached 8 days after plating. Cell numbers increased logarithmically over the first five days (insert), peaking at day 8 followed by an apparent decline over the next 8 days. When protein content was expressed as a function of DNA content (Figure 2) the data indicated a relatively stable protein/DNA ratio between 0.035 and 0.041 mg protein/μg DNA for the first 10 days in culture. As cultures aged the ratio increase to a peak of 0.059 mg protein/μg DNA 14 days after plating.

As shown in Figure 3, the cytosolic marker enzyme LDH, increased dramatically during the growth phase. Normalized for protein content, LDH activity displayed a 14-fold increase by day 8. Cellular LDH stabilized after the cells had reached confluence. LDH levels then remained elevated up to 15 days in culture. The brush border enzyme marker AP exhibited a decreased rate in activity which was maximal during the growth phase. Although the rate of decline diminished as cells reached confluence, there was a consistent decline from day 8 through day 15 in culture. The absolute drop in AP activity was 18-fold. During the growth phase the lysosomal enzyme marker NAG displayed a 2-fold increase which peaked when the cells reached confluence. NAG exhibited an additional 19% decline from day 10 through day 15. These events coincided with an increase in cellular vacuolization and loss of brush border which has been demonstrated by electron microscopic studies [22].

The Phase I metabolic function was determined by measuring cytochrome P-450 content and associated MFO activities in microsomes derived from rabbit kidney cortex and in 10,000 x g supernatant derived from proximal tubule cells in culture. Values from renal cortex microsomes compared favorably with previously reported literature values shown in Table 1. However, cytochrome P-450 content and MFO activities were undetectable in proximal tubule cells after 14 days in culture. The levels reported for cells in culture represent the lower limits of detection for each assay.

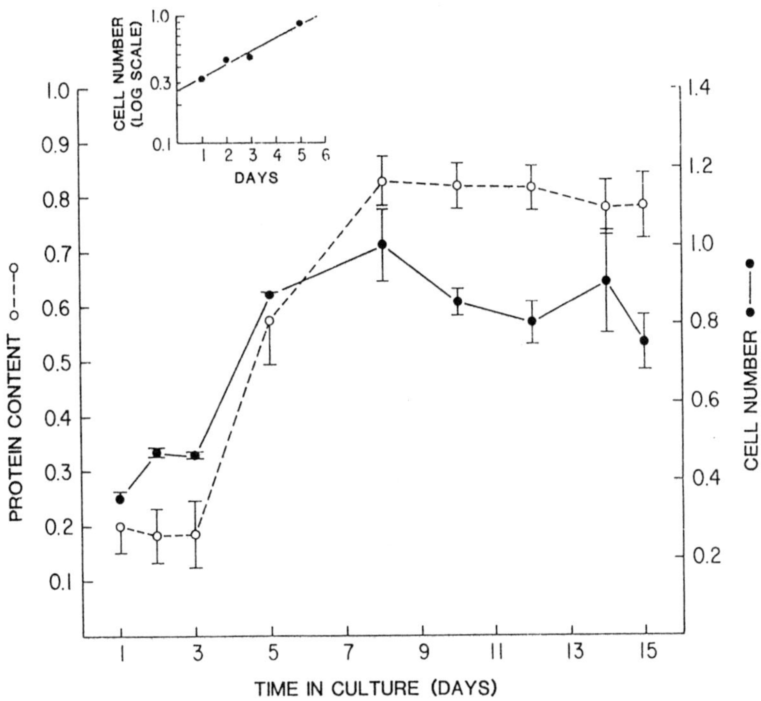

Figure 1. Time course for the growth of renal proximal tubule cells in primary culture. The cell number x 10^6/plate (●——●) and protein content in mg/plate (o---o) were plotted against time in culture (Days) after the initial plating of FIPT. The insert represents a logarithmic plot of the cell number data. Each point represents the Mean ± S.E.M. (N = 6).

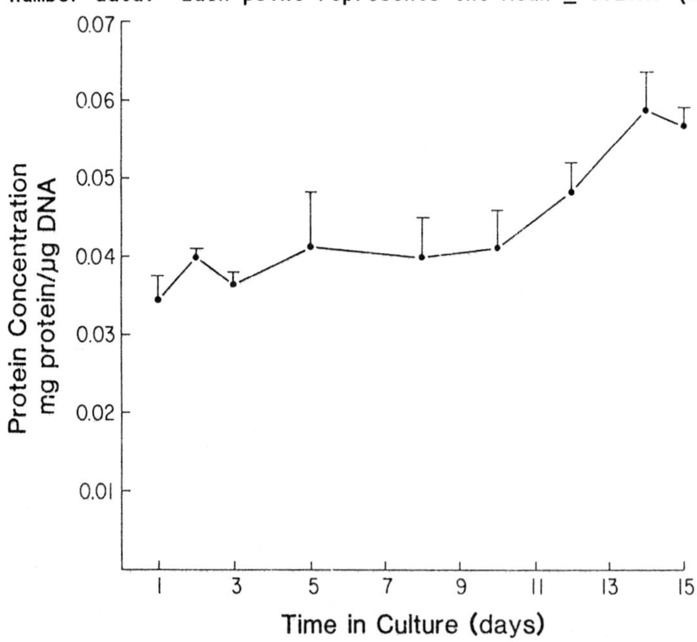

Figure 2: Time course for protein content of renal proximal tubule cells relative to cellular DNA. The protein content of renal proximal tubule cells was expressed as a function of their DNA content over a 15 day period in culture. Each point represents the Mean ± S.E.M. (N = 6).

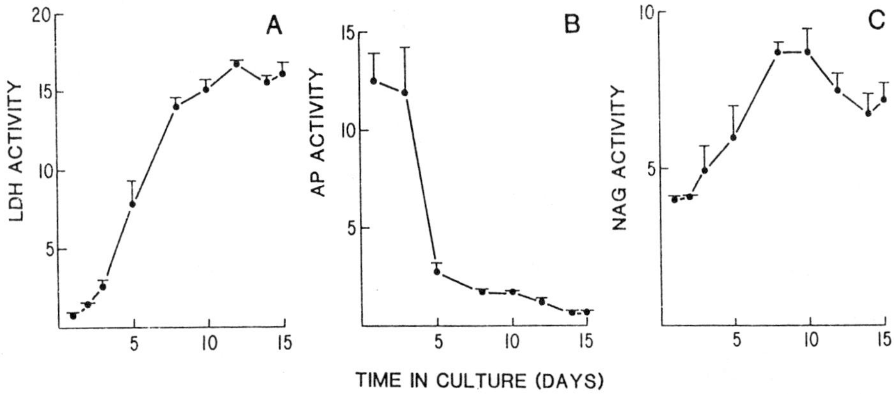

Figure 3. Time course for cellular enzyme activity in renal proximal tubule cells in primary culture. The activities of LDH, AP, and NAG were plotted as a function of time in culture. LDH activity was expressed in Wroblewski Units/mg protein x 10^3 (2.08 μmoles substrate conversion/min/mg protein x 10^3 at 25 °C). One Unit of AP activity represented the liberation of 0.25 μmoles p-nitrophenol/30 min/mg protein at 37 °C. One Unit of NAG activity was defined as the liberation of 1 μmole p-nitrophenol/hr/mg protein at 37 °C. Each value represents the Mean ± S.E.M. (N = 6).

Glutathione and Phase II glutathione dependent metabolic functions were maintained relatively well in culture. As shown in Table 2, the TGS concentration in FIPT was 2.8 μg TGS/mg total protein. This level was 2 to 3 times less than that observed in cultured proximal tubule cells maintained in antibiotic-free medium which had levels ranging from 8.9 to 20.6 μg TGS/mg total protein. When normalized for cell count, proximal tubule cells in culture maintained stable levels of TGS throughout a 3 wk period. Furthermore, when compared to freshly isolated rat kidney cortex cells or established kidney cell lines, primary cultures of rabbit proximal tubule cells consistently exhibited a higher TGS content.

The form in which glutathione exists intracellularly is important in maintaining membrane integrity and metabolic functions. The redox state of glutathione intracellularly was compared to FIPT (Figure 4). FIPT not only lost significant amounts of cellular glutathione (Table 2), but 37% of the glutathione remaining was found in its oxidized form. As TGS levels rebounded in culture (Table 2), this ratio was quickly re-established to normal levels in pre-confluent and confluent cultures, such that 87-94% of cellular TGS was maintained in its reduced form.

GST activity was monitored as an indicator of glutathione dependent Phase II metabolic activity. When FIPT and proximal tubule cells in culture were evaluated for GST activity (Table 3), FIPT displayed a remarkably high level of GST activity of nearly 4 Units/mg protein. The levels of GST activity were diminished in cultured cells to 50% of the level in FIPT. The levels found in FIPT were 2-fold higher than that reported for rabbit kidney cortex. Although there was a decline of GST levels in proximal tubule cells in culture compared to FIPT, the levels maintained were at least 10-fold higher than those found in established kidney cell lines.

TABLE 1

Cytochrome P-450 Content and Mixed-Function Oxidase Activities of Rabbit Kidney Cortex Microsomes and Proximal Tubule Cells in Culture

	Cytochrome P-450[a]	BND[b]	ECOD[c]	EROD[d]
Kidney Cortex Microsomes[e]	189 ± 9	468 ± 118	61 ± 26	4 ± 1
Kidney Cortex Microsome Data Liem *et al.* [38]	180 ± 10	---	---	<10
Kidney Cortex Microsome Data Kuo *et al.* [39]	112 ± 25	236 ± 6	97 ± 36	---
Kidney Cortex Microsome Data Rush *et al.* [40]	120 ± 10	190 ± 20	170 ± 20	11 ± 3
Proximal Tubule Cells in Culture[f]	< 10	< 60	< 2	< 1

a Pmoles P-450/mg protein.
b Benzphetamine N-Demethylase activity (pmoles of formaldehyde formed/min/mg protein).
c Ethoxycoumarin O-Deethylase activity (pmoles of 7-hydroxycoumarin formed/min/mg protein).
d Ethoxyresorufin O-Deethylase activity (pmoles of resorufin formed/min/mg protein).
e Values are the Mean ± S.E.M. of triplicate determinations in kidneys obtained from 5 individual rabbits.
f Assays were performed in 10,000 x g supernatant from proximal tubule cells after 14 days in culture grown in antibiotic-supplemented medium.

γ-GTP, an enzyme of critical importance in conserving and maintaining normal levels of glutathione within proximal tubule cells, was measured as a function of time in culture (Table 4). FIPT had 1.5 Units of activity per mg protein. This high level of activity was, however, not maintained in culture. Cells exhibited a 60% reduction in γ-GTP within 4 days and a further loss of 64% through 15 days in culture. Despite this decrease, the levels retained in culture were consistently higher than those reported for the LLC-PK_1 cell line. The levels of γ-GTP activity found in FIPT closely matched those found in the rabbit S_3 (pars recta) segment of the nephron. This segment is higher in γ-GTP activity than any other proximal tubule segments [48].

The release of toxicologically useful enzyme markers into culture medium from proximal tubule cells in culture are presented in Figure 5. Release of LDH, AP, NAG, and protein into the culture medium was highest in freshly isolated tubules and then tended to stabilize after the cells had reached confluence. There was a trend toward increased output of enzymes into medium as the cells aged in culture. Of the enzymes studied, LDH expressed the least change in enzyme output after cells had reached confluence. The generalized increase in enzymes in culture with aging was consistent with an increase in total protein in the medium.

TABLE 2
Total Glutathione Levels in FIPT,
Proximal Tubule Cells in Culture, and Established Cell Lines

	Total Glutathione Content[a]	
	μg/mg protein	nmoles/10^5 cells
FIPT	2.8 ± 3.4	ND[b]
Proximal Tubule Cells in Culture		
4 Days	20.6 ± 6.6	ND
8 Days	11.5 ± 3.4	6.68 ± 0.84
11 Days	10.9 ± 3.0	ND
15 Days	8.9 ± 3.8	6.71 ± 0.51
21 Days	ND	6.90 ± 0.57
Freshly Isolated Rat Kidney Cortex Cells	4.44 ± 1.66[c]	2.89 ± 1.08[d]
Cell Lines		
MDBK[e]	0.95 ± 0.22	---
RAG[f]	8.05 ± 1.33	---
BHK[g]	3.26 ± 0.68	---

a Values represent the Mean ± S.D. (N = 6-9).
b Not Determined.
c Calculated data of Ormstad *et al*. [41] and Ormstad *et al*. [42].
d From Ormstad *et al*. [41].
e From Bracken and Sharma [43].
f From Summer and Wiebel [44].

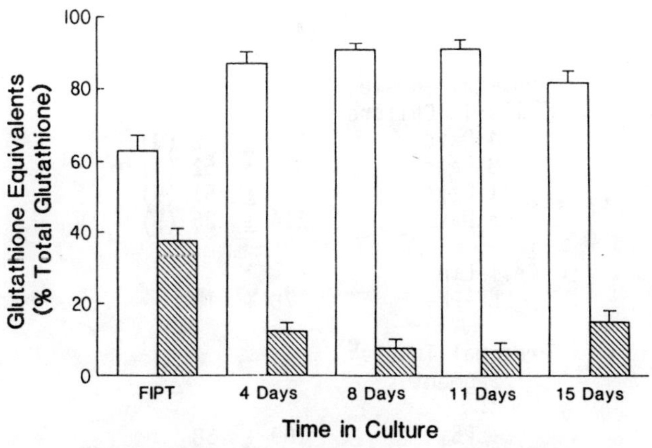

Figure 4. Glutathione status of renal proximal tubule cells in primary culture. Reduced (open bars) and oxidized (shaded bars) glutathione was plotted as a percentage of total glutathione on the culture dish for freshly isolated proximal tubules (FIPT) and cells grown for 4, 8, 11, and 15 days in culture. Each values represents the Mean ± S.E.M. (N = 9-12).

TABLE 3
Glutathione S-Transferase Levels in FIPT, Proximal Tubule Cells in Culture, and Established Cell Lines

	Glutathione S-Transferase[a] Units/mg protein
FIPT	4.059 ± 0.225
Proximal Tubule Cells in Culture	
4 Days	1.933 ± 0.439
8 Days	1.666 ± 0.168
11 Days	1.954 ± 0.218
15 Days	2.083 ± 0.333
Rabbit Kidney[b] Cortex	2.470 ± 0.171
Cell Lines	
RAG[c]	0.147 ± 0.028
BHK[c]	0.066 ± 0.006
$LLC\text{-}PK_1$[d]	0.041 ± 0.003

a Values represent the Mean ± S.E.M. (N = 9-12).
b Data from Mohandas *et al.* [45].
c Data from Summer and Wiebel [44].
d Data from Stevens *et al.* [46].

TABLE 4
Gamma-Glutamyltranspeptidase Levels in FIPT, Proximal Tubule Cells in Culture, and an Established Cell Line

	Gamma-Glutamyltranspeptidase[a] mU/mg protein
FIPT	1499 ± 83 (9)
Proximal Tubule Cells in Culture	
4 Days	610 ± 72 (9)
8 Days	636 ± 62 (9)
11 Days	413 ± 51 (9)
15 Days	214 ± 26 (9)
Cell Line[b]	
$LLC\text{-}PK_1$	70 ± 10
Proximal Tubule[c] Segment	
PS_1	100 ± 38
PS_2	712 ± 212
PS_3	1352 ± 94

a Values represent the Mean ± S.E.M. (N = 9).
b Data from Stevens *et al.* [46].
c Data from Shimada *et al.* [47].

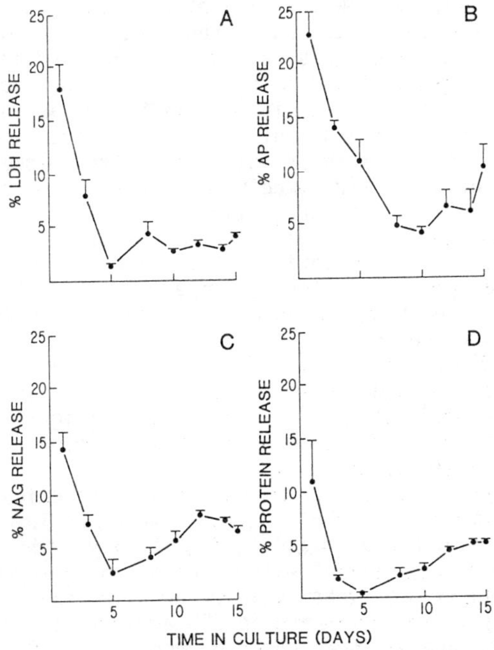

Figure 5. Time course for release of cellular marker enzymes and protein into culture medium from renal proximal tubule cells. LDH, AP, NAG, and protein content in culture medium was expressed as a percentage of the total activity on the culture dish over a 15 day time course. Each point represents the Mean ± S.E.M. (N = 6).

DISCUSSION

Primary cultures of rabbit renal proximal tubule cells maintained in serum-free hormonally-defined medium offer a number of advantages for studying chemical-induced nephrotoxicity. Since the proximal tubule is an extremely sensitive area of the nephron to chemical-induced injury, the development and characterization of a tissue culture model that utilizes this particular cell type may have broad implications to the study of renal toxicology. Having cultures obtained from a defined area of the mammalian proximal tubule not only provides excellent opportunities to the study of renal toxicology but differentiation, metabolism, and transport properties on a cellular and molecular level. Although there are a number of established kidney cell lines, they may have undefined cellular origins or express a multiplicity of differentiated functions from various nephronic cell types. For example, the MDBK cell line has an unknown cellular origin while the LLC-PK_1 cell line expresses a glucose transport system [8,9,48] typical of the proximal tubule [49], an adenylate cyclase activity sensitive to arginine-vasopressin and calcitonin [6] like the medullary thick ascending limb [50,51] and a high transepithelial resistance [9,52] that resembles the distal nephron [53]. Other kidney cell lines such as RAG and BHK do not express an epithelial-like morphology in culture. Primary cultures of proximal tubule cells are epithelial in origin and express transport and biochemical functions characteristic of the proximal tubule cell *in vivo* [13-16]. Additionally, the use of serum-free hormonally-defined medium successfully eliminates fibroblast overgrowth and deters the loss of highly differentiated functions [13,17].

The present study revealed dramatic differences between proximal tubule cells grown in antibiotic-free medium and cells grown in antibiotic-supplemented medium. We have noted, along with Chung *et al*. [13], that proximal tubule cells grown in antibiotic-supplemented medium required 2 weeks of growth before cells reached confluence compared to 8 days when grown in antibiotic-free medium. Proximal tubule cells grown in antibiotic-free medium reached a higher degree of confluency with cell numbers within culture plates as much as 2-fold higher. These differences in growth and confluency were noted even though the initial plating densities used in these studies were 2-fold lower than Chung *et al*. [13]. The use of antibiotic-free medium not only allows one to obtain confluent cultures in half of the time, but also avoids the confounding presence of antibiotics in the medium. This is an important consideration in the application of this system to toxicological screening or mechanistic studies. The time course for protein content of renal proximal tubule cells in culture indicates that after reaching confluence, the protein content per plate was more stable than measured cell number (Figure 1). Owing to the stability of the protein content after reaching confluence, this parameter was selected to normalize subsequent biochemical data reported here. The increase in protein content to DNA observed after 12 days in culture (Figure 2) argue for limiting the useful testing period of these cells from the time of cellular confluence (day 8) to 12 days after plating.

We noted major adaptive changes in the biochemical characteristics of primary cultured proximal tubule cells. Increases in cellular LDH and NAG activity were found with a decrease in AP activity. The increase in cellular LDH activity would be consistent with a change in energy metabolism. Proximal tubule cells typically use Krebs cycle products as energy sources and are even gluconeogenic [54]. The increase in LDH activity is evidence of increased glucose dependence, and has been observed recently by Dickman and Mandel [55] and Tang and Tannen [56]. The apparent increase in glucose dependence coincided with a loss of brush border enzymes and an increase in lysosomal enzyme activity. These biochemical changes coincided with a change in cellular morphology. Loss of brush border microvilli and lysosomal vacuoles were noted previously by Aleo *et al*. [22]. These changes may all be attributed to adaptation to culture conditions.

The cytochrome P-450 mixed-function oxidase enzyme system, is normally present within the proximal tubule cell [57,58] and can be found in rabbit renal cortex microsomes [38-40,59]. Cytochrome P-450 and mixed-function oxidases were undetectable in confluent primary cultures. This was not unexpected considering the rapid loss of MFO activity in primary cultured hepatocytes plated on tissue culture plastic [60]. The absence of MFO activity, however, does allow this system to be used to study the direct effects of xenobiotics on renal proximal tubule cells in the absence of Phase I metabolism. It may also be possible to study the effects of Phase I metabolism by the addition of S_9 microsomal fractions to the culture medium. This approach has been used successfully in other tissue culture systems [61,62].

Total cellular glutathione content was notably stable after the cells reached confluence. The difference in TGS content between FIPT and cultured cells is consistent with a loss of TGS during the tubule isolation procedure and is comparable to the value of 3.4 μg reported by O'Conner and Humes [63] for FIPT. It is well known that glutathione is quite unstable in biological samples unless fixed with a high concentration of reducing equivalents [33]. This suggests that oxidative stress may cause loss of glutathione from proximal tubules during the isolation procedure. This is supported by the shift to a high proportion of GSSG relative to GSH in FIPT. The glutathione redox state was re-established and well maintained within culture and resembled the ratio of reduced to oxidized glutathione reported in kidney cortex [64].

The absolute concentration of TGS is higher in proximal tubule cells in culture is higher than what might be expected from whole cortex TGS content. This is to be expected since proximal tubules were selectively isolated for culture, and the proximal straight and convoluted tubule are reported to contain the highest concentration of glutathione along the entire nephron [65]. This may explain the lower thiol content reported by Ormstad *et al*. [42] (Table 2) who used an unpurified preparation of freshly isolated rat kidney cortex cells obtained from the entire cortex. The large differences in TGS content between the renal proximal tubule culture system and established kidney cell lines argue for the use of primary cultures of rabbit renal proximal tubule cells to study glutathione related phenomena.

Although the activities of GST and -GTP in primary cultured proximal tubule cells were not maintained at levels comparable to FIPT, these enzyme functions were retained in culture, albeit at $<\frac{1}{2}$ the levels found in FIPT. These enzyme levels are however consistently much higher than those found in established kidney cell lines. Cellular maintenance of TGS content and redox state and the retention of γ-GTP and GST activity were of considerable importance since Phase II glutathione conjugation can either detoxify xenobiotics and their metabolites or lead to the formation of reactive intermediates that are nephrotoxic [66-68].

Release of cytosolic, brush border, and lysosomal enzyme markers as well as protein was fairly stable after the cells reached confluence. This would indicate that these particular enzymes may be useful indicators of cytotoxicity in primary cultured proximal tubule cells exposed to model nephrotoxins. Studies with several metals support this contention [28]. Because of the induction of LDH and NAG and decrease in AP activity within these cells, LDH and NAG may prove more useful in detecting mild toxic or cytotoxic effects than AP.

A tentative identification of the proximal tubule section isolated during purification can be drawn from Table 4. Evidence based on levels of -GTP activity in FIPT alone would suggest an enriched preparation of S_3. However, definitive conclusions cannot be drawn without further enzymatic and electron microscopic verification.

These data indicate that primary cultures of rabbit renal proximal tubule cells offer a novel tissue culture system for use in *in vitro* toxicology. Presently, this culture system is being used to study the toxicity and mechanisms of action of proximal tubule poisons.

ACKNOWLEDGMENTS

The authors thank the technical assistance of S. Kulbacki and D. Handley and technical graphics by T. Atkinson. This work was supported by grants GM 07145, The Johns Hopkins Center for Alternatives to Animal Testing, and a Sigma Xi Grants-in-Aid of Research Award.

Requests for reprints should be sent to Dr. Paul J. Kostyniak, SUNY at Buffalo, Department of Pharmacology and Therapeutics, Toxicology Research Center, 127 Farber Hall, Buffalo, New York 14214.

REFERENCES

1. Grisham, J.W. and Smith, G.J. (1984). Predictive and mechanistic evaluation of toxic responses in mammalian cell culture systems. *Pharmacol. Rev.* **36**: 151s-171s.

2. Rowan, A.N. (1984). The search for alternatives. *Fundam. Appl. Toxicol.* **4**: 508-516.

3. Rowan, A.N. and Goldberg, A.M. (1985). Perspectives on alternatives to current animal testing techniques in preclinical toxicology. *Ann. Rev. Pharmacol. Toxicol.* **25**: 225-247.

4. Rowan, A.N. (1987). Scientific perspectives in the development of alternatives in toxicology. *Comments on Toxicology* **1**: 275-288.

5. Misfeldt, D.S., Hamamoto, S.T. and Pitelka, D.R. (1976). Transepithelial transport in cell culture. *Proc. Natl. Acad. Sci. USA* **73**: 1212-1216.

6. Goldring, S.R., Dayer, J-M., Ausiello, D.A. and Krane, S.M. (1978). A cell strain cultured from porcine kidney increases cyclic AMP content upon exposure to calcitonin or vasopressin. *Biochem. Biophys. Res. Commun.* **83**: 434-440.

7. Rindler, M.J., Chuman, L.M., Shaffer, L. and Saier, M.H. (1979). Retention of differentiated properties in an established dog kidney epithelial cell line (MDCK). *J. Cell Biol.* **81**: 635-648.

8. Mullin, J.M., Weibel, J., Diamond, L. and Kleinzeller, A. (1980). Sugar transport in the LLC-PK_1 renal epithelial cell line: Similarity to mammalian kidney and the influence of cell density. *J. Cell. Physiol.* **104**: 375-389.

9. Misfeldt, D.S. and Sanders, M.J. (1981). Transepithelial transport in cell culture: D-glucose transport by a pig kidney cell line (LLC-PK_1). *J. Membr. Biol.* **59**: 13-18.

10. Woodhall, P.B., Tisher, C.C., Simonton, C.A. and Robinson, R.R. (1978). Relationship between para-aminohippurate secretion and cellular morphology in rabbit proximal tubules. *J. Clin. Invest.* **61**: 1320-1329.

11. Becker, J.H. and Willis, J.S. (1979). Properties of Na-K pump in primary cultures of kidney cells. *J. Cell. Physiol.* **99**: 427-440.

12. Mullin, J.M. and Kleinzeller, A. (1985). Sugar transport in the renal epithelial cell culture. In: *Tissue culture of epithelial cells*, M. Taub Ed.) Plenum Press, New York, 71-86.

13. Chung, S.D., Alavi, N., Livingston, D., Hiller, S. and Taub, M. (1982). Characterization of primary rabbit kidney cultures that express proximal tubule functions in a hormonally defined medium. *J. Cell Biol.* **95**: 118-126.

14. Sakhrani, L.M., Badie-Dezfooly, B., Trizna, W., Mikhail, N., Lowe, A.G., Taub, M. and Fine, L.G. (1984). Transport and metabolism of glucose by renal proximal tubular cells in primary culture. *Am. J. Physiol.* **246**: F757-F764.

15. Fine, L.G., Badie-Dezfooly, B., Lowe, A.G., Hamzeh, A., Wells, J. and Salehmoghaddam, S. (1985). Stimulation of Na^+/H^+ antiport is an early event in hypertrophy of renal proximal tubular cells. *Proc. Natl. Acad. Sci. USA* **82**: 1736-1740.

16. Waqar, M.A., Seto, J., Chung, S.D., Hiller-Grohol, S. and Taub, M. (1985). Phosphate uptake by primary renal proximal tubule cell cultures grown in hormonally defined medium. *J. Cell. Physiol.* **124**: 411-423.

17. Taub, M. and Sato, G. (1980). Growth of functional primary cultures of kidney epithelial cells in defined medium. *J. Cell. Physiol.* **105**: 369-378.

18. Møller, J.V. and Sheikh, M.I. (1983). Renal organic anion transport system: Pharmacological, physiological, and biochemical aspects. *Pharmacol. Rev.* **34:** 315-358.

19. Schwarze, P.E. and Seglen, P.O. (1981). Effects of antibiotics on protein synthesis and degradation in primary cultures of rat hepatocytes. *In Vitro* **17**: 71-76.

20. Cook, W.F. and Pickering, G.W. (1958). A rapid method for separating glomeruli from rabbit kidney. *Nature* **182**: 1103-1104.

21. Brendel, K. and Meezan, E. (1975). Isolation and properties of a pure preparation of proximal kidney tubules obtained without collagenase treatment. *Fed. Proc.* **34**: 803.

22. Aleo, M.D., Taub, M.L., Olson, J.R., Nickerson, P.A. and Kostyniak, P.J. (1987). Cellular uptake and response of primary cultures of rabbit renal proximal tubule cells exposed to mercuric chloride and methylmercury chloride. In: *In Vitro Toxicology: Approaches to Validation*, A.M. Goldberg (Ed.) Vol 5, Mary Ann Liebert, Inc., New York, 211-226.

23. Bradford, M.M. (1976). A rapid and sensitive method for the quantitation of microgram quantities of protein utilizing the principle of protein-dye binding. *Anal. Biochem.* **72**: 248-254.

24. Labarca, C. and Paigen, K. (1980). A simple, rapid, and sensitive DNA assay procedure. *Anal. Biochem.* **102**: 344-352.

25. Mitchell, D.B., Santone, K.S., and Acosta, D. (1980). Evaluation of cytotoxicity in cultured cells by enzyme leakage. *J. Tissue Culture Methods* **6**: 113-116.

26. Linhardt, K. and Walter, K. (1965). Phosphatases: Determination in serum with p-nitrophenyl-phosphate. In: *Methods of Enzymatic Analysis*, H-U. Bergmeyer (Ed.) 2nd Edn., Academic Press, New York, 779-785.

27. Maruhn, D. (1976). Rapid colorimetric assay of ß-galactosidase and N-acetyl-ß-glucosaminidase in human urine. *Clin. Chim. Acta* **73**: 453-461.

28. Aleo, M.D. and Kostyniak, P.J. Use of enzyme markers as general measures of cytotoxicity in sub-confluent cultures of rabbit renal proximal tubule cells. In preparation.

29. Guengerich, F.P. (1982). Microsomal enzymes involved in toxicology - analysis and separation. In: *Principles and Methods of Toxicology*, A.W. Hayes (Ed.) Raven Press, New York, 609-634.

30. Omura, T. and Sato, R. (1964). The carbon monoxide-binding pigment of liver microsomes: I. Evidence for its hemoprotein nature. *J. Biol. Chem.* **239**: 2370-2378.

31. Prough, R.A., Burke, M.D. and Mayer, R.T. (1978). Direct fluorometric methods for measuring mixed-function oxidase activity. In: *Methods in Enzymology*, S. Fleischer and L. Packer (Eds.) Vol. LII, Academic Press, New York, 372-377.

32. Tietze, F. (1969). Enzymic method for quantitative determination of nanogram amounts of total and oxidized glutathione: Applications to mammalian blood and other tissues. *Anal. Biochem.* **27**: 502-522.

33. Mulder, K.M. and Kostyniak, P.J. (1985). Stabilization of glutathione in urine and plasma: Relevance to urinary metal excretion studies. *J. Anal. Toxicol.* **9**: 31-35.

34. Habig, W.H., Pabst, M.J. and Jakoby, W.B. (1974). Glutathione S-transferases: The first enzymatic step in mercapturic acid formation. *J. Biol. Chem.* **249**: 7130-7139.

35. Orlowski, M. and Meister, A. (1963). Gamma-glutamyl-p-nitroanilide: A new convenient substrate for determination and study of L- and D-gamma-glutamyltranspeptidase activities. *Biochim. Biophys. Acta* **73**: 679-681.

36. Meister, A., Tate, S.S. and Griffith, O.W. (1981). Gamma-glutamyl transpeptidase. In: *Methods in Enzymology*, W.B. Jakoby (Ed.) Vol. 77, Academic Press, New York, 237-253.

37. Smith, P.K., Krohn, R.I., Hermanson, G.T., Mallia, A.K., Gartner, F.H., Provenzano, M.D., Fujimoto, E.K., Goeke, N.M., Olson, B.J. and Klenk, D.C. (1985). Measurement of protein using bicinchoninic acid. *Anal. Biochem.* **150**: 76-85.

38. Liem, H.H., Muller-Eberhard, U. and Johnson, E.F. (1980). Differential induction by 2,3,7,8-tetrachlorodibenzo-p-dioxin of multiple forms of rabbit microsomal cytochrome P-450: Evidence for tissue specificity. *Mol. Pharmacol.* **18**: 565-570.

39. Kuo, C-H., Rush, G.F. and Hook, J.B. (1982). Renal cortical accumulation of phenobarbital in rats and rabbits: Lack of correlation with induction of renal microsomal monooxygenases. *J. Pharmacol. Exp. Ther.* **220**: 547-551.

40. Rush, G.F., Wilson, D.M. and Hook, J.B. (1983). Selective induction and inhibition of renal mixed function oxidases in the rat and rabbit. *Fundam. Appl. Toxicol.* **3**: 161-168.

41. Ormstad, K., Jones, D.P. and Orrenius, S. (1980). Characteristics of glutathione biosynthesis by freshly isolated rat kidney cells. *J. Biol. Chem.* **255**: 175-181.

42. Ormstad, K., Orrenius, S. and Jones, D.P. (1981). Preparation and characteristics of isolated kidney cells. In: *Methods in Enzymology*, W.B. Jakoby (Ed.) Vol. 77, Academic Press, New York, 137-146.

43. Bracken, W.M. and Sharma, R.P. (1985). Biochemical responsiveness of a bovine kidney cell line to inorganic mercury. *Arch. Environ. Contam. Toxicol.* **14**: 509-515.

44. Summer, K-H. and Wiebel, F.J. (1981). Glutathione and glutathione S-transferase activities of mammalian cells in culture. *Toxicol. Lett.* **9**: 409-413.

45. Mohandas, J., Marshall, J.J., Duggin, G.G., Horvath, J.S. and Tiller, D.J. (1984). Differential distribution of glutathione and glutathione-related enzymes in rabbit kidney: Possible implications in analgesic nephropathy. *Biochem. Pharmacol.* **33**: 1801-1807.

46. Stevens, J., Hayden, P. and Taylor, G. (1986). The role of glutathione conjugate metabolism and cysteine conjugate ß-lyase in the mechanism of *S*-cysteine conjugate toxicity in LLC-PK_1 cells. *J. Biol. Chem.* **261**: 3325-3332.

47. Shimada, H., Endou, H. and Sakai, F. (1982). Distribution of gamma-glutamyl transpeptidase and glutaminase isoenzymes in the rabbit single nephron. *Japan. J. Pharmacol.* **32**: 121-129.

48. Rabito, C.A. and Ausiello, D.A. (1980). Na^{+}-dependent sugar transport in a cultured epithelial cell line from pig kidney. *J. Membr. Biol.* **54**: 31-38.

49. Ullrich, K.J. (1976). Renal tubular mechanisms of organic solute transport. *Kidney Int.* **9**: 134-148.

50. Chabardès, D., Imbert-Teboul, M., Montégut, M., Clique, A. and Morel, F. (1976). Distribution of calcitonin-sensitive adenylate cyclase activity along the rabbit kidney tubule. *Proc. Natl. Acad. Sci. USA* **73**: 3608-3612.

51. Imbert, M., Chabardès, D., Montégut, M., Clique, A. and Morel, F. (1975). Vasopressin dependent adenylate cyclase in single segments of rabbit kidney tubule. *Pflügers Arch.* **357**:, 173-186.

52. Handler, J.S., Perkins, F.M. and Johnson, J.P. (1980). Studies of renal cell function using cell culture techniques. *Am. J. Physiol.* **238**: F1-F9.

53. Boulpaep, E.L. and Seely, J.F. (1971). Electrophysiology of proximal and distal tubules in the autoperfused dog kidney. *Am. J. Physiol.* **221**: 1084-1096.

54. Klahr, S. and Hammerman, M. (1985). Renal metabolism. In: *The Kidney: Physiology and Pathophysiology*, D.W. Seldin and G. Giebisch (Eds.) Raven Press, New York, 699-718.

55. Dickman, K. and Mandel, L.J. (1986). Early onset of metabolic alterations in cultured rabbit proximal tubules (RPTs). In: *Abstracts of The American Society of Nephrology*, 19th Annual Meeting, 6A.

56. Tang, M.J. and Tannen, R.L. (1986). The primacy of glycolytic induction in the adaptation of proximal tubule cells to the culture environment. In: *Abstracts of The American Society of Nephrology*, 19th Annual Meeting, 245A.

57. Cojocel, C., Maita, K., Pasino, D.A., Kuo, C-H. and Hook, J.B. (1983). Metabolic heterogeneity of the proximal and distal kidney tubules. *Life Sci.* **33**: 855-861.

58. Endou, H., Koseki, C., Hasumura, S., Kakuno, K., Hojo, K. and Sakai, F. (1982). Renal cytochrome P450; Its localization along a single nephron and its induction. In: *Biochemistry of Kidney Functions*, F. Morel (Ed.) INSERM Symposium No. 21, Elsevier Biomedical Press, Amsterdam, 319-327.

59. Zenser, T.V., Mattammal, M.B. and Davis, B.B. (1978). Differential distribution of the mixed-function oxidase activities in rabbit kidney. *J. Pharmacol. Exp. Ther.* **207**: 719-725.

60. Guzelian, P.S., Bissell, D.M. and Meyer, U.A. (1977). Drug metabolism in adult rat hepatocytes in primary monolayer culture. *Gastroenterology* **72**: 1232-1239.

61. Williams, P.D., Hottendorf, G.H. and Laska, D.A. (1986). The role of desacetylation in the detoxification of cephalothin. *The Toxicologist* **6**: 144.

62. Borenfreund, E. and Puerner, J.A. (1987). Short-term quantitative in vitro cytotoxicity assay involving an S-9 activating system. *Cancer Lett.* **34**: 243-248.

63. O'Connor, R.P. and Humes, H.D. (1986). Exogenous glutathione (G) supplementation augments cellular G levels and ameliorates oxidative injury in rabbit proximal tubule segments (PTS). In: *Abstracts of The American Society of Nephrology*, 19th Annual Meeting, 215A.

64. Stein, A.F., Dills, R.L. and Klaassen, C.D. (1986). High-performance liquid chromatographic analysis of glutathione and its thiol and disulfide degradation products. *J. Chromatogr.* **381**: 259-270.

65. Brehe, J.E., Chan, A.W.K., Alvey, T.R. and Burch, H.B. (1976). Effect of methionine sulfoximine on glutathione and amino acid levels in the nephron. *Am. J. Physiol.* **231**: 1536-1540.

66. Elfarra, A.A. and Anders, M.W. (1984). Renal processing of glutathione conjugates: Role in nephrotoxicity. *Biochem. Pharmacol.* **33**: 3729-3732.

67. Rush, G.F., Smith, J.H., Newton, J.F. and Hook, J.B. (1984). Chemically induced nephrotoxicity: Role of metabolic activation. *CRC Crit. Rev. Toxicol.* **13**: 99-160.

68. Igwe, O.J. (1986). Biologically active intermediates generated by the reduced glutathione conjugation pathway: Toxicological implications. *Biochem. Pharmacol.* **35**: 2987-2994.

Poster A2

Structure-Activity Relationships of Inorganic Metals, Organometals, and Organic Test Agents Determined *In Vitro* with the Neutral Red Assay

H. BABICH[1,2] and E. BORENFREUND[1]

[1]*Laboratory Animal Research Center*
The Rockefeller University
New York, NY 10021
[2]*Department of Biological Sciences*
Yeshiva University, Stern College
New York, NY 10016

ABSTRACT

The neutral red (NR) in vitro cytotoxicity assay was applied for the determination of structure-activity relationships (SARs) among related test agents. Groups of chemical agents, with SARs reported in the literature and based on in vivo LD_{50} and LC_{50} assays, were selected for tests with the NR assay, using a variety of target cells, such as BALB/c mouse 3T3 fibroblasts, bluegill sunfish BF-2 fibroblasts, and mouse N_2a neuroblastoma cells, as the bioindicators. SARs similar to those established in vivo were determined with the 24 hr NR assay and were found applicable to the various cell types examined. The sequence of cytotoxicity for a series of substituted phenolics and of chlorinated toluenes, benzenes, and anilines was observed to be a function of their lipophilicity as described by their logarithmic octanol/water partition coefficients (log P). For a series of diorganotins the relationship was a function of lipophilicity based on Hansch π parameters; and for a series of divalent cationic metals it was based on chemical softness σ_p parameters. Dinitrotoluenes were "outliers", in that their cytotoxicities were greater than predicted based solely on log P values. It could thus be demonstrated that the NR assay, which is a rapid, quantitative, and semi-automated test, can be most useful in determining SARs for series of test agents.

INTRODUCTION

The large number of synthetic chemicals in commerce in the United States coupled with the annual synthesis of novel xenobiotics, has necessitated the development of various mechanisms to predict the biological activity of many of these poorly studied and novel chemicals. However, given the volume of such chemicals that require biological analysis, present resources do not permit an empirical determination for each compound (24). One mechanism for predicting the biological effects of xenobiotics has been the development of structure-activity relationships (SARs). This approach encompasses two aspects: (1) the quantitative measurement of a specific biological effect, which is usually derived from a concentration-response correlation and (2) the selection of a descriptor(s) of the physicochemical properties of the test agents that most govern their biological activity (26). For example, the biological effects considered when developing SARs have included acute toxicity, mutagenicity, and carcinogenicity measurements and the physicochemical parameter most utilized has been the hydrophobic parameter - the logarithmic octanol/water partition coefficient (log P). Such SARs, once established and quantitated, can then permit the prediction of the biological activity of a similar, but untested, chemical.

SARs utilizing acute toxicity as the biological index have relied primarily on LD_{50} and LC_{50} assays with laboratory animals and fish (14,20,27,29), although some research has been directed to <u>Daphnia</u> (12,15), protozoa (26), algae (31,32), and bacteria (16) as the test organisms. Little research, however, has utilized "<u>in vitro</u> tissue culture alternative assays" for quantitating and establishing SARs. Dillingham <u>et al</u>. (13), using growth inhibition of mouse fibroblast L-cells as the endpoint, were able to correlate the toxicity of a series of methyl- and halogen-substituted alcohols with their log P values. Using the highest-tolerated dose (HTD) assay with BALB/c 3T3 mouse fibroblasts, hamster CH V79 fibroblasts, mouse RAW 264.7 macrophages, and human hepatoma $HepG_2$ cells, Borenfreund and coworkers (1,11) demonstrated a correlation between the acute toxicity of series of alkyl alcohols and their log P values. The present paper reports on the applicability of the neutral red (NR) cytotoxicity assay for SAR determinations of a series of inorganic metals, organometals, and organic test agents. The principles governing the dynamics of the NR assay have been previously reported (8-10).

MATERIALS AND METHODS

<u>Cell lines</u>: BALB/c mouse 3T3 fibroblasts, mouse N_2a neuroblastoma cells, and bluegill sunfish BF-2 fibroblasts were propagated in Dulbeccos's modified Eagle's medium supplemented with 10% fetal bovine serum, 100 U/ml penicillin G, 100 µg/ml streptomycin, and 1.25 µg/ml Fungizone. All cells were maintained in a humidified 5.5% CO_2 incubator. The mammalian cell lines were maintained at 37°C. Initial studies with the BF-2 cell line were at 26°C, the temperature at which optimal replication was reported to occur (30). In subsequent studies, the temperature of incubation was increased to 34°C, as the cell line apparently adapted to cell culture conditions with optimal replication now occurring at 33-34°C (3,21). The mammalian cell lines were trypsinized with 0.05% trypsin-0.02% EDTA, whereas for the BF-2 cells a milder solution, consisting of 0.8% NaCl, 0.058% $NaHCO_3$, 0.04% KCl, 0.1% glucose, 0.05% trypsin, and 0.02% EDTA, was used.

<u>Experimental</u>: BALB/c 3T3 fibroblasts (9×10^3), neuroblastoma N_2a cells (1.5×10^4), and bluegill BF-2 fibroblasts (2×10^4 - 34°C; 3.2×10^4 - 26°C) were seeded into 96-well tissue culture plates and allowed to form monolayers of about 60-70% confluency after 24 hr incubation. Test agents diluted into medium in a range of concentrations were added at 0.2 ml per well, with 4 to 8 replicates per concentration, and were incubated for 24 hr as described (8-10). Briefly, medium was then removed and 0.2 ml of fresh medium containing 50 µg/ml of the supravital dye, neutral red (NR), was added to each well with a multichannel pipette. Two wells at

the top of the first row received medium without NR and served as blanks for subsequent spectrophotometric analysis. The dye-containing medium had been prepared 24 hr earlier and was centrifuged before use to remove fine crystalline precipitates. After 3 hr of incubation, the NR containing medium was removed from the culture plates and the cells were rapidly washed with a mixture of 1% formalin-1% $CaCl_2$. The dye, incorporated into the lysosomes of viable cells, was then extracted into the supernatant with 0.2 ml of solution of 1% acetic acid-50% ethanol. The plates were placed for a few seconds on a plate shaker and 10 minutes later were transferred to a microtiter plate reader where absorbance was measured at 540 nm. Data were expressed as percent of the control and presented as midpoint cytotoxicity (i.e., NR_{50}) values. All experiments were performed at least 3 times.

RESULTS AND DISCUSSION

Organics:

The *in vitro* cytotoxicities to bluegill BF-2 fibroblasts for a series of substituted phenolics were determined with the NR assay. For monosubstituted phenolics the sequence of potency was chlorophenol > nitrophenol > methylphenol > phenol and for a series of multiple chlorinated phenolics it was pentachlorophenol > tetrachlorophenol > trichlorophenol > dichlorophenol > monochloropheonol > phenol. The cytotoxic potencies of these substituted phenolics was a direct function of their partition coefficients: i.e., cytotoxicity increased with increasing log P values (Table 1) (2). Similar results were obtained when the NR assay was used with BALB/c 3T3 mouse fibroblasts as the target cell type (1), indicating that the relationship between phenolic cytotoxicity and log P was not cell-type specific.

Bols *et al*. (6), using inhibition of attachment of rainbow trout RTG-2 fibroblasts to a substratum when in the presence of test agents, noted the sequence of toxicity for a series of substituted phenolics to be pentachlorophenol > p-methylaminophenol > 2,4-dinitrophenol > p-chlorophenol > p-cyanophenol > p-nitrophenol > p-methylphenol > phenol > p-methoxyphenol. This sequence of potency was also noted to correlate with log P values of the test agents.

For a series of chlorinated toluenes the sequence of cytotoxicity, as determined with the NR assay using BF-2 fibroblasts, was α,α,2,6-tetrachlorotoluene > 2,4-dichlorotoluene > o-, m-, and p-chlorotoluene > toluene. As noted with the chlorinated phenolics, this sequence of potency was a direct function of the lipophilicity of the substituted toluenes (Table 1). However, within the toluene series, the nitro-substituted toluenes were outliers, in that their cytotoxicities were greater than would be predicted on the basis of log P values alone. Apparently, the mechanism of cytotoxicity of the nitrotoluenes differed from that of the chlorotoluenes. Furthermore, the ring position of the nitro-group on the ring structure had a strong influence on the cytotoxicity of the molecule, as noted by the greater potency of 2,3-dinitrotoluene than of 2,4- and 2,6-dinitrotoluene (Table 1) (1,2). These findings were also noted when BALB/c mouse 3T3 cells were the target cells (1).

The NR assay with BF-2 fish cells as the targets was utilized to establish SARs for a series of chlorinated benzenes and anilines. In both series the parent molecules were the least cytotoxic, with potencies progressively enhanced by the incorporation of chlorine atoms into the ring structure. The sequence of cytotoxicities for the chlorinated benzene and aniline series was a direct function of the partition coefficients of the test agents. Furthermore, the incorporation of an amino-group into the ring structure apparently enhanced toxicity, as noted by the greater potency of the aniline, than of the benzene, chlorinated series (Table 2) (4).

From the above-mentioned studies with the four chlorinated series or organic test agents, the following generalizations were established:

a. sequentially increasing the extent of chlorination on the parent molecule progressively increased the cytotoxicity of the molecule;

b. the presence of a chlorine atom on the ring structure was more critical in affecting cytotoxicity than was its position on the ring structure. Thus, for example, 1,2,3-, 1,2,4-, and 1,3,5-trichlorobenzene exhibited similar cytotoxicities as did o-, m-, and p-chlorotoluene.

c. increasing the chlorination on the molecule resulted in a concomitant increase in its partition coefficient and the sequence of cytotoxicity for each chlorinated series was a function of the log P values of the individual test agents.

The correlations noted between the potencies of the substituted phenolic series and of the chlorinated toluene, benzene, and aniline series with their partition coefficients that were demonstrated *in vitro* with the NR assay have also been shown using *in vivo* acute toxicity (LD_{50} and LC_{50}) assays. Using guppies as the test system, Konemann and Musch (23) and Lipnick *et al*. (25) correlated the acute toxicities of substituted phenolics and Konemann (22) of chlorinated toluenes with their log P values. The sequence of the acute toxicities for a series of chlorinated benzenes towards guppies (22), fathead minnows (14,27), *Daphnia magna* (15), and freshwater algae (32) and for chlorinated anilines to guppies (17) were directly correlated with their partition coefficients.

Organometals:

Toxicity studies with freshwater algae (31), *Daphnia magna* (20), and larvae of a marine mud crab (24) demonstrated that the sequence of toxicity for a series of organotins was a direct function of their lipophilicities. For the organotins, lipophilicity could be described either as log P values or, in the absence of such data, as Hansch π parameters, which describe the partitioning behavior of the R groups attached to the tin atom.

Using either BALB/c 3T3 fibroblasts or mouse N_2a neuroblastoma cells in the NR assay, the sequence of cytotoxicity for a series of diorganotin salts was dibutyltin > dibenzyltin > diphenyltin > dipropyltin > diethyltin > dimethyltin. For the dialkyltins there was a direct relationship between the length of the carbon chain of the R group and the potency of the test agent. Futhermore, the sequence of cytotoxic potencies of the diorganotin series was a direct function of the lipophilicities of the molecules, as noted by their Hansch π parameters (Table 3) (7). Similar correlations were noted when the NR assay was performed with bluegill BF-2 fibroblasts (Table 3) (4).

TABLE 1

Cytotoxicity of substituted phenolics and toluenes

Phenolic Series	log P	NR_{50} (mM)	Toluene Series	log P	NR_{50} (mM)
pentachlorophenol	5.01	0.17	α, α,2,6-tetrachlorotoluene	4.64	0.21
2,3,5,6-tetrachlorophenol	4.33	0.27	2,4-dichlorotoluene	3.98	0.64
2,3,5-trichlorophenol	3.69	0.33	o-chlorotoluene	3.42	1.6
2,4,6-trichlorophenol	3.69	0.48	m-chlorotoluene	3.42	1.6
2,4-dichlorophenol	3.30	0.51	p-chlorotoluene	3.42	1.7
4-chloro-3-methylphenol	3.10	0.70	toluene	2.69	7.4
4-chlorophenol	2.35	1.6			
2,4-dimethylphenol	2.30	2.4	"outliers"		
2-chlorophenol	2.15	2.4	2,3-dinitrotoluene	1.98	0.41
3-methylphenol	1.95	5.3	2,4-dinitrotoluene	1.98	1.4
4-nitrophenol	1.91	4.3	2,6-dinitrotoluene	1.98	1.6
2,4-dinitrophenol	1.54	4.1			
phenol	1.48	6.9			

Exposure of BF-2 cells to test agents was at 26°C
NR_{50} is midpoint toxicity expressed as percent of control
Data from references 1 and 2

TABLE 2

Cytotoxicity of substituted benzenes and anilines

Benzene Series	log P	NR_{50} (mM)	Aniline Series	log P	NR_{50} (mM)
1,2,3,4-tetrachlorobenzene	4.94	0.34	2,4,6-trichloroaniline	3.41	0.51
1,3,5-trichlorobenzene	4.20	0.63	3,5-dichloroaniline	2.90	0.65
1,2,4-trichlorobenzene	4.20	0.64	4-chloroaniline	2.02	1.90
1,2,3-trichlorobenzene	4.20	0.77	aniline	0.90	16.5
1,3-dichlorobenzene	3.53	1.37			
1,2-dichlorobenzene	3.53	1.53			
monochlorobenzene	2.81	5.69			
benzene	2.13	19.5			

Exposure of BF-2 cells to test agents was at 34°C
Cytotoxicity data from reference 4

Inorganic cationic metals:

There has been some effort to relate the acute *in vivo* toxicities of cationic metal ions with some physicochemical parameter of the metals (14,19). Once such property, which is based on the hard and soft classification of metals, is the chemical softness σ_p parameter. Strong correlations have been noted between LD_{50} acute toxicity data towards rats (19), mice (18,29), and *Drosophila* (18) and softness σ_p parameters of metals.

Using the NR assay either with BF-2 (5) or 3T3 (10) fibroblasts, there were strong correlations between the sequence of cytotoxicities of a series of divalent cationic metals and their chemical softness parameters (Table 4). Previous studies by Hsie *et al.* (18), using a cloning efficiency assay with Chinese hamster ovary cells, also noted a correlation between metal toxicity and chemical softness parameters.

SUMMARY

The neutral red cytotoxicity assay has been applied to the determination of structure-activity relationships. The *in vitro* cytotoxic potency of a series of substituted phenolics and of chlorinated toluenes, anilines, and benzenes could be directly correlated with the lipophilicity of the molecules, expressed in terms of their log octanol/water partition coefficients. Dinitrotoluenes were outliers, in that their cytotoxic effects were underestimated by consideration only of their partition coefficient values. The sequence of cytotoxicity for a series of diorganotins could be directly correlated with the lipophilicity of the molecules, expressed in their Hansch π parameters. The sequence of cytotoxicity for a series of divalent cationic metals was a function of their chemical softness σ_p parameters. The development of these SARs was independent of the cell line used (BALB/c mouse 3T3 fibroblast; bluegill sunfish BF-2 fibroblast; mouse N_2a neuroblastoma). The SAR models developed with the neutral red assay were consistent with similar models developed *in vivo*, using LD_{50} and LC_{50} acute toxicity assays.

ACKNOWLEDGMENT

Portions of the research were supported, in part, by grant 813760 from the U.S. Environmental Protection Agency. The views expressed are not necessarily those of the Agency.

TABLE 3

Cytotoxicities of a series of diorganotin salts

Tin salt	Hansch π parameter	NR_{50} (mM) 3T3	N_2a	BF-2
dimethyltin	0.56	64.0	25.0	39.9
diethyltin	1.02	18.0	6.0	17.1
dipropyltin	1.55	8.0	1.8	11.6
diphenyltin	1.96	2.3	1.4	1.2
dibenzyltin	2.01	1.6	0.6	-
dibutyltin	2.13	0.4	0.1	0.8
dicyclohexyltin	2.51	-	-	0.3

Exposure of 3T3 and N_2a was at 37°C and of BF-2 was at 34°C
Data from references 3 and 7

TABLE 4

Cytotoxicities of a series of divalent cationic metals

Metal cation (salt)	σ_p	NR_{50} (mM) 3T3	BF-2
mercury ($HgCl_2$)	0.064	0.02	0.02
cadmium ($CdCl_2$)	0.081	0.02	0.08
copper ($CuCl_2$)	0.104	0.4	0.6
zinc ($ZnCl_2$)	0.115	0.2	0.2
manganese ($MnCl_2$)	0.124	0.4	6.2
nickel ($NiCl_2$)	0.126	1.8	2.0
cobalt ($CoCl_2$)	0.130	0.9	0.6
lead ($Pb(NO_3)_2$)	0.131	1.8	2.7
tin ($SnCl_2$)	0.145	-	4.7

Exposure of 3T3 was at 37°C and of BF-2 was at 26°C
Data from references 1, 5, and 10

REFERENCES

1. BABICH, H. and BORENFREUND, E. (1987). Structure-activity relationship (SAR) models established in vitro with the neutral red cytotoxicty assay. Toxic. In Vitro 1:3-9.

2. BABICH, H. and BORENFREUND, E. (1987). In vitro cytotoxicity of organic pollutants to bluegill sunfish (BF-2) cells. Environ. Res. 2:229-237.

3. BABICH, H. and BORENFREUND, E. (1987). Fathead minnow FHM cells for use in in vitro cytotoxicity assays of aquatic pollutants. Ecotoxicol. Environ. Saf. (in press).

4. BABICH, H. and BORENFREUND, E. (1988). Structure-activity relationships for diorganotins, chlorinated benzenes, and chlorinated anilines established with bluegill sunfish BF-2 cells. Fundam. Appl. Toxicol. (in press).

5. BABICH, H., PUERNER, J.A. and BORENFREUND, E. (1986). In vitro cytotoxicity of metals to bluegill (BF-2) cells. Arch. Environ. Contam. Toxicol. 15:31-37.

6. BOLS, N.C., BOLISKA, S.A., DIXON, D.G., HODSON, P.V. and KAISER, K.L.E. (1985). The use of fish cell cultures as an indication of contaminant toxicity to fish. Aquat. Toxicol. 6:147-155.

7. BORENFREUND, E. and BABICH, H. (1987). In vitro cytotoxicity of heavy metals, acrylamide, and organotin salts to neural cells and fibroblasts. Cell Biol. Toxicol. 3:63-73.

8. BORENFREUND, E. and PUERNER, J.A. (1984). A simple quantitative procedure using monolayer cultures for cytotoxicity assays (HTD/NR-90). J. Tiss. Cult. Meth. 9:7-9.

9. BORENFREUND, E. and PUERNER, J.A. (1985). Toxicity determined in vitro by morphological alterations and neutral red absorption. Toxicol. Lett. 24:119-124.

10. BORENFREUND, E. and PUERNER, J.A. (1986). Cytotoxicity of metals, metal-metal and metal-chelator combinations assayed in vitro. Toxicology 39:121-124.

11. BORENFREUND, E. and SHOPSIS, C. (1985). Toxicity monitored with a correlated set of cell culture assays. Xenobiotica 15: 705-711.

12. DEVILLERS, J. and CHAMBON, P. (1986). Acute toxicity and QSAR of chlorophenols in Daphnia magna. Bull. Environ. Contam. Toxicol. 37:599-605.

13. DILLINGHAM, E.O., MAST, R.W., BASS, G.E. and AUTIAN, J. (1973). Toxicity of methyl- and halogen-substituted alchohols in tissue culture relative to structure-activity models and acute toxicity in mice. J. Pharm. Sci. 62:22-30.

14. HALL, L.H., KIER, L.B. and PHIPPS, G. (1984). Structure-acivity relationship studies on the toxicities of benzene derivatives: An additivity model. Environ. Toxicol. Chem. 3:355-365.

15. HERMENS, J., BROEKUYZEN, E., CANTON, H. and WEGMAN, R. (1985). Quantitative structure activity relationships and mixture toxicity studies of alcohols and chlorohydrocarbons: effects on growth of Daphnia magna. Aquat. Toxicol. 6: 209-217.

16. HERMENS, J., BUSSER, F., LEEUWANGH, P. and MUSCH, A. (1985). Quantitative structure-activity relationships and mixture toxicity of organic chemicals in Photobacterium phosphoreum: the Micotox test. Ecotoxicol. Environ. Saf. 9:17-25.

17. HERMENS, J., LEEUWANGH, P. and MUSCH, A. (1984). Quantitative structure-activity relationships and mixture toxicity studies of chloro- and alkylanilines at an acute lethal toxicity level to the guppy (Poecilia reticulata). Ecotoxicol. Environ. Saf. 8:388-394.

18. HSIE, A.W., SCHENLEY, R.L., TAN, E.-L., PERDUE, S.W., WILLIAMS, M.W., HAYDEN, T.L. and TURNER, J.E. (1984). The toxicity of sixteen metallic compounds in Chinese hamster ovary cells: a comparison with mice and Drosophila. Alternative Methods in Toxicology Vol. 2, A.M. Goldberg (Ed.). Mary Ann Liebert Inc., Publishers, NY, 115-124.

19. JONES, M.M. and VAUGHN, W.K. (1978). HSAB theory and acute metal ion toxicity and detoxification processes. J. Inorg. Nucl. Chem. 40:2081-2088.

20. KAISER, K.L.E. (1985). Correlation of metal ion to toxicities to mice. Sci. Total Environ. 46:113-119.

21. KOCAN, R.M., LANDOLT, M.L., BOND, J. and BENEDITT, E.P. (1981). In vitro effect of some mutagens/carcinogens on cultured fish cells. Arch. Environ. Contam. Toxicol. 10:663-671.

22. KONEMANN, H. (1981). Quantitative structure-activity relationships in fish toxicity studies. Part 1: Relationship for 50 industrial pollutants. Toxicology 9:209-221.

23. KONEMANN, H. and MUSCH, A. (1981). Quantitative structure-activity relationships in fish toxicity studies. Part 2: The influence of pH on the QSAR of chlorophenols. Toxicology 19:223-228.

24. LAUGHLIN, R.B., JOHANNSEN, R.B., FRENCH, W., GUARD, H. and BRINCKMAN, F.E. (1985). Structure-activity relationships for organotin compounds. Environ. Toxicol. Chem. 4:343-351.

25. LIPNICK, R.L., BICKINGS, C.K., JOHNSON, D.E. and EASTMOND, D.A. (1985). Comparison of QSAR predictions with fish toxicity screening data for 110 phenols. Aquatic Toxicology and Hazard Assessment: Eigth Symposium, A.C. Bahner and D.J. Hansen (Eds.). American Society for Testing and Materials, Philadelphia, 153-176.

26. SCHULTZ, T.W. and MOULTON, B.A. (1985). Structure-activity relationships for nitrogen-containing aromatic molecules. Environ. Toxicol. Chem. 4:353-359.

27. VEITH, G.D., CALL, D.J. and BROOKE, L.T. (1983). Structure-toxicity relationships for the fathead minnow, Pimephales promelas: narcotic industrial chemicals. Can. J. Fish. Aquat. Sci. 40:743-748.

28. VIGHI, M. and CALAMARI, D. (1985). QSARs for organotin compounds in Daphnia magna. Chemosphere 14:1925-1932.

29. WILLIAMS, M.W., HOESCHELE, J.D., TURNER, J.E., JACOBSON, K.B., CHRISTIE, N.T., PATON, C.L., SMITH, L.H., WITSCHI, H.R. and LEE, E.H. (1982). Chemical softness and acute metal toxicity in mice and Drosophila. Toxicol. Appl. Pharmacol. 63:461-469.

30. WOLF, K. and MANN, J.A. (1980). Poikilotherm vertebrate cell lines and viruses: a current listing for fishes. In Vitro 16:168-179.

31. WONG, P.T.S., CHAU, Y.K., DRAMAR, O. and BENGERT, G.A. (1982). Structure-activity relationships of tin compounds on algae. Can. J. Fish. Aquat. Sci. 39:483-488.

32. WONG, P.T.S., CHAU, Y.K. RHAMEY, J.S. and DOCKER, M. (1984). Relationship between water solubility of chlorobenzenes and their effects on a freshwater green alga. Chemosphere 13:991-996.

Poster A3

An Improved CAM Assay for Predicting Ocular Irritation Potential

D.M. BAGLEY, P.Y. RIZVI, B.M. KONG, and S.J. DE SALVA

Colgate-Palmolive Company
909 River Road
Piscataway, NJ 08854

ABSTRACT

The Chorioallantoic membrane (CAM) surrounding fertile chicken eggs has been evaluated by various investigators as a model system for predicting eye irritation potential. Kong et al. (In Vitro Toxicology - Approaches to Validation, Vol, 5, A. M. Goldberg (Ed.), M. A. Liebert, Inc., NY (1986)) reported on a CAM assay method which used a single quantifiable endpoint for assessing the CAM response to test materials. Although this method showed promise as a model for in vivo eye irritation potential, a number of materials were found to give a false-positive response. These false-positive responses were primarily due to three classes of materials; Tweens, PEG-Fatty Acids and products containing quaternary ammonium compounds (Quats). We have now modified the CAM assay to improve its usefulness and to reduce the incidence of false-positives. This modification of the CAM assay involves evaluation of the CAM response at a much earlier time point (30 min.) after treatment. The response of the CAM at this early time is vascular hemorrhaging. Probit analysis of the incidence of hemorrhaging is used to determine an RC_{50} value (concentration which gives a reaction in 50% of the treated eggs) which provides the basis of ranking for irritation potential. Tweens and products containing Quats are not false-positives in the modified CAM assay. This modification offers the advantages of a better correlation with Draize scores, obtaining results in 30 minutes instead of 3 days and using a simpler endpoint for establishing a positive response. In applying Cooper's criteria for describing the validity of a screening test (Cooper et al. (1979), Br. J. Cancer 39:87), this modification of the CAM assay has a sensitivity of 100%, a specificity of 90% and a predictive value of 88%. Therefore, this assay is a more useful way to reduce animal usage for eye irritation testing compared to previously described CAM methods.

Introduction

Finding an alternative to the Draize rabbit eye test for evaluating the ocular irritancy potential of materials has been a prime goal of researchers and public animal rights groups who are interested in reducing or eliminating animal use. An alternative method being investigated in our labs at Colgate-Palmolive Co. is an assay which utilizes the chorioallantoic membrane (CAM), a well vascularized membrane which surrounds a developing chick embryo. The original procedure used in our labs was modified from Leighton et al. (1) and has been described (2). Briefly, this procedure involves application of the test article onto the CAM on day 14. The CAM response is evaluated on Day 17. This evaluation involved measuring the longest length of a lesion formed on the CAM. A lesion length greater than 2 mm is defined as a positive response. Using the incidence of positive responses and probit analysis a PC_{50} value can be determined for each material. The PC_{50} value is the concentration of test material which results in 50% of the eggs showing a positive response. Correlation of PC_{50} values with *in vivo* Draize results shows that the primary limitation of this method is that certain samples give a false-positive response. However, more importantly, there are no false-negatives in this assay. We directed our research towards understanding the nature of the false-positive response in order to reduce the incidence of its occurrence. This paper describes the current approach to this aspect of the assay and the results of our studies.

Method

Test Sample Preparation

Test materials are dissolved or suspended in either sterile deionized distilled water or soybean oil. Both vehicles have been shown to be innocuous to the CAM but are run as controls in each assay. Serial dilutions are made of each material on a percentage basis. The concentrations used should encompass the concentration expected to result in a positive response in 50% of the eggs.

CAM Preparation and Treatment

Fertile hen eggs (DeKalb XL strain) are maintained at 99 $\pm$ 1°F and 50-60% relative humidity. On day 4 of development, 2.5 ml of albumen are removed through the pointed end of the eggs using a needle and syringe. A wheel bit on a dentist drill is used to cut a rectangular window in the side of the shell over the position of the embryo. The shell window is removed and the hole covered with transparent tape. On day 14 the window tape is peeled back, a Teflon ring is placed on the CAM and 40 ul of the test material are pipetted onto the CAM within the ring. The window is resealed with tape and the eggs returned to the incubator.

Evaluation of CAM Response

Thirty minutes after treatment the eggs are removed from the incubator and the tape and surrounding shell peeled away to expose the CAM. In this modified CAM method, the presence of vascular hemorrhaging or ghost vessels is considered a positive response. The concentration of test material which results in 50% of the eggs showing such a response is calculated using probit analysis. This value is referred to as an RC_{50}, analogous to the PC_{50} used in the original CAM method.

Results & Discussion

Products and ingredients which gave a false-positive response in the original CAM assay fall into 3 classes of materials:

- Tweens
- Polyethylene glycol (PEG) - Fatty Acids
- Products containing quaternary ammonium compounds

As part of our research to understand why false-positives occur and how they could be reduced, we looked at the time course of effects of an irritant on the CAM. The initial response of the CAM to an irritant is vascular hemorrhaging. Between 24 and 48 hours postdosing, this vascular hemorrhaging progresses to the lesion formation which is used as the endpoint in the original CAM procedure. Two materials originally tested in this time course were Tween 80 and a liquid detergent. Both materials resulted in significant lesion formation at 72 hrs (Fig. 1) but only the liquid detergent is an eye irritant. However, at 30 mins after treatment the liquid detergent caused significant CAM hemorrhaging while Tween 80 had little effect (Fig. 2). This suggested that 30 min. may be more appropriate than 3 days for assessment of the CAM response. Testing more samples by this method indicated that the incidence of CAM bleeding or ghost vessels (blood vessels devoid of blood flow) can be used as the endpoint for a positive response. Probit analysis is used to calculate the test article concentration which results in 50% of the eggs showing this reaction. This value is referred to as an RC_{50} and is used to quantitate and rank the ocular irritation potential of test materials.

Another method using the effects of test materials on the CAM vasculature was previously reported by Luepke (3). However, his method differs considerably from the Modified CAM assay reported here. In the Luepke method, CAM's are treated on day 10 and then the vasculature evaluated for hyperemia, hemorrhage and coagulation at 0.5, 2 and 5 minutes post treatment. A score is assigned to each observed effect based on its time to appearance (i.e. the earlier the effect is manifested, the higher the score assigned to it). Our studies show that a 10 day old CAM is much more sensitive than a 14 day old CAM and reacts to test materials with a more severe response than would be expected from <u>in vivo</u> studies. Also, evaluation of the endpoint in the Luepke method is more time consuming and subjective than that used in the Modified CAM assay. The Luepke method involves examination of each CAM at three different time points and determining the presence of three different vascular effects. The Modified CAM assay involves one examination of each CAM (at 30 min.) and one simple determination: the presence or absence of hemorrhaging. Our studies show that evaluating the CAM response at times earlier than 30 mins. results in a high level of variability from CAM to CAM and poor dose response curves.

To compare RC_{50} values from the Modified CAM assay and PC_{50} values

FIGURE 1
RESPONSE AT 72 HOUR POSTDOSING

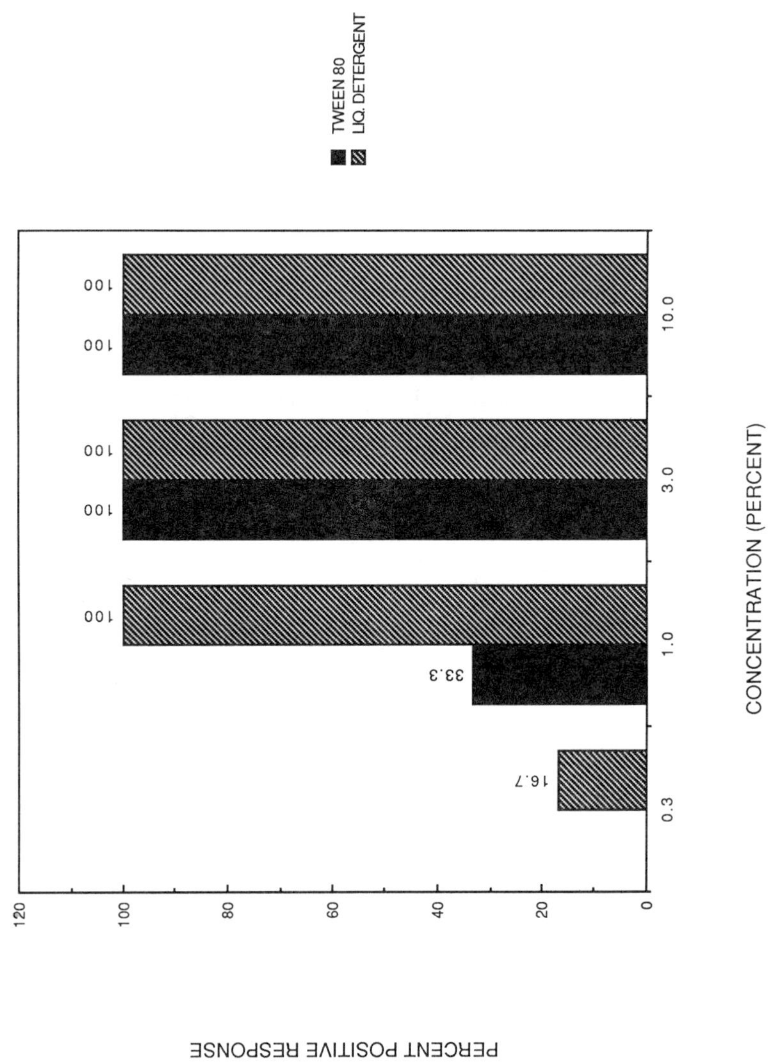

FIGURE 2

RESPONSE AT 30 MIN POSTDOSING

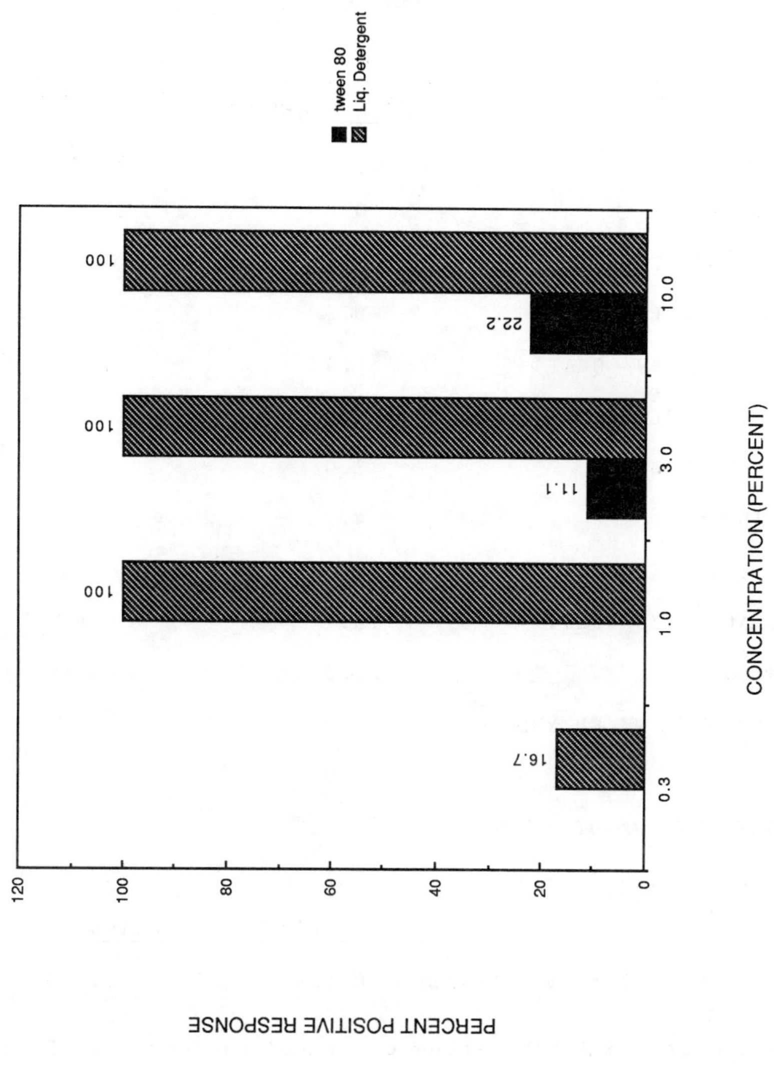

Table 1

CORRELATION OF CAM ASSAY RESULTS TO IN VIVO DRAIZE SCORES

SAMPLE	MAXIMUM AVERAGE DRAIZE SCORES	RC50 (%)	PC50 (%)
BABY SHAMPOO	0	3.0	2.6
TWEEN 80	0	22.5	1.4
PEG-8-LAURATE	0	0.7	2.8
TALLOW ALKYL AMIDE	0.3	85 - 100	6.0
HAIR COND. (W/ QUAT)	1.0	>100	0.5
METHYL ALKYL AMIDE	1.2	13.9	16.8
DISH DETERGENT	2.0	3.2	3.2
LIQUID APC	4.7	1.6	6.0
LIQ. LAUNDRY DET. - A	14.0	0.03	0.15
LIQ. AUTO DISH DET.	18.7	0.43	0.9
SHAMPOO A	25.2	0.56	1.8
POWDER DET. W/ ENZYME	33.0	0.08	1.4
SHAMPOO B	37.0	0.4	0.3
POWDER DET. W/OUT ENZYME	39.0	0.3	0.1
LIQ. LAUNDRY DET. - B	39.7	0.3 - 1.0	0.5

SPEARMAN RANK CORRELATIONS

RC50 vs. DRAIZE = 0.8 PC50 vs. DRAIZE = 0.6

from the original CAM method described by Kong et. al (2) to *in vivo* Draize eye irritation scores, test materials evaluated in all 3 assays were ranked and a Spearman Rank Correlation coefficient calculated (Table 1). The test material population included samples from all the classes of false-positive materials in addition to true positive and true negative materials. The comparison indicates that the Modified CAM assay correlates better with *in vivo* Draize scores.

A primary use of the Draize rabbit eye test is to comply with regulatory requirements such as those stated in the Federal Hazardous Substances Labelling Act (FHSLA) (4). The FHSLA does not directly depend on Draize scores for determining irritation potential but uses the frequency of animals showing a positive response. If at least 4/6 animals exhibit a positive reaction

Table 2

DRAIZE SCALE FOR SCORING OCULAR LESIONS

	Possible Scores*
1. Cornea	
(A) Opacity	0, 1, 2, 3, 4
(B) Area Involved	1, 2, 3, 4
Score = A x B x 5	Total Maximum = 80
2. Iris	0, 1, 2
Score = A x 5	Total Maximum = 10
3. Conjunctivae	
(A) Redness	0, 1, 2, 3
(B) Chemosis	0, 1, 2, 3, 4
(C) Discharge	0, 1, 2, 3
Score = (A + B + C) x 2	Total Maximum = 20

Maximum Total Score = Cornea + Iris + Conjuctivae = 110

*UNDERLINED VALUES = POSITIVE SCORES

Table 3

COMPARISON OF IRRITANT CLASSIFICATION BETWEEN THE DRAIZE EYE TEST AND THE MODIFIED CAM ASSAY

Number of Samples	Draize Rabbit Test	Modified CAM Assay
7	+	+
8	-	- (7) + (1)

(Table 2) the substance is considered an irritant. Comparing RC_{50} values to the frequency of positive *in vivo* responses shows that an RC_{50} threshold could be determined to distinguish irritants from nonirritants as defined under the FHSLA. Based on this threshold, the Tweens and products containing Quats would not be false positives as in the original CAM assay. Only the PEG-Fatty Acids remain as false-positives.
The criteria of Cooper et al. (5) were used to determine the specificity, sensitivity and predictive value of the Modified CAM vs. the standard CAM assays.

	Standard CAMA	Modified CAMA
Sensitivity	100%	100%
Specificity	36%	90%
Predictive Value	72%	88%

Sensitivity is the ability of the assay to correctly identify positives. Since neither assay gives a false negative response the sensitivity of each is 100%. The specificity is the assay's ability to correctly identify nonirritants. The higher specificity of the modified CAM reflects the reduction in false-positives. The predictive value reflects the proportion of eye irritants among the materials which give a positive response in the CAM assay. These values support the position that the Modified CAM assay is an improvement over the standard CAM assay for discriminating between eye irritants and nonirritants.

Conclusions

An improved method for using the CAM of a fertile chicken egg has been developed for predicting ocular irritation potential. This method offers the following advantages over previously reported CAM assay methods:

- Better correlation with Draize scores.
- Reduces the incidence of false-positives responses.
- Shortens assay time from 17 days to 14 days.
- Uses a more easily defined endpoint.

This modified CAM assay is a valuable prescreen for determining ocular irritation potential of products and ingredients and can be used to significantly reduce animal usage.

REFERENCES

[1] Leighton, J. Nassauer, J., Tchao, R. and Verdone, J. (1983), Development of a procedure using the chick egg as an alternative to the Draize rabbit test, Alternative Methods in Toxicology Testing, Vol. 1; Product Safety Evaluation, A. M. Goldberg(Ed.), M. A. Liebert, Inc., New York, 163-77

[2] Kong, B., Viau, C., Rizvi, P., and De Salva, S. (1987) The development and evaluation of the Chorioallantoic Membrane (CAM) assay, In Vitro Toxicology-Approaches to Validation - Vol. 5; A. M. Goldberg (Ed.), M. A. Liebert Inc., New York, 59-73.

[3] Luepke, N. (1985) Hen's egg Chorioallantoic Membrane test for irritation potential, Fd. Chem. Toxic. 23:287-91.

[4] Consumer Products Safety Commission (1973), Federal Hazardous Substances Act Regulations, Section 1500.42, Vol. 38, No. 187.

[5] Cooper, J. II, Saracci, R., and Cole P. (1979), Describing the validity of carcinogen screening tests, Br. J. Cancer, 39:87-89.

Poster A4

The Effects of Hyperoxic and Hypoxic Exposure on Catalase in Mouse Skin Explants

M.G. BIRD,[1] G. WITZ,[2] R.A. SCALA,[1] and D.V. PARKE[3]

[1]*Exxon Biomedical Sciences, Inc.*
East Millstone, NJ
[2]*UMDNJ Robert Wood Johnson Medical School*
Piscataway, NJ
[3]*Surrey University, Guilford, Surrey, UK*

ABSTRACT

As our previous studies with phorbol ester tumor promotors using mouse skin explants indicated greater basal catalase activity in vitro than in vivo, we investigated whether this might be due to the greater availability of oxygen to the explant tissue under in vitro incubation conditions compared with mouse skin in vivo. Groups of 4 dorsal skin explants from CD_1 mice were incubated in Dulbecco's MEM and fetal bovine serum for 30 minutes while exposed to the following oxygen/nitrogen mixtures (%): 5/95, 10/90, 21/79 (standard air), 40/60, 60/40, 80/20.

Catalase activity (K/mg protein) showed a dose-related increase from 10.9 $\pm$ 1.7 at 5/95 (% O_2/N_2) to 14.9 $\pm$ 2.7 at 80/20 (% O_2/N_2). This maximum in vitro value at 80/20 (% O_2/N_2) was 185% of mouse skin exposed in vivo to laboratory air (20.8% O_2) and which had a catalase activity of 8.14 $\pm$ 1.6 K/mg protein. Normal structural integrity and Trypan Blue exclusion of the skin explants were seen in all groups post-exposure.

The above elevation of catalase activity is consistent with the finding by others of increased catalase and superoxide dismutase in lung tissue of rats following hyperoxic exposure. Such an increase may be a compensatory response to O_2 toxicity. It also suggests that the effects of nonphysiological incubation conditions should be considered when interpreting in vitro studies of tissue enzymes which are often conducted under high (95%) oxygen-containing atmospheres.

INTRODUCTION

Verma and Boutwell[1] established the skin explant system, using skin from adult CD_1 mice, to study the effects of the tumor promoter phorbol 12,13-myristate acetate (PMA) on viable explants over a 48-hour period. The incorporation of ^{3}H-thymidine into DNA and the induction of epidermal ornithine decarboxylase occurred to a similar extent and had a similar time course as those seen in the intact mouse receiving topical application of PMA, however they also noted a large increase in epidermal ornithine decarboxylase activity in incubated skin pieces without the PMA treatment.

Our previous studies(2) involved the topical application of PMA to CD_1 mouse skin with subsequent maintenance of the excised skin in vitro over 24 hours. This treatment produced an unpredicted dose-dependent elevation in catalase compared with the untreated skin maintained under the same in vitro conditions, which in turn was higher than untreated skin in vivo. This elevation in the catalase activity of the control tissue led to the hypothesis that the incubation conditions (e.g., circulating atmosphere of 95% air; 5% CO_2) may be implicated in this response and that hyperoxic conditions may have a significant effect on basal catalase activity.

METHOD

Ethanol-swabbed skin was excised in a sterile hood from the shaved backs of female CD1 mice, aged 6 weeks, which had been killed by cervical dislocature. The subcutaneous fat and muscle were scraped off with a sterile scalpel blade under aseptic conditions. Skin explants (approximately 2 x 2 cm and 2 per animal) were transferred to sterile tissue culture plates containing Dulbecco's MEM medium and 10% fetal bovine serum and gentamycin (0.1 mg/ml).

Each explant was placed within a 10 ml well and laid upon a mesh supporting platform, such that the medium subsequently added totally surrounded the tissue. The lid of the incubation tray was deliberately omitted and the plate was placed on the perforated floor of a 1 cubic liter dessicator.

Sets of 4 explants per group were exposed for 30 minutes to oxygen/nitrogen mixtures (%): 5/95, 10/90, 21/79 (standard air), 40/60, 60/40, 80/20. These atmospheres were obtained premixed and with certified analyses (MG Industries Ref. #15-14). However, an Oxygen Indicator (Model OX-80 Gastech Inc. CA) was placed in the dessicator to verify the oxygen content of the incubation atmosphere. A group of 4 animals remained untreated and exposed in vivo to laboratory air (20.8% O_2).

The pH of the medium post-exposure was measured, since earlier studies had indicated that a pH change might be occurring as seen by a slight color change of the medium pH sensitive dye. Oxygen tension measurements of the medium during exposure were erratic (and discontinued), because of the inability to ensure homogeneity of the medium with respect to oxygen tension in the absence of agitation of the medium. At the end of the incubation period total catalase was determined in replicate by the modified method of Cohen et al.(3) and expressed as the first order reaction constant, K/mg protein. The protein content of each explant was determined by the method of Lowry et al.(4).

VIABILITY

The following viability tests were also carried out on retained tissue or culture medium:

- Examination of morphological appearance under phase contrast microscopy.
- Ability of explant cells to exclude Trypan Blue.
- Ability of explant cells to reduce tetrazolium chloride to formazan.
- Retention of the intracellular enzymes - lactate dehydrogenase, aspartate aminotransferase and alanine aminotransferase, otherwise appearing in the culture medium (method of Kao et al(5)).

TABLE 1

EFFECT OF HYPEROXIA AND HYPOXIA ON CATALASE IN MOUSE SKIN EXPLANT

SKIN TYPE	NOMINAL EXPOSURES (%)		CATALASE ACTIVITY (K/mg Protein ± SE)
	OXYGEN	NITROGEN	
Explant	5.0	95.0	10.88 ± 1.75
Explant	10.0	90.0	12.46 ± 2.26
Explant	21.0[A]	79.0	13.28* ± 2.45
Explant	40.0	60.0	14.46 ± 2.50
Explant	60.0	40.0	14.80 ± 2.98
Explant	80.0	20.0	14.90 ± 2.73
In vivo	20.8[B]	n.d.	8.14 ± 1.62

[A] Standard air

[B] Laboratory air

n.d. = Not determined

* $p \leq 0.05$ from *in vivo* value

Catalase activities are means ± SE of duplicate determinations on 4 skin explants (or for the *in vivo* group, 4 mice).

RESULTS

Catalase activity (K/mg protein) showed a dose-related increase from 10.9 ± 1.7 at 5/95 (% O_2/N_2) to 14.9 ± 2.7 at 80/20 (% O_2/N_2). This maximum *in vitro* value at 80/20 (% O_2/N_2) was 185% of mouse skin exposed *in vivo* to laboratory air (20.8% O_2) and which had a catalase activity of 8.14 ± 1.6 K/mg protein. (See Figure and Table 1)

Normal structural integrity and Trypan Blue exclusion of the skin explants were seen in all groups post-exposure. Leakage of intracellular enzymes was minimal. Actual oxygen concentrations were within ± 2% of nominal indicated in Table 1. The pH of the medium was found to increase slightly with increasing oxygen concentration as indicated in Table 2.

DISCUSSION

The finding of increased total catalase in skin explants from exposure to increasing concentrations of oxygen is analogous to those reported by others for lung tissue. Stevens and Autor[6] found a three-fold increase in catalase, and two-fold increase in mitochondrial superoxide dismutase of rat pulmonary macrophages following 24 hours of either *in vivo* or *in vitro* hyperoxic exposure.

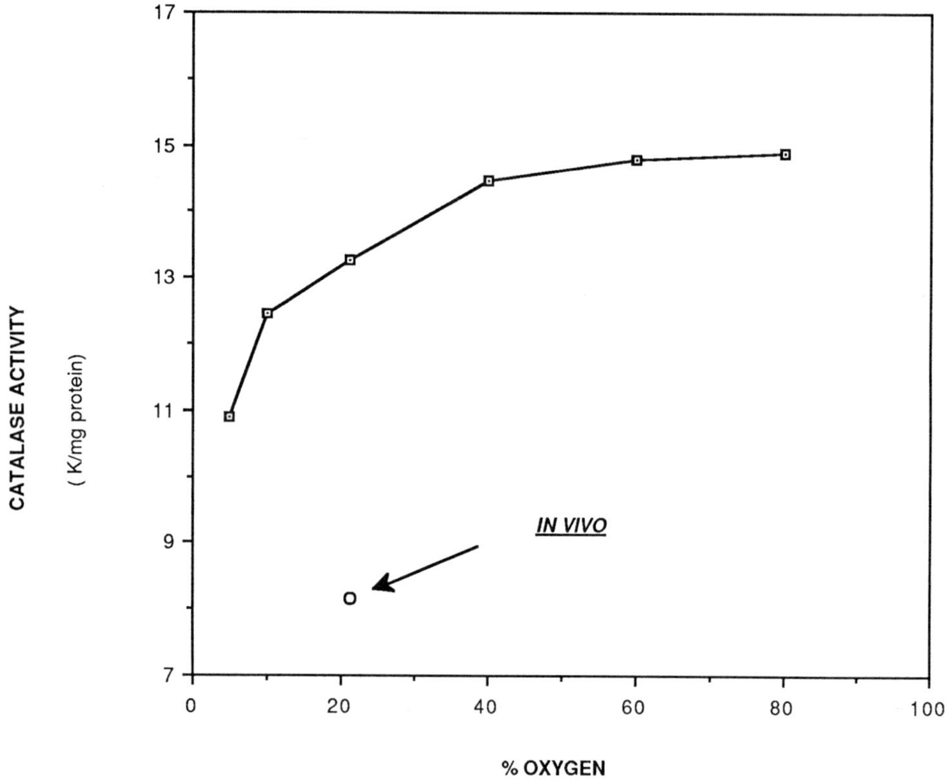

FIGURE: EFFECT OF OXYGEN EXPOSURE ON CATALASE IN MOUSE SKIN EXPLANT

TABLE 2

pH OF EXPLANT MEDIUM POST EXPOSURE

EXPOSURE GROUP (O_2%/N_2)	pH OF MEDIUM
MEDIUM *per se*	7.50
5/95	7.50
10/90	7.52
21/79	7.56
40/60	7.56
60/40	7.64
80/20	7.75

They noted that the superoxide dismutase and catalase responses were found to be age dependent in rat, the neonatal animal having more catalase than the adult; this correlated with the extraordinary resistance of this neonate to oxygen toxicity. They also reported that the enzymes were localized specifically in the pulmonary macrophages and the result of induced protein synthesis. With regard to the latter however, the short observed response time (30 minutes) in the present studies seems too rapid for much protein synthesis to occur. This is supported by the similar values for catalase obtained whether expressed as protein weight or by weight of wet tissue.

Our data suggest that hyperoxia may in some way contribute to an increase in enzyme activity such as has been observed by Verma and Boutwell(1) who reported a dramatic 20-fold increase in ornithine decarboxylase of PMA-treated mouse skin explants incubated in an atmosphere of 95% oxygen and 5% CO_2. While ornithine decarboxylase induction from PMA treatment has been reported in vivo by O'Brien[7] the dramatic increases reported by Verma and Boutwell[1] may be due in part to the hyperoxic incubation conditions. It would also suggest that such biochemical studies of explants in vitro should be carried out at two different incubation atmospheres to ensure differentiation of the effects observed in hyperoxia versus a true induction. If viability can be maintained, the oxygen tension of the explant medium should better mimic that of body fluids in vivo (approximately 2-3% oxygen).

CONCLUSION

The findings that total catalase in the skin explants increased from exposure to increasing concentrations of oxygen, support the hypothesis that elevated catalase activity is due in part to the unphysiological oxygen concentration used during incubations. These findings are consistent with the observations by Stevens and Autor[1] of increased catalase in pulmonary macrophages during hyperoxic exposure.

The elevation in catalase in response to hyperoxic conditions underlines the need for caution in interpreting biochemical responses of explant or isolated cell systems incubated with oxygen concentrations different from those that would be experienced in vivo.

ACKNOWLEDGEMENTS

The studies were made possible through the Exxon Corporation. The authors would like to thank Linda Viebrock for her excellent secretarial assistance.

REFERENCES

1. VERMA, A.K. and BOUTWELL, R.K. (1980), An organ culture of adult mouse skin: an in vitro model for studying the molecular mechanism of skin tumor promotion. Biochem. Biophys. Res. Commun. 96:854-862

2. BIRD, M.G., TRAUL, K.A., WITZ, G. and GOLDSTEIN, B.D. (1984), The effect of tumor promotor phorbol-12-myristate-13-acetate (PMA) on cultured mouse skin explants. Toxicologist 4 (1)#155.

3. COHEN, G., DEMBIEC, D., and MARCUS, J. (1973), Measurement of catalase activity in tissue extracts. Anal. Biochem. 34:30-38.

4. LOWRY, O.H., ROSEBROUGH, N.J., FARR, A.L., and RANDALL, R.J. (1951), Protein measurement with the folin phenol reagent. J. Biol. Chem. 193:265-275.

5. KAO, J., HALL, J., and HOLLAND, J.M. (1983), A quantification of cutaneous toxicity: an in vitro approach using skin in organic culture. Toxicol. & Appl. Pharmacol. 68:206-217.

6. STEVENS, J.B. and Autor, A.P. (1977), Superoxide dismutase in pulmonary macrophages. Lab. Invest. 37:470-478

7. O'BRIEN, T.G. (1976), The induction of ornithine decarboxylase as an early possibly obligatory, event in mouse skin carcinogenesis. Cancer Res. 36, 2644-2653.

Poster A5

Prediction of the Eye Irritation Potential for Surfactant-Based Household Cleaning Products Using the SIRC Cell Toxicity Test

J. DEMETRULIAS and H. NORTH-ROOT

The Dial Corporation
Dial Technical Center
Scottsdale, AZ 85254

ABSTRACT

Eight surfactants or surfactant-based products were evaluated using the SIRC cell toxicity test in the Soap and Detergent Association-sponsored program to identify alternatives to the Draize test for ocular irritancy. Different concentrations of the test materials were added to SIRC cells in culture. Number of surviving cells was determined by enumerating colonies seven days post treatment. The probit method was then used to establish LC_{50} concentrations. Ocular irritation in vivo was measured by the Draize method and by a low volume method in which 0.01 ml or g of material was applied to the cornea and the resulting irritation monitored until it subsided. Relative cytotoxicities were compared to the relative maximum average scores (Draize) and median days to clear (low volume) by rank correlation. The in vitro test predicted the relative ocular irritation of the test materials as measured by either in vivo method (r = 0.8 and 0.7 respectively). These results add to the growing evidence that indicates the SIRC cell toxicity test adequately predicts ocular irritation and support its use as a pre-screen of surfactant-based products prior to animal testing.

INTRODUCTION

Predicting the ocular irritation potential of surfactant-based household cleaning products largely relies upon the results of the Draize eye irritation test in albino rabbits. Although the test has been criticized due to inherent problems with interlaboratory inconsistency and apparent limited correlation with human experience, it has been useful in identifying severely irritating substances. Unfortunately, in such instances the test is likely to cause pain and possibly permanent damage to the eyes of test rabbits. Several investigators have developed alternative methods to supplant the Draize test (1). Recently, the Soap and Detergent Association sponsored a pilot study to identify in vitro methods that show promise for use in testing surfactant-based products for their potential to cause eye irritation through accidental exposure. The SIRC cell toxicity test, a clonal assay utilizing an established rabbit corneal cell line, accurately predicted the relative irritation ranking of several surfactants and shampoos (2-4) and was therefore included in the SDA pilot study.

This paper presents results of the test materials selected by the SDA as assessed using the SIRC cell toxicity test and correlates the relative cytotoxicities with the relative *in vivo* ocular irritation measured by the Draize test and by a modified, *i.e.*, *low* volume, method in rabbits. Griffith and co-workers have shown that the low volume test in which a smaller volume of test material is applied on the cornea and the subsequent irritation monitored until it subsides, better predicts the irritation observed from accidental ocular exposure in humans than does the Draize test (5). Correlations of cytotoxicity with the results of both *in vivo* methods is warranted since historical Draize test results are *available* for a large number of chemicals and products enabling the *in vitro* data to be placed into perspective with a large *in vivo* data base *while the* low volume test results have demonstrated better *correlation* with human exposure (5-8).

EXPERIMENTAL MATERIALS

Product formulations were considered proprietary. Consequently, generic formulas with ingredient ranges are reported. Sodium Lauryl Sulfate, 92.2% active; Liquid Laundry Detergent 1: water 50-74%, alkyl ethoxylate 10-24%, ethanol 10-24%, ditallow dimethyl ammonium chloride 1-4%; Liquid Laundry Detergent 2: water 50-74%, linear alkylbenzene sulfonate 25-49%, alkyl ethoxylate 10-24%, ethanol 5-9%, triethanolamine 1-4%, coconut fatty acid 1-4%, magnesium hydroxide 1-4%; Light Duty Liquid Household Cleaner: water 75-99%, 2-butoxyethanol 1-4%, trisodium phosphate 1-4%, linear alkylbenzene sulfonate 1-4%; Light Duty Liquid Detergent: water 50-74%, magnesium alkyl ethoxylate sulfate 25-49%, magnesium alkyl sulfate 5-9%, ethanol 5-9%, ammonium chloride 1-4%, ammonium xylene sulfonate 1-4%, alkylamine oxide 1-4%; Granular Laundry Detergent 1: complex sodium phosphates 25-49%, sodium sulfate 25-49%, sodium carbonate 10-24%, water 5-9%, sodium alkyl sulfate 5-9%, sodium alkyl ethoxylate sulfate 5-9%, sodium linear alkylbenzene sulfonate 1-4%, sodium silicate 1-4%; Granular Laundry Detergent 2: sodium sulfate 40-50%, sodium carbonate 25-35%, sodium linear alkylbenzene sulfonate 10-15%, moisture 3-5%; and Tween 20.

EXPERIMENTAL METHODS

SIRC CELL TOXICITY TEST

Cells and Cell Culture: The SIRC cell line was derived from the cornea of a normal rabbit (*Orycytologus cuniculus*) by M. Volkert of the Staatens Seruminstitute, Copenhagen, Denmark, 1957. The cell line has since undergone over 400 passages and was obtained from the American Type Culture Collection (CCL 60). Cell stocks are stored in liquid nitrogen. The cells were grown in Ham's F12 media (KC Biological, Inc., Lenexa, Kans.) supplemented with 10% heat-treated (30 min., 56°C) fetal calf serum (Flow Laboratories, Inc., Inglewood, Calif.) at 37°C in a humidified atmosphere containing 5% CO_2 in air.

Preparation of cells: The media was removed from the 100-mm tissue culture dishes containing the growing cells. The attached cells were washed with 1 ml and exposed for five minutes to 2 ml of saline D1 (9) containing 0.05% trypsin (1:300 Gibco Laboratories, Santa Clara, Calif.) and 0.02% disodium ethylendiamine tetraacetic acid in the incubator. Cell clumps were broken with a Pasteur pipette. Two ml Ham's F12 media supplemented with 10% fetal calf serum (F12S) were added to the dish to stop the action of trypsin, and the cells were thoroughly dispersed with a Pasteur pipette. Cell numbers were determined with an Elzone particle counter (Particle Data, Inc., Elmhurst, Ill.).

Preparation of test solutions: Assay test solutions were prepared weight/volume at a 1% concentration in sterile Ham's F12 without serum (F12) and filter sterilized (0.2 micron filter). Further dilutions were prepared volume/volume in sterile F12.

Cell Treatment: The cells were adjusted to 1 x 10^4 cells/ml in F12. Forty microliters of the cell suspension were added to 60-mm dishes containing 4 ml F12S. The dishes were incubated at 37°C in the humidified incubator containing 5% CO_2 in air for 18 hours to allow the cells to attach to the dish. The media was removed and the dishes were washed twice with 2 ml F12. Four ml of each concentration of test material were added to dishes in triplicate. Dishes were incubated for one hour. The test solutions were removed from the dishes and the dishes washed twice with two ml F12S. Five ml of F12S were added to each dish. The dishes were placed in the 37°C humidified incubator containing 5% CO_2 in air for seven to eight days. The media was changed once during the incubation period. The media was removed and the cells were fixed with 10% formalin and stained with 0.1% crystal violet. Clones containing ten or more cells were counted using a dissecting microscope.

Appropriate concentrations of one of the samples, sodium lauryl sulfate, were included in the assay of the remaining test samples to serve as an internal control to measure reproducibility of the assay and to serve as a positive control to ensure the responsiveness of the test system.

The LC_{50} value, i.e., the concentration allowing 50% cell survival, was determined by the probit method (10). The response rate was corrected for the natural response rate determined by two control samples of 3 plates each.

The LC_{50} values were assigned ranks from one to eight (least to most toxic). Confidence intervals were established for the LC_{50} concentrations of each assay. Assays were not considered acceptable unless the mean absolute cell survival of the six control dishes was at least 8%, each data point was represented by the mean of at least two replicates, three data points were within 100% and 10% relative survival, and the positive control LC_{50} was within two sigma variations of the historical value.

IN VIVO EXPERIMENTS

DRAIZE OCULAR IRRITATION TEST

Draize test results were supplied as part of the sponsored program. The tests were conducted by a contract laboratory using the standard Draize eye irritation protocol and grading system (1, 10). Irritation was ranked by the maximum average score (MAS) obtained from the group of animals administered each test material. The results, assigned ranks one to eight (least to greatest irritation), and MAS confidence intervals were supplied to our laboratory for comparison with the SIRC cell test results.

LOW VOLUME OCULAR IRRITATION TEST

Animals: New Zealand albino rabbits (Orycytologus cuniculus) of both sexes were obtained from Bell Rabbitry, Clovis, N. Mex., and housed individually in self-flushing Hoeltge wire mesh cages. They received 12 hours of light and 12 hours of darkness daily. Purina rabbit chow (Ralston Purina, St. Louis, Mo.) and tap water were supplied ad libitum. The rabbits were identified with metal ear tags and were acclimated to the laboratory for a minimum of one week prior to testing.

Test Material Preparation/Administration: Liquid test materials were administered as received. Powders were ground to less than 125 micron particulate size. One hundredth (0.01) ml liquid or 0.01 g of powder was administered directly to the cornea of the test eye. Each animal was then fitted with a plastic flexible Elizabethan-type collar that remained in place until the first observation. Irritation was observed at 24, 48 and 72 hours and daily thereafter. Observations were scored according to the system described by Draize, Woodard and Calvery (11). However, the samples were assigned ranks by determining the median days to clear (MDC) as described by the proposed ASTM ocular irritation method (12). Ranks one to eight (least to greatest irritation) were assigned to the test samples.

STATISTICAL COMPARISONS

Relative LC_{50} values were correlated with MAS and MDC, values using the Spearman rank correlation analysis (13).

RESULTS

The results from the tests, LC_{50}, MAS and MDC, are summarized in Table 1 as are the ranks assigned to test samples by each method. The materials are ranked according to their cytotoxicity (1 being the least cytotoxic) and the severity of the ocular irritation observed by each method (smallest MAS and shortest MDC being the least irritating). The ranks of ocular irritation differ depending upon the test method.

TABLE 1

SUMMARY OF IN VITRO AND IN VIVO TEST RESULTS

TEST MATERIAL	SIRC RANK	SIRC LC_{50}[a]/CI[b]	DRAIZE RANK	DRAIZE MAS[c]/CI[b]	LOW VOLUME RANK	LOW VOLUME MDC[d]/CI[b]
Sodium lauryl sulfate	5	24.8[e] 22.4-26.4	4	23.2 17.8-28.6	7	13.0 ND
Liquid laundry detergent 1	7	16.4 8.9-22.6	5	24.2 11.9-36.5	5	5.0 ND
Liquid laundry detergent 2	8	8.5 8.0-8.9	8	52.2 23.3-81.1	8	16.0 ND
Light duty liquid cleaner	1	812.0 653.5-860.9	2	3.0 1.0-5.0	2	3.0 ND
Light duty liq. detergent	3	57.5 55.6-60.5	3	24.3 18.2-30.4	6	9.0 ND
Granular detergent 1	4	34.4 30.3-36.3	7	33.7 29.3-38.1	3.5	3.5 ND
Granular detergent 2	6	24.0 ND	6	30.0 28.0-32.0	3.5	3.5 ND
Tween 20	2	135.1 125.6-143.4	1	0.0 -	1	2.5 ND

a in parts per million
b 95% confidence intervals
c maximum average score
d median days to clear
e mean of seven control values = 27.6 ± 1.69
ND not determined

Correlation of the cytotoxicity rank scores with the in vivo rank scores is illustrated in figures 1 and 2. The correlation coefficients indicate good agreement between the relative LC_{50} and MAS or MDC values (0.8 and 0.7 respectively).

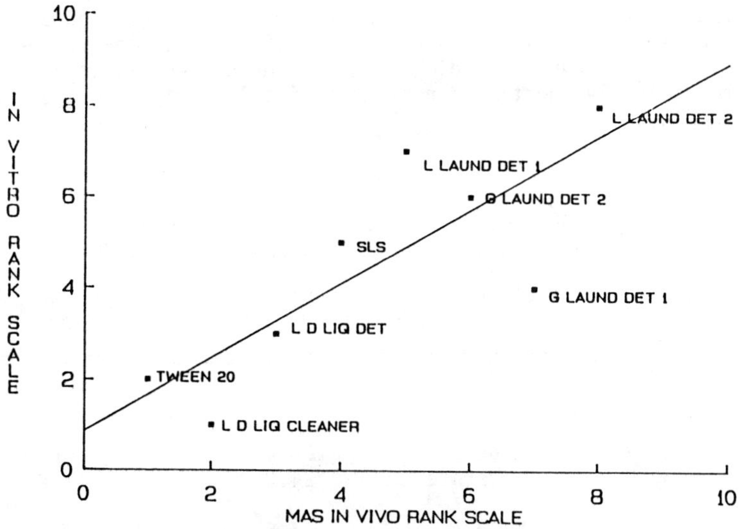

Figure 1. LC $_{50}$ vs MAS ranks,
1 being the least cytotoxic/irritating.
Spearman correlation coefficient = 0.8.

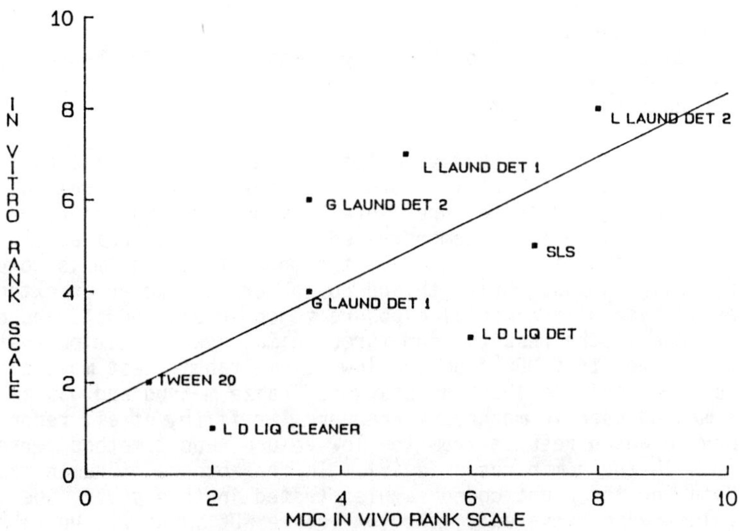

Figure 2. LC $_{50}$ vs MDC ranks,
1 being the least cytotoxic/irritating.
Spearman correlation coefficient = 0.7.

DISCUSSION

The relative cell toxicity test results demonstrate good correlation with the relative ocular irritation measured by both Draize and low volume methods. Draize descriptive ratings coinciding with the MAS scores, Table 2, show that the Draize test clearly identified non- to minimally irritating and severely irritating samples.

TABLE 2

COMPARISON OF DRAIZE TEST RESULTS AND DESCRIPTIVE CLASSIFICATIONS TO LC_{50} AND MDC RESULTS

Test Sample	Draize MAS[a]	Description Classification[b]	SIRC LC_{50}[c]	Low Volume MDC[d]
L Laund Det 2	52.2	Severe	8.5	16
G Laund Det 1	33.7	Moderate	34.4	3.5
G Laund Det 2	30.0	Moderate	24.0	3.5
L D Liq Det	24.3	Mild	57.5	9
L Laund Det 1	24.2	Mild	16.4	5
SLS	23.2	Mild	24.8	13
L D Liq Cleaner	3.0	Minimal	812.0	3
Tween 20	0.0	Non	135.1	2.5

a maximum average score
b descriptive classification based upon maximum average score
c in parts per million
d median days to clear

No actual resolution of the five mild to moderate irritants was observed (Table 1). Clearly, the SIRC cell cytotoxicity test serves as well as the Draize test in identifying these three levels of ocular irritation. Although the SIRC cell toxicity test has demonstrated the ability to adequately predict ocular irritation in rabbits, the goal of the model test system is to predict ocular responses in humans. Griffith and co-workers conducted an extensive historical evaluation of accidental exposure to consumer products and compared those observations to the results from three animal eye irritation testing methods. They showed that MDC from the low volume rabbit test more closely related to human experience than the standard Draize method and was as good as the eye test method used in monkeys. Freeberg, Griffith, et al. reported a clinical study in which results from the low volume rabbit method correlated significantly with the human response (8). In the absence of human ocular irritation data for the eight coded samples tested in this study, the *in vitro* LC_{50} values were compared to the low volume MDC values. The rank correlation was good. The ocular irritation potential of the samples for which the LC_{50} and MDC scores were the most discrepant, the granular detergents, was apparently overestimated by the *in vitro* test. Further, there were no LC_{50} results that would be interpreted as false negatives thereby breaching the margin of safety required by a model test system.

Testing granular samples poses the additional problem of retention of the test material in the eye. The Draize test utilizes the conjunctival cul-de-sac to retain the sample in the rabbit's eye. Directly applying the sample on the cornea as in the low volume test inevitably allows an undetermined amount of the material to be blinked from the eye, much as would be expected in accidental human exposure (14). Both the SIRC cell and Draize tests allow equivalent exposure of powders and liquids to the test system and the values obtained from these methods are in better relative agreement than with the low volume, direct corneal application values. Previous SIRC cell test results have been correlated with irritation rankings developed by studying different concentrations of each surfactant or shampoo and determining the concentration that would result in a Draize score of 20 (ED_{20})(2-4). Ranking was based on the ED_{20} values. The nearly perfect correlation shown in the earlier studies may be explained by the in vivo testing of the materials only as solutions.

Sodium lauryl sulfate (SLS) was assayed previously in the SIRC cell test (2). The LC_{50} value reported (8.5 ppm) differs considerably from the value reported here (24.8 ppm); however, the earlier study tested a commercial grade material which may have contained contaminants that influenced the cytotoxicity of the sample. The results from the repeated assay of SLS as a control in this study (27.6 ppm ± 1.69 ppm) underscores the reproducibility of the test.

In summary, the SIRC cell toxicity test is relatively easy to conduct, inexpensive to perform (2) and does not involve the use of live animals as tissue donors. The SIRC cell line has been shown to be a suitable test system for predicting the irritation caused by surfactants and promises to be useful in screening prototype formulations of surfactant-based consumer products prior to animal testing.

REFERENCES

1. Frazier, J. M., Gad, S. C., Goldberg, A. M., McCulley, J. P. and Meyer, R. D., (1987), A critical evaluation of alternatives to acute ocular testing. Alternative Methods in Toxicology 4, Alan Goldberg (Ed.) Mary Ann Liebert, Inc., New York, NY.

2. North-Root, H., Yackovich, F., Demetrulias, J., Gacula, Jr., M., and Heinze, J. E., (1983), Evaluation of an in vitro cell toxicity test using rabbit corneal cells to predict the eye irritation potential of surfactants, Safety Evaluation and Regulation of Chemicals, F. Homburger (Ed.) S. Karger, Basel, 259-269.

3. North-Root, H., Yackovich, F., Demetrulias, J., Gacula, Jr., M. and Heinze, J. E., (1983), Evaluation of an in vitro cell toxicity test using rabbit corneal cells to predict the eye irritation potential of surfactants and surfactant-based products. Toxicologist, 3:197.

4. North-Root, H., Yackovich, F., Demetrulias, J., Gacula, Jr., M., and Heinze, J. E., (1985), Prediction of the eye irritation potential of shampoos using the in vitro SIRC cell toxicity test. Fd. Chem. Toxicol. 23(2):271.

5. Griffith, J. F., Nixon, G. A., Bruce, R. D., Reer, P. J. and Bannan, E. A., (1980), Dose-response studies with chemical irritants in the albino rabbit eye as a basis for selecting optimum testing conditions for predicting hazard to the human eye. Toxicol. Appl. Pharmacol. 55:501.

6. Freeberg, F. E., Griffith, J. H. F., Bruce, R. D. and Bay, P. H. S., (1984), Correlation of animal test methods with human experience for household products. J. Toxicol.-Cut. and Ocular Toxicol. 1(3):53.

7. Freeberg, F. E., Hooker, D. T. and Griffith, J. F., (1986), Correlation of animal eye test data with human experience for household products: An Update. J. Toxicol.-Cut. and Ocular Toxicol. 5(2):115.

8. Freeberg, F. E., Nixon, G. A., Reer, P. J., Weaver, J. E., Bruce, R. D., Griffith, J. F. and Sanders, L. W., (1986), Human and rabbit eye response to chemical insult. Fund Appl. Toxicol. 7:626.

9. O'Neil, J. P. and Hsie, A. W., (1979), Phenotypic expression time of mutagen induced 6-thioguanine resistance in Chinese hamster ovary cells. Mut. Res. 59:109.

10. Finney, D. J., (1971), Probit Analysis. 3rd Ed., p. 125, Cambridge University Press, Cambridge.

11. Draize, J. H., Woodard, G. and Calvery, H. O., (1944), Methods for the study of irritation and toxicity of substances applied to the skin and mucous membranes. J. Pharmac. Exp. Ther. 82:377.

12. Evaluation of eye irritation in albino rabbits, E1055-85, American Society for Testing and Materials, Section 11, volume 11.04, p. 764.

13. Steel, R. G. D. and Torrie, J. H., (1960), Principles and Procedures of Statistics, p. 409, McGraw-Hill, NY.

14. Chrai, S. S., Patton, A. M. and Robinson, J. R., (1973), Lacrimal and instilled fluid dynamics in rabbit eyes. J. Pharm. Sci. 62:1112.

Poster A6

Differential Response of *In Vitro* Vaginal Tissue to Various Test Agents

N.H. DUBIN, R.B. GHODGAONKAR, and T.H. PARMLEY

Department of Gynecology and Obstetrics
Johns Hopkins University School of Medicine
Baltimore, MD

ABSTRACT

An in vitro assay for vaginal irritancy has been developed. Since prostaglandins are mediators of the inflammatory process, we have measured prostaglandin release by in vitro rat vaginal segments after exposure to various test agents. Exposure to long chain alcohols (butanol and isoamyl alcohol) caused prostaglandin release at lower doses than short chain alcohols (ethanol and methanol). Ethanol exposure had no effect on LDH release from tissues suggesting that the increase in prostaglandin release was not due to membrane leakage. Exposure of vaginal tissue to octanol and the detergents, nonoxynol-9 and sodium dodecyl sulfate, caused decreased prostaglandin synthesis suggestive of acute toxicity. Only nonoxynol exposure elevated LDH levels. It may be possible to differentiate between inflammatory responses and acute cytotoxicity by prostaglandin measurements alone or in conjunction with other end points.

INTRODUCTION

The role of prostaglandins as a mediator in the inflammatory process has been widely reviewed (Higgs, 1984; Davies et al, 1984). We have hypothesized that prostaglandin production in vitro might be used as an index of inflammation or cytotoxicity and thus may serve as an alternative to currently used live animal toxicologic assays. The model we have used is an in vitro vaginal tissue assay which was designed as a possible alternative for the presently used rabbit vaginal toxicity assay (Kaminsky and Willigan, 1982) or mucosal membranes in general.

We have demonstrated that, PGE_2, PGF_{2a}, 6-Keto-PGF_{1a} and TXB_2, as detected radioimmunologically, are all released into buffer following incubation of vaginal segments and release of these prostanoids increases in response to ethanol (Dubin et al, 1984). The current study examines the response of vaginal tissue to other alcohols and detergents.

METHODS

Rats in the diestrus stage of their cycles were injected intraperitoneally with sodium pentobarbital (5 mg/100 gm body weight) and exsanguinated via the abdominal aorta with a needle and syringe. Vaginal tissue were removed and placed in cold saline. The tissue was then cut into small full thickness segments weighing between 20 and 30 mg. Each segment was placed into a pre-wetted 12 mm Multicell (Millipore, Bedford, MA) which was inserted into a well of a tissue culture plate containing 1 ml Minimum Essential Media (Eagles). The tissue culture plate was secured in a Dubanoff incubator at 37°C and shaken at a slow speed for a 5 min equilibration period. The tissue was transferred via the Multicell carrier into a test well containing either a test substance or control media. The time of exposure to the test agent was 30 seconds. The tissue was then transferred to a third well containing fresh media and rinsed for 30 seconds. The tissue was then transferred to the final well containing fresh media and was incubated for 30 minutes under 95% O_2/5%CO_2. At the end of the incubation period, the media was removed and analyzed for PGF_{2a} and/or lactate dehydrogenase (LDH). Tissues treated with control media and tissues treated with test substances were processed for light microscopy and their histology were evaluated and compared.

Previous experiments demonstrated a good correlation in response between PGE_2 and PGF_{2a}, thus only PGF_{2a} is reported in this study. Prostaglandin F_{2a} was assayed by radioimmunoassay as previously described in detail (Dubin et al, 1979). LDH was assayed by following NADH formation spectrophotometrically at 340 nm during the conversion of lactate to pyruvate (Sigma Diagnostics LD-L procedure No. 226-UV).

RESULTS

The effect of exposure to various alcohols on in vitro vaginal segments is shown in Figure 1. Ethanol and methanol exposure resulted in an increase in PGF_{2a} release into the media at approximately a 10 M concentration. Butanol and isoamyl alcohol caused release at a 1 M concentration.

In contrast to previously tested alcohols, a longer chain alcohol, octanol, did not cause any increase in PGF_{2a}, but at the highest concentration (99%;6.4 M) a decrease in PGF_{2a} was observed (Figure 2). An anionic detergent used in shampoos, sodium dodecyl sulfate (S.D.S.) was also studied. S.D.S. resulted in a significant reduction in PGF_{2a} at a concentration of 100 mM. Nonoxynol-9, a nonionic detergent used in spermacides, also caused a reduction of PGF_{2a} at 100% concentration (~ 2M).

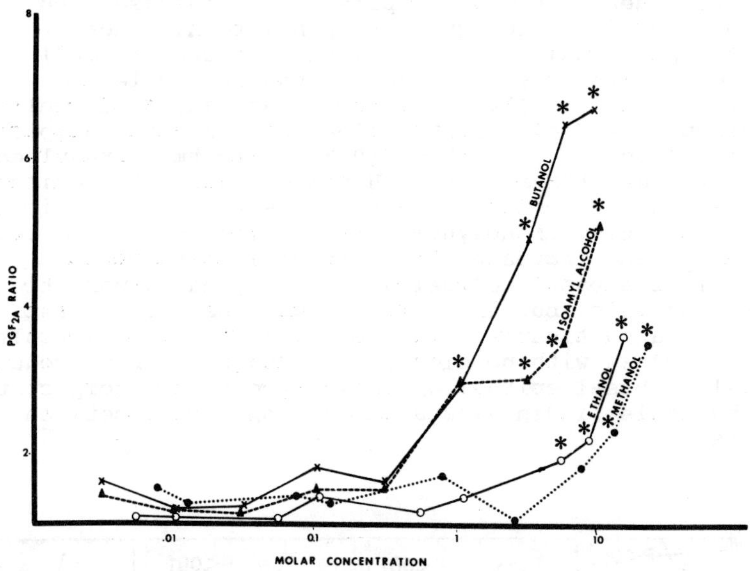

Figure 1: Dose-response curves for the effect of various alcohols on PGF_{2a} release by vaginal tissue segments in vitro. PGF_{2a} ratio is the ratio of prostaglandin released by the test drug divided by the amount released by untreated control tissue from the same rat. * P <0.05 vs untreated controls.

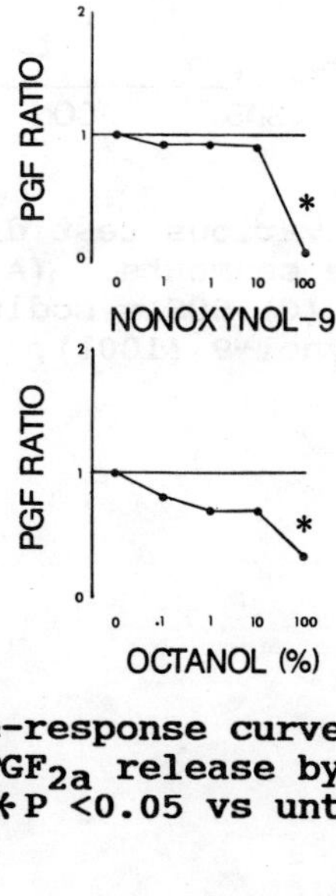

Figure 2: Dose-response curve for the effect of various agents on PGF_{2a} release by vaginal tissue segments in vitro. * P <0.05 vs untreated controls.

In a subsequent study we compared PGF_{2a} release, LDH release, and vaginal histology in response to high doses of some of the agents previously tested. Seventy percent ethanol increased PGF_{2a} without significant change in LDH levels (Figure 3). Histologically the intermediate and basal cells of the epithelium showed cytoplasmic clearing and basal displacement of the nuclei (Figure 4). S.D.S. (0.3 M) treatment resulted in decreased PGF_{2a} and LDH release. Histologically, the epithelial layer has been separated from underlying stroma. The epithelial cells were autolyzed. Nonoxynol-9 (100%) treatment resulted in decreased PGF_{2a} and increased LDH release into the media. Histologically the basal epithelial cells appeared more tightly packed than controls, but this finding was less consistent between the treated tissues. Octanol (99%) treatment resulted in a decrease in PGF_{2a} with no significant change in LDH production. Histologically, basal epithelial cells appear more compact than controls, but this finding was also not consistent between treated tissues.

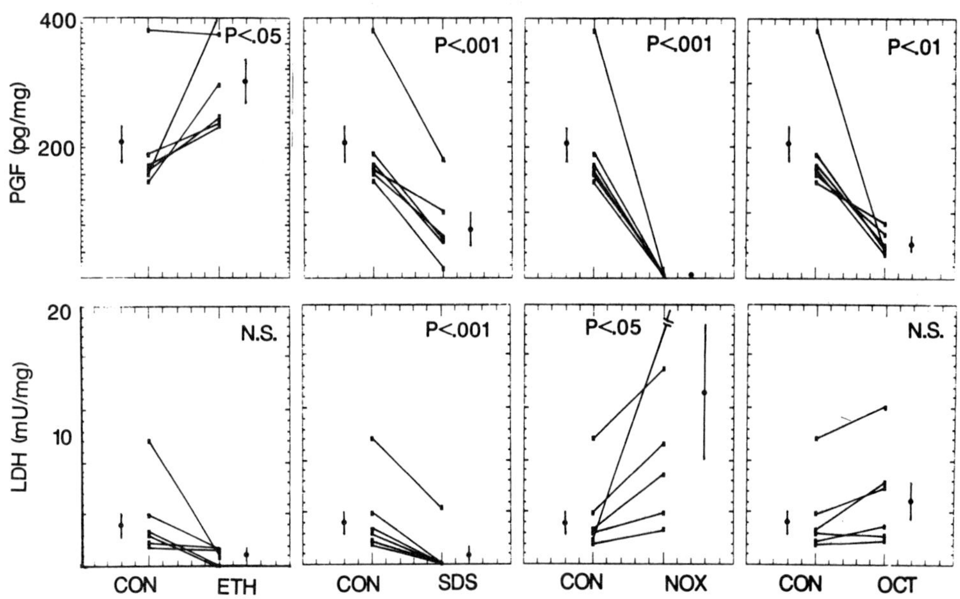

Figure 3: Effect of various test drugs on PGF_{2a} and LDH release by vaginal tissue segments. (A) CON = control (B) ETH = ethanol (70%); (C) SDS = sodium dodecyl sulfate (0.3 M); (D) NOX = nonoxynol-9 (100%); (E) OCT = octanol (99%)

Figure 4: Effect of various test drugs on the morphologic appearance of vaginal tissue after treatment.

A) control
B) ethanol (70%)
C) sodium dodecyl sulfate (0.3 M)
D) nonoxynol-9 (100%)
E) octanol (99%)

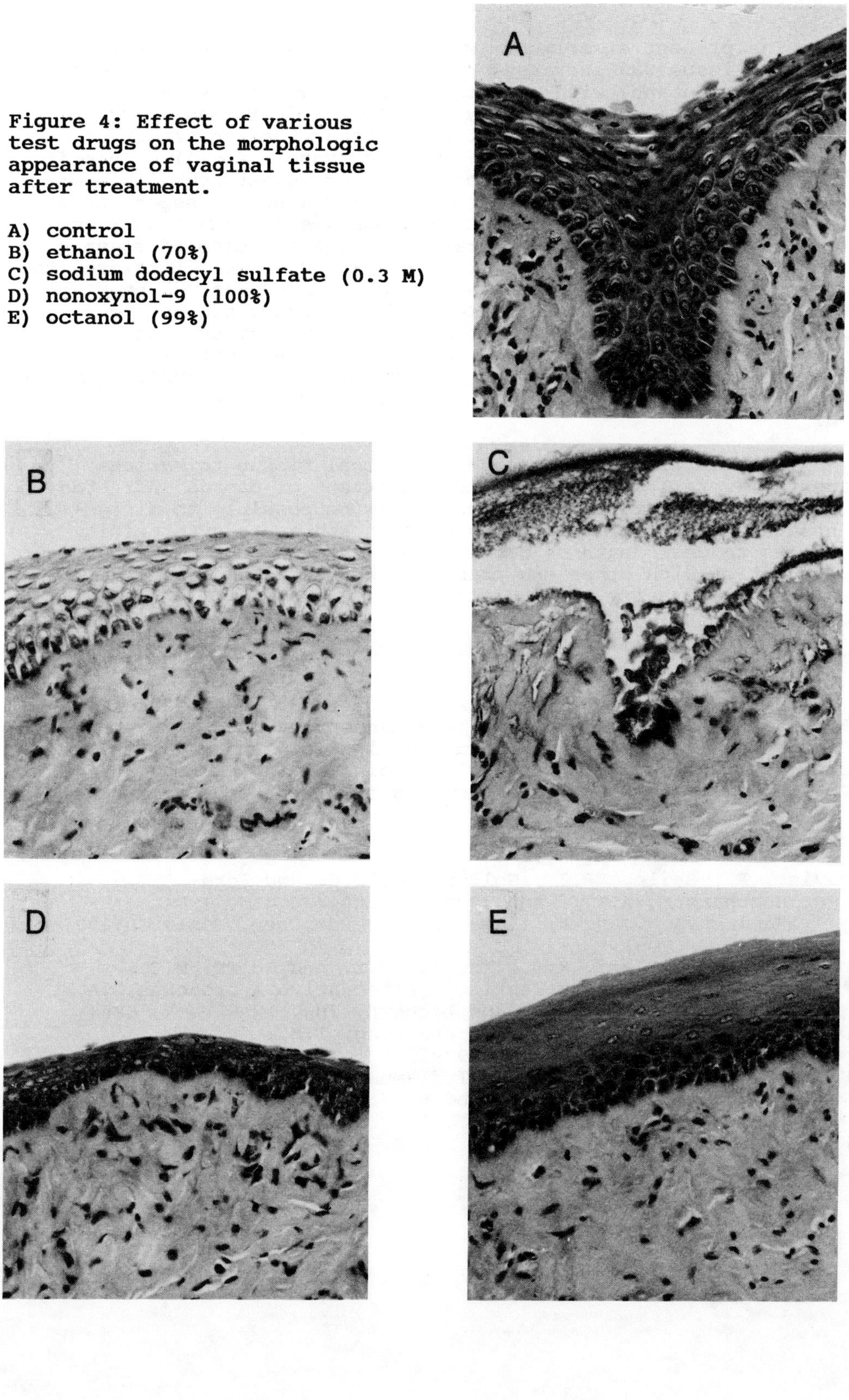

DISCUSSION

The present experiments indicate that PGF_{2a} release by vaginal tissue was increased by 30 second exposure to various alcohols. Butanol with a carbon chain length (C) equal to 4 and isoamyl alcohol (C = 5) caused significant increases in PGF_{2a} release at lower molar concentrations than the shorter chain length alcohols, ethanol (C = 2) and methanol (C = 1). This is in accordance with known toxicity of these substances. However, a longer chain alcohol, octanol (C = 8) did not cause an increase in PGF_{2a} release, and in fact there was a significant decrease. This might be due to a denaturation or inactivation of enzymes or co-factors in the prostaglandin synthetic pathway. Likewise, the detergents reduced PGF_{2a} release. Nonoxynol-9 was the only agent tested which caused an increase in LDH release, suggesting a breach in membrane integrity. S.D.S., on the other hand, resulted in a decrease in LDH activity. This might also represent altered function of this enzyme, since histologically it is apparent that the epithelial cells are completely disrupted.

The differential response of vaginal tissue to various agents may reflect the mechanism or extent of damage inflicted upon mucous membranes. Indeed, it may be possible to differentiate between inflammatory responses and acute cytotoxicity leading to cell death by prostaglandin measurement alone, or in conjunction with other end points. More detailed studies are required to clarify this point.

ACKNOWLEDGMENTS

We thank Mr. Robert Noorami for technical assistance and Ms. Fran Karas for preparation of this manuscript. We also thank the Center for Alternative to Animal Testing for support of these studies. We thank Dr. Masami Tsuboshima of Ono Pharmaceutical Co., Osaka, Japan for the generous gift of the prostaglandins.

REFERENCES

Davies, P., Bailey, P.J., Goldenberg, M.M. and Ford-Hutchinson, A.W.: Ann. Rev. Immunol. 2:335, 1984. Kaminsky, M. and Willigan, D.A.: Fd. Chem. Toxic 20:193, 1982.

Dubin, N.H., DiBlasi, M.C., Thomas, C.L. and Wolff, M.C.: In: Acute Toxicity Testing: Alternative Approaches. A.M. Goldberg (Eds.), Mary Ann Liebert, Inc., New York, 1984.

Dubin, N.H., Ghodgoankar, R.B. and King, T.M.: Endocrinology, 105:47, 1979.

Higgs, G.A.: In: Advances in Inflammation Research, I. Otterness, R. Capetola, and S. Wong (Eds.), Vol. 7, Raven Press, New York, 1984, p 223.

Kaminsky, M. and Willigan, D.A.: Fd. Chem. Toxic 20:193, 1982.

Poster A7

Use of Isolated Hepatocytes for Studying the Biochemical Mechanisms of Steatosis and Cholestasis

FABIENNE GOETHALS, DOMINIQUE DEBOYSER, CONCEPCIÓN GONZÁLEZ and MARCEL ROBERFROID

Unit of Biochemical Toxicology and Cancerology
Université Catholique de Louvain
73 Av. Mounier, Box 73.69
B-1200 Brussels, Belgium

Abstract

Within the scope of the evaluation of drug-mediated hepatotoxicity, steatosis (fat accumulation) and cholestasis (reduction of bile flow) are common pathologies.
The present work is focused on the study of those specific hepatotoxicities using isolated hepatocytes in suspension. Secretory processes of the hepatocytes are indeed among the most active hepatocytic functions and may thus be the targets of the cytotoxic action of chemical.
With regard to the evaluation of the mechanisms leading to steatosis, the effects of tetracycline which is known to induce steatosis in vivo, were studied on triglycerides synthesis and secretion, protein synthesis and secretion. Tetracycline was shown to induced a concentration-dependent inhibition of lipoprotein secretion but did affect neither protein secretion nor triglycerides synthesis. In addition, the effect of tetracycline or protein synthesis is slight and appears only at 10^{-3}M. In conclusion we suggest that the mechanism of tetracycline-induced steatosis could be a specific interference with the association of the lipid part and the protein part of lipoprotein.

With regard to the use of isolated hepatocytes to study the alterations of bile secretion, a methodology for measuring the uptake of ^{14}C taurocholate (TC) by hepatocytes was developped and the effects of chlorpromazine (CPZ) which is known to be cholestatic were analysed. The uptake of ^{14}C-taurocholate is linear during 2 min.; then the intracellular content of TC reaches a plateau which reflects an equilibrium between uptake and secretion of TC. The kinetic parameters of this transport have been determined: Km = 43.2 uM and Vmax: 2.83 nmol/min/mg protein.
In the aim to investigate the biochemical mechanisms of cholestasis induced by CPZ, hepatocytes were incubated in the presence of various concentrations of CPZ (10-100 uM). CPZ was shown to inhibit both the initial velocity and the intracellular level of accumulation of TC.

INTRODUCTION

Secretory processes are among the most active hepatocytic functions.

Alterations of the secretory processes resulting **steatosis** (fat accumulation) or **cholestasis** (reduction of bile flow) occur as the last stage of various metabolic impairment which are the mechanistic events of such pathologies.

Isolated hepatocytes is an in vitro model well recognized for assessing drug toxicity. It can be used both to screen for general cytotoxicity and to study the biochemical events related to drug-mediated toxicity (1,2).

Our study was aimed to demonstrate the applicability of such an experimental model for evaluating specific hepatotoxicity like steatosis and cholestasis.

As steatosis and cholestasis may result from an impairment, at any step, in the secretion of lipoprotein or bile respectively, it was necessary first to develop adequate methods for controlling each of those steps and thus for determining the cellular target of drug action. The effects of tetracycline, which is known to produce steatosis in man, and chlorpromazine, which is known to be cholestatic, were therefore analysed.

MATERIALS AND METHODS.

Chemicals

Collagenase was purchased from Worthington, (Freehold, NY, USA); Dulbecco's modified Eagle medium from Flow Laboratories (Irvine, Scotland). Taurocholate and bovine serum albumin (BSA) (fraction V) were purchased from Sigma Chemical Co. (St Louis, MO,USA). Cycloheximide was obtained from Boehringer (Manheim, Germany); Colchicine from Calbiochem (San Diego,CA,USA); tetracycline hydrochloride and chlorpromazine hydrochloride from Federa (Brussels, Belgium). Silicone oils AR 20 et AR 200 were obtained from Wacker Chemie (Munich, Germany).
All the other reagents were of the purest analytical grade available from Merck (Darmstadt, Germany).
(U - ^{14}C) Leucine (339 mCi/nmol) and Tauro[carbonyl-^{14}C]cholic acid, sodium salt (56 mCi/nmol) were purchased from Amersham International (Amersham, England). [1 - ^{14}C] palmitic acid (5.7 mCi/nmol) was provided by New England Nuclear Co (USA).
Aquasol (New England Nuclear Co, USA) and NA (Beckman, Geneva,Switzerland) were used as liquid scintillation cocktails.

Palmitate-albumin bound solution stock solutions of [1-^{14}C] palmitate (0.5 mM)-BSA (0.75 mM) and unlabelled palmitate (1.70 mM) - BSA (1.13 mM) were each prepared by addition of BSA solution to a warmed solution (70°C) of palmitate.

Isolation and incubation of hepatocytes Male Wistar rats (Iffa Credo, Lyon, France) weighing from 240 to 260 g, were housed two per cage, on a 6am/6pm light schedule and fed ad libitum until time of perfusion. Hepatocytes were isolated by an "in situ" perfusion with collagenase as previously described (3).

They were incubated in suspension in a Dulbecco medium supplemented with 1.5% bovine serum albumin at a cell concentration of 0.5 10^6 cells/ml (4). Cellular viability was controlled by measuring the LDH leakage (4).

Biochemical assays.

Protein synthesis was evaluated by measuring incorporation of ^{14}C-leucine (94 uCi/nmol) into $HClO_4$ precipitable proteins (5).

Protein secretion was estimated by measuring the incorporation of ^{14}C-leucine into extracellular proteins. In experiments with prelabelled proteins, hepatocytes were preincubated for 1h with ^{14}C-leucine (627uCi/nmol). The cells were then washed, resuspended in fresh medium and incubated in the presence or the absence of the tested compound. The secretion of prelabelled proteins was quantified by measuring the amount of ^{14}C-proteins in the incubation medium.

Triglyceride synthesis was evaluated by measuring the incorporation of ^{14}C-palmitate into triglycerides. Hepatocytes were incubated in the presence of a mixture of ^{14}C-palmitate and non radio-labelled palmitate at a final concentration of 0.04 mM (710 uCi/nmol).

Aliquots of 1.5 ml of cell suspension were centrifuged (400 rpm/1 min). The supernatant was kept aside for the determination of triglycerides secretion. Intracellular triglycerides were extracted with isopropanol-heptane (4/1). After 60 min at room temperature, heptane and water were added in order to separate the two phases. After 2 washings with ethanol/NaOH 1N / H_2O (50/5/45), an aliquot of the organic phase was mixed with NA Beckman Liquid Scintillation and counted. In order to evaluate triglycerides secretion, the extracellular medium (supernatant of the centrifugation) was lyophilized in a Lyovac GT2 (Leybold-Heraeus) lyophilisator.

The glyceride fraction present in the lipoproteins secreted by the hepatocytes was extracted and counted as described above.

Uptake of taurocholate

After 30 min preincubation in the presence or in the absence of the tested compound, a mixture of ^{14}C-taurocholate and nonlabelled taurocholate was added to the incubation medium to yield final concentration of taurocholate of 10 - 900 uM. Uptake reaction was stopped by separating the cells from the medium by centrifugal filtration through a silicone layer (6). Duplicate samples of the cell suspension were removed at 0.5; 2; 4; 10 and 20 min after addition of taurocholate and placed in polypropylene microfuge tubes previously layered with 100 ul of 14% $HClO_4$ and 350 ul of silicone oil (mixture of silicone oils AR 20 and AR 200 1/3; density:1.020). The samples were then centrifuged for 10 sec in a Beckman microfuge.

The cells , being more dense than the silicone oils, move through the oil into the $HClO_4$ within 1-2 sec. Each polypropylene tube was cut just above the oil - $HClO_4$ interface and placed in a scirtillation vial. After the cell pellet has been dissolved in 500 ul of 0.3N NaOH for 2h, 10 ml of aquasol liquid scintillation were added and each sample was counted in a Berthold (BF 5000) liquid scintillator counter.

All the results obtained for these biochemical assays are expressed per mg of cellular protein. The amount of protein was determined by the method of Lowry (7) using bovine serum albumin as a standard.

Statistical analysis

Most of the data are reported as means ± S.E.M. of at least three separate experiments.

The evolution of the treatments during the incubation time was tested by analysis of variance (ANOVA). The Snedecor's test was used to compare the evolution of two treatments.

The Student's t-test was used to evaluate the significance level of differences between mean values at the same incubation time.

RESULTS

1. Isolated hepatocytes as a model to test for the effects of steatogenic agents. Investigation into the mechanism of tetracycline induced steatosis.

Steatosis is a very common consequence of drug-mediated hepatotoxicity. It may result from an alteration at any step in the sequence from protein and triglycerides synthesis to lipoprotein secretion.

Previous results (8) have shown that, in our experimental conditions, isolated hepatocytes are a suitable model to test for the effects of steatogenic agents. The validation was realized by incubating the cells in the presence of well-known steatogenic compounds, i.e. cycloheximide and colchicine. By analysing the effects of those reference compounds on the different biochemical pathways involved in lipoprotein secretion, we demonstrated that it was possible to locate in vitro their site of action : protein synthesis for cycloheximide and secretory processes for colchicine.

The aim of the present study was to investigate the mechanism of tetracycline induced steatosis. Administration of high doses of tetracycline may indeed produce microvesicular steatosis of the human liver resulting in severe hepatic dysfunctions. However, the biochemical mechanisms by which tetracycline induces that pathology are still unclear.

1.a. Effect of tetracycline on triglycerides synthesis and secretion

Isolated hepatocytes were incubated in the presence of various concentrations of tetracycline (10^{-5}, 10^{-4}, and 10^{-3}M). The secretion of triglycerides was inhibed by tetracycline in a concentration-dependent way (Fig.1a). At 10^{-4} and 10^{-3}M, tetracycline induced 41% and 74% inhibition respectively after 150 min of incubation, whereas 10^{-5}M had no effect.

The inhibition of triglycerides secretion resulted in an accumulation of triglycerides within the cells (Fig.1b). The magnitude of that increase in the intracellular triglycerides level is comparable to the degree of inhibition of their secretion.

1.b Effect of tetracycline on protein synthesis and secretion.

At 10^{-3}M, tetracycline reduced the rate of incorporation of ^{14}C-leucine into protein (29% inhibition after 150 min of incubation). The secretion of protein assayed by measuring the $HClO_4$ precipitable radioactivity in the medium was decreased to the same extent (26% inhibition after 150 min), suggesting that such an effect results from the inhibition of protein synthesis.

When it was added at a concentration of 10^{-4}M, tetracycline did modify neither protein synthesis nor protein secretion (Fig.2).

1.c Discussion.

Tetracycline is known to inhibit protein synthesis (9, 10, 11) and such an effect is often proposed to be responsible for the microvesicular steatosis induced by this antibiotic.

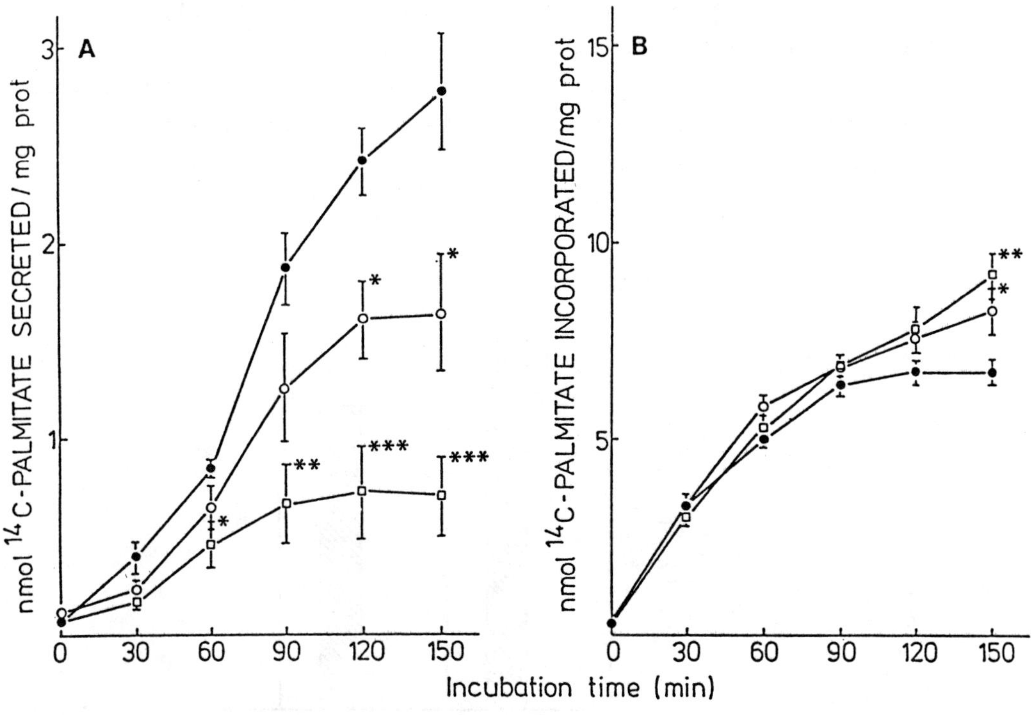

Fig.1.
Incorporation of ^{14}C-palmitate into extracellular (A) or intracellular (B) triglycerides in the absence (●) or in the presence of 10^{-4} M (○) and 10^{-3} M (□) tetracycline.
Data are expressed as means ± S.E.M. ($3 \leqslant n \leqslant 7$).

*, **, *** indicate a statistically significant difference between treated and control cells ($p \leqslant 0.05$, $p \leqslant 0.01$ and $p \leqslant 0.001$).

Our results however demonstrate that the effect of tetracycline on protein synthesis cannot explain its capacity to inhibit lipoprotein secretion. Indeed, 10^{-4}M tetracycline did not inhibit protein synthesis within the incubation time (150 min) whereas it significantly inhibited triglycerides release. Moreover, at 10^{-3}M tetracycline only inhibited protein synthesis by 29% eventhough it caused a 74% inhibition of lipoprotein secretion.

Since the amount of triglycerides which were not secreted when hepatocytes were exposed to tetracycline, was similar to the excess amount of triglycerides which were accumulated into the cells our results also prove that tetracycline does not modify the total esterification of palmitate.

In conclusion, we suggest that an impaired outward transport of triglycerides could be the major factor responsible for the development of the hepatic steatosis induced by tetracycline.

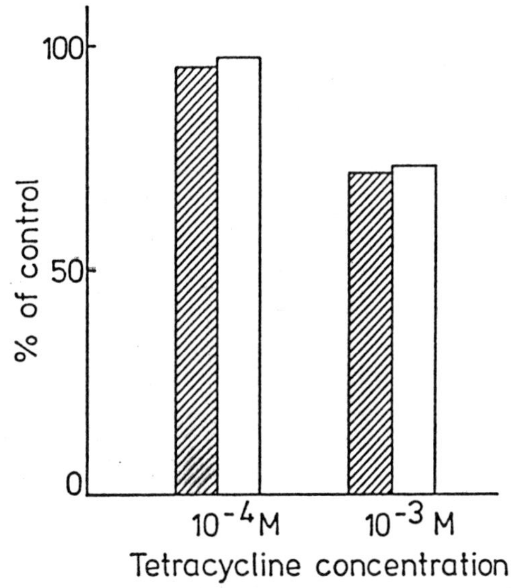

Fig.2.
Effect of tetracycline on protein metabolism
▨ intracellular incorporation of ^{14}C-leucine,
☐ extracellular ^{14}C-protein.

Data are expressed as % of control value after 150 min. of incubation.

To inquire further into the mechanism which causes that pathology, studies on the effects of tetracycline on the apoproteintriglyceri des association and on the mechanism of lipoprotein secretion mechanism are in progress.

2. Isolated hepatocytes as a model to test for the effects of cholestatic agents.

Cholestasis is a bile flow stagnation which may result from obstruction of extrahepatic bile ducts (extrahepatic cholestasis) intralobular obstruction or secretory failure by the hepatocyte (intrahepatic cholestasis). Bile formation is the final result of a number of transports across the baso-lateral membrane (mainly uptake processes), within the hepatocytes (intracellular transport) and across the canalicular membrane (12). Drug-induced cholestasis is mostly due to alterations at any step of those transport systems. Our study was aimed to develop the use of isolated hepatocytes as a reliable in vitro model for assessing the biochemical events related to cholestasis.

2.a Characteristics of taurocholate uptake.

The primary cellular event in bile formation appears to involve the uptake of bile acids at the baso lateral membrane of the hepatocyte, which plays an important role in the regulation of bile secretion.

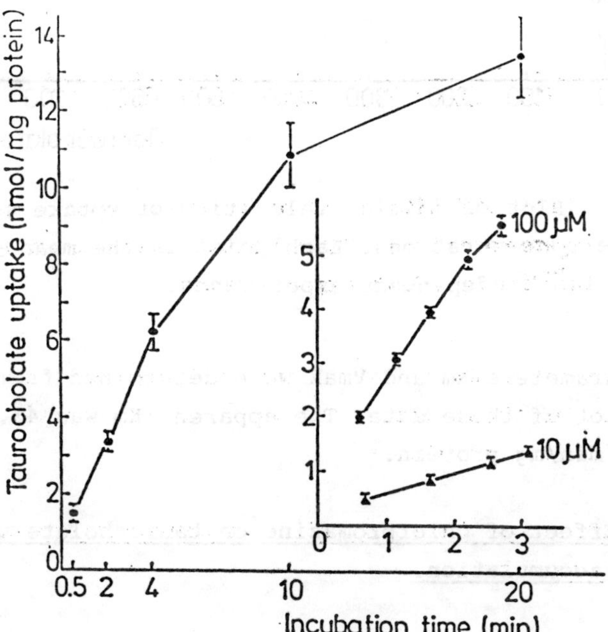

FIG. 3 Time course of Taurocholate uptake by isolated hepatocytes. Hepatocytes were suspended in the presence of 10μM (▲) or 100μM (●) of Taurocholate.

The time course of taurocholate uptake by isolated hepatocytes is shown in Fig.3. The uptake process was extremely rapid and it was linear for at least 2 min for the two concentrations of taurocholate tested (10 and 100 uM). Thereafter, it gradually decreased and reached a plateau which probably reflects an equilibrium between uptake and secretion of taurocholate.

The initial rate of taurocholate uptake, calculated from the difference between the intracellular amount of bile acid at 0.5 and 2 min was plotted against each taurocholate concentration (Fig.4).

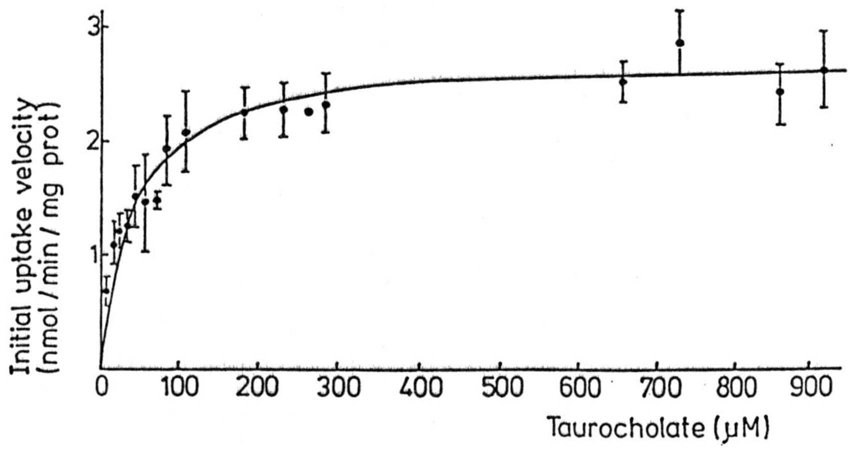

FIG. 4 Plot of initial velocities of uptake vs Taurocholate concentrations. Each point is the mean ± S.E.M. of three to four independant experiments.

The kinetic parameters Km and Vmax were determined from the Hanes-Woolf plot of these data. The apparent Km was 43.2 uM and Vmax was 2.83 nmol/min/mg protein.

2.b Effect of chlorpromazine on taurocholate uptake and accumulation.

To assess the biochemical events related to an impairment of bile acid dependent secretion, it is important to evaluate the effects of the cholestatic drug on both, the initial rate of taurocholate uptake (which reflects mainly the entry of taurocholate in the cell) and the steady-state level of accumulation of taurocholate

within the hepatocyte (which represents an equilibrium between the inward and the outward transport systems of taurocholate).
Therefore, we studied the effects of chlorpromazine on both the initial uptake velocity (measured between 0.5 and 2 min) and the accumulation of taurocholate in the hepatocytes.
Isolated hepatocytes were preincubated for 30 min in the presence of various concentrations of the drug, namely 2.5 10^{-5}, 5.10^{-5}, 7.5 10^{-5} and 10^{-4}M. Then, a mixture of ^{14}C-taurocholate and nonlabelled taurocholate was added to the culture medium at a final concentration of 100 uM.

Chlorpromazine reduced the initial rate of taurocholate uptake by the hepatocytes in a concentration dependent way (Table 1.).

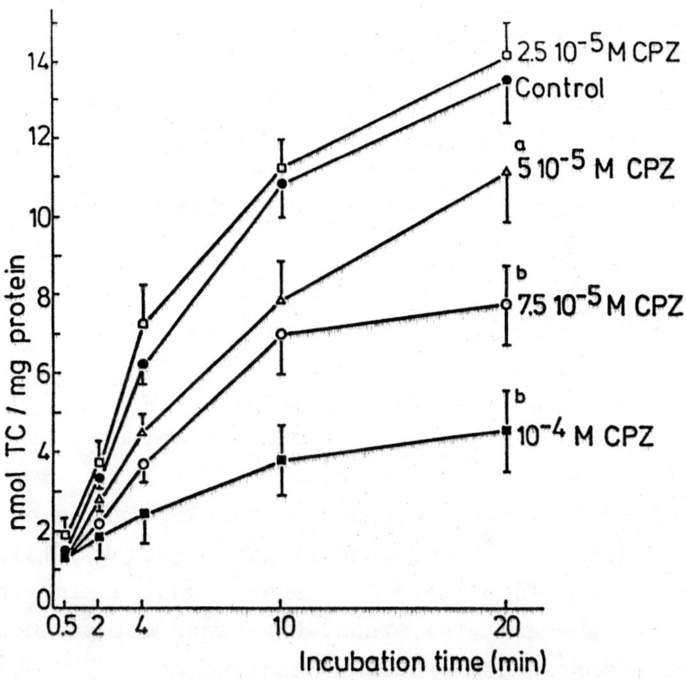

FIG. 5 Effect of Chlorpromazine on Taurocholate accumulation in hepatocytes. a and b indicate that the treatment is significantly different from the control treatment ($p \leq 0.05$ and $p \leq 0.01$ respectively).

That effect was statistically significant at 7.5 10^{-5}M (37.8% inhibition) and at 10^{-4}M (65.7% inhibition).

	Control	2.5 10^{-5} M CPZ	5.10^{-5} M CPZ	7.5 10^{-5} M CPZ	10^{-4} M CPZ
$\bar{X}$ ±S.E.M.(n) nmol/min/ mg protein	1.24 ±0.11 (13)	1.10 ±0.25 (5)	1.04 ±0.16 (7)	0.67 ±0.14* (7)	0.37 ±0.01** (3)
% inhibition	—	11.1	16.1	45.9	70.1

TABLE 1. Effect of Chlorpromazine on initial rate of Taurocholate uptake. * and ** indicate a statistically significant difference from the control value ($p \leq 0.05$ and $p \leq 0.01$ respectively).

Chlorpromazine also modified the accumulation of taurocholate within the hepatocyte (Fig.5). At 2.5 10^{-5}M it had no effect, whereas a concentration dependent inhibition which was statistically significant, was observed from 5 10^{-5}M upward. After 20 min of incubation, it reached 17%, 37.8% and 65.7% inhibition at 5 10^{-5}M, 7.5 10^{-5}M and 10^{-4}M respectively.

2.c Discussion.

Intrahepatic cholestasis associated with CPZ administration is largely known in man and in laboratory animals, but the mechanism of that pathogenesis remains unknown (13, 14).

CPZ is an amphiphatic cation tertiary amine detergent that is rapidly adsorbed into hepatocellular membranes (15). The drug may interdigitate within biliary lipids and cause a disturbance of the membrane architecture (16). Thus, the transport process across the hepatocyte membrane are probably impaired.

Our results demonstrate that chlorpromazine inhibited taurocholate transport into hepatocytes in a concentration dependent manner. Such effect was observed on both, the initial rate of taurocholate uptake, and the taurocholate intracellular accumulation. This inhibition may be one of the mechanisms of chlorpromazine-induced cholestasis, because bile acids are the principal component of bile and because they are the major determinants of bile secretion. Thus,

a decreased biliary acids uptake would be responsible for the bile flow reduction present
in cholestasis.

CONCLUSIONS.

That research supports the relevance of isolated hepatocytes as an in vitro model for studying the mechanisms of drug-induced hepatotoxicity, particularly steatosis and cholestasis.
An integrated analysis of the effects on the metabolic pathways and transport processes involved in secretion of either lipoprotein or bile, had permit to more occurently define the biochemical mechanisms of those pathologies. Isolated hepatocytes appeared thus as being helpful in analysing the biochemical mechanisms of those pathologies.

ACKNOWLEDGMENTS.

This research was supported by the John Hopkins Center for Alternatives to Animal Testing. (USA).

REFERENCES

1. Goethals F., Krack G., Deboyser D. and Roberfroid M.(1983) Effects of diethylmaleate on protein synthesis in isolated hepatocytes.
Toxicology, 26, 47-54

2. Goethals F., Krack G., Deboyser D., Vossen P., and Roberfroid M. (1984)
Critical biochemical functions of isolated hepatocytes as sensitive indicators of chemical toxicity.
Fund.Appl.Toxicol., 4, 441-450

3. Krack G., Gravier O., Roberfroid M. and Mercier M. (1980 a)
Subcellular fractionation of isolated rat hepatocytes. A comparison with liver homogenate.
Biochim.Biophys.Acta., 632, 619-629.

4. Krack G., Goethals F., Deboyser D., and Roberfroid M. (1980 b)
Interference of chemicals with glycogen metabolism in isolated hepatocytes.
Toxicology 18, 213-223.

5. Seglen P.O., and Solheim A.E. (1978)
Incorporation of radioactive aminoacids into protein in isolated hepatocytes.
Biochim.Biophys.Acta, 442, 391-404

6. Schwarz L.R., Burr R., Schwenk M., Pfaff E. and Greim H. (1975).
Uptake of taurocholic acid into isolated rat liver cells.
Eur.J.Biochem., 55, 617-623.

7. Lowry O.H., Rosenbrough N.J.,Farr A.L., and Randall R.J. (1951)
Protein measurement with Folin phenol reagent.
J.Biol.Chem., 193, 265-273.

8. Krack G., Vossen P., Deboyser D., Goethals F. and Roberfroid M. (1985)
An in vitro model for acute toxicity screening using hepatocytes freshly isolated from adult mammals.
in : Alternative methods in toxicology.
Vol.3 : In vitro Toxicology, 143-162.

9. Hansen C.H., pearson L.H., Schenker S. and Combes,B. (1986)
Impaired secretion of triglycerides by the liver; a cause of tetracycline-induced fatty liver.
Proc.Soc.Exp.Biol.med., 128, 143-146

10. Breen K.J., Schenker S. and Heimberg M. (1975)
Fatty liver induced by tetracycline in the rat.
Gastroenterology, 69,714-723

11. Hopf G., Bocker R. and Estler C.J. (1985)
Comparative effects of tetracycline and doxycycline on liver function of young adult and old mice.
Arch.Int.Pharmacodyn., 278, 157-168

12. Erlinger S. (1986)
Mechanisms of drug-induced cholestasis
In: hepatotoxicity of drugs (J.P.Fillastre, ed.)
INSERM 246

13. Ishak K.G., Irey N.S. (1972)
Hepatic injury associated with the phenothiazines
Arch.Pathol., 93, 283-304

14. Ros E., Small D.M., Carey M.C. (1979)
Effects of chlorpromazine hydrochloride on bile salt synthesis, bile formation and biliary secretion in the Rhesus monkey: a model for chlorpromazine-induced cholestasis.
Eur.J.Clin.Investg., 9, 29-41.

15. Sahab A.S., Dujovne C.A. (1979).
Chlorpromazine uptake by isolated rat heaptocytes.
Proc.Soc.Exp.Med., 161, 270-274.

16. Jung W., Gebhart R., Robenek H. (1985)
Primary culture of rat hepatocytes as a model system of canalicular development; biliary secretion and intrahepatic cholestasis. V. Disturbance of the cellular membrane and bile canalicular ultrastructure induced by chlorpromazine.
Virchows Arch.B., 49, 349-363

Poster A8

The Use of Freshly Isolated Hepatocytes for Studying Toxicity of Drug Mixtures

FABIENNE GOETHALS, PIERRE VOSSEN, MARIE-NOËLLE BLAUDE, and MARCEL ROBERFROID

Unit of Biochemical Toxicology and Cancerology
Université Catholique de Louvain
73 Av. Mounier
B-1200 Brussels, Belgium

Abstract

It is well recognized that the human population is exposed to many toxicants simultaneously rather than as individual toxicants. However, practically no effort has been devoted to adress the detection and characterization of toxicant interactions in toxicity testing.

The present study demonstrates the applicability of isolated hepatocytes for studying the toxicity of chemicals alone or in combination in an attempt to evaluate their potential interaction. The biochemical endpoints were LDH leakage, glycogen content, RNA and protein synthesis.

Two associations were studied : aflatoxin B1-oxytetracycline and retinol acetate-butylated hydroxytoluene butylated hydroxyanisole. Oxytetracycline which was shown in vivo to protect against the hepatotoxic effect of aflatoxin B1 did not modify the effects of aflatoxin in vitro on isolated rat hepatocytes. Indeed the inhibition of protein, RNA and glycogen synthesis induced by aflatoxin B1 (10^{-7} to 10^{-4} M) was not modified by the concommitant addition of oxytetracycline (10^{-4} or 10^{-3} M).

Since retinol acetate is often combined in pharmaceutical

preparations with antioxydants like BHT or BHA, the effects of those compounds either alone or in combination were investigated on isolated hepatocytes. We observed that the impairment of glycogen metabolism and protein synthesis was more pronounced when the hepatocytes were incubated in the presence of the 3 drugs in comparison with the effect obtained with each drug alone.
In conclusion, these studies support the feasibility of utilizing isolated hepatocytes as an in vitro model for investigating drug interactions. Biochemical processes like glycogen and protein synthesis appear as useful criteria to detect toxic joint actions.

INTRODUCTION

It is well recognized that the human population is exposed to mixture of toxicants rather than to pure compounds. Likewise, many pharmaceutical preparations contain more than one component. However, practically no effort has been devoted to address the detection and characterization of toxicant interactions in toxicity testing. According to the classical toxicological procedure, it is difficult to evaluate the toxicity of mixtures as compared to single products. In vitro test systems should be useful tools to identify toxicant joint actions.

The present report will illustrate the applicability of isolated hepatocytes for comparing the toxicity of chemicals alone or in combination, in an attempt to evaluate their potential interactions (additive, synergistic or antagonistic). Two mixtures were studied: aflatoxin B_1-oxytetracycline and retinol acetate-butylated hydroxytoluene-butylated hydroxyanisole.

MATERIALS AND METHODS

Materials

Oxytetracycline chlorhydrate was purchased from Certa Belgium, Aflatoxin B_1 from Aldrich, West-Germany. Retinol acetate, butylated hydroxytoluene (BHT), butylated hydroxyanisole (BHA) and bovine serum albumin were obtained from Sigma Chemical Co, USA. Glucagon was provided by Novo Industri (Copenhagen, Denmark). Collagenase (type I) was purchased from Worthington (Freehold, NJ, USA); Dulbecco's modified Eagle's Medium from Flow Laboratories (Irvine, Scotland). L-(U-^{14}C)-leucine (specific activity: 348 mCi/mmol), and (6-^{14}C)-orotic acid (specific activity: 61 mCi/mmol) were provided by Amersham International (Amersham, England).

Animals

Male Wistar rats (250-300 g) were purchased from Iffa Credo (Lyon, France) and maintained on commercial rodent chow and water *ad libitum*.

Isolation and incubation of hepatocytes

Hepatocytes were prepared by a two step perfusion technique (1). Briefly, rats were anesthetized with sodium pentobarbital (60 mg/kg, i.p.) and the liver flushed with calcium free media. Connective tissue was digested by a 15 min perfusion with collagenase (150 U/ml). Hepatocytes were dispersed, filtered, washed and incubated in suspension in a Dulbecco medium supplemented with 1.5% BSA at a concentration of 0.5 10^6 cells/ml. Incubation was performed at 37°C under an atmosphere of 95% O_2- 5% CO_2.
Aflatoxin B_1 was dissolved in DMSO, oxytetracycline in water. Retinol acetate, BHT and BHA were first dissolved in ethanol and then diluted twice with DMSO. Non treated hepatocytes were incubated in the presence of the solvant at the same concentration (always $<$ 1%).

Evaluation of cytotoxicity

Cell viability was evaluated by leakage of lactate dehydrogenase (LDH).

Control of metabolic competence of the hepatocytes was used as an index of cellular alteration (2). The intracellular glycogen content was measured as a function of the incubation time (3). Protein synthesis was estimated by incorporation of ^{14}C-leucine into $HClO_4$ precipitable proteins (4). RNA synthesis was assayed by the incorporation of ^{14}C-orotic acid into $HClO_4$ precipitable material (5). Protein content was determinated by the method of Lowry et al. (6) using bovine serum albumin as a standard.

Statistical analysis

Mean values ± S.E.M. given in figures and table were obtained from at least three separate experiments. The data were analyzed using Student's t test.

RESULTS

1. Interaction between aflatoxin B_1 and oxytetracycline

Aflatoxin B_1 is one of the most toxic and carcinogenic mycotoxin. Some in vivo investigations, with the rabbit and the goat, have shown that oxytetracycline protects against the hepatotoxic effect of chronic and acute aflatoxicosis (7,8). The present work was aimed at studying a possible interaction between these two chemicals using freshly isolated rat hepatocytes.

Hepatocytes were first incubated in the presence of each compound alone, and then the effects of their association were also evaluated. As sensitive criteria of cellular perturbations, LDH leakage, glycogen, protein and RNA synthesis were measured during the incubation time.

1.a. Biochemical effects of aflatoxin B_1

Even at the highest concentration tested (10^{-4}M), aflatoxin B_1 did not induce LDH leakage during the 3h of incubation.

Incorporation of ^{14}C-leucine into protein was significantly reduced after incubation of hepatocytes with

10^{-6}, 10^{-5} or 10^{-4}M aflatoxin B_1 for 90, 60 and 30 min respectively whereas 10^{-7}M and 10^{-8}M aflatoxin had no effect (Fig.1).

Aflatoxin B_1 also affected RNA synthesis in a concentration-dependent way. A significant decrease of ^{14}C-orotic acid incorporation into RNA was observed as early as 30 min of incubation for 10^{-7}M and 10^{-6}M aflatoxin B_1. 10^{-8}M aflatoxin did not impair that metabolic process (Fig.1).

Aflatoxin B_1 impaired glycogen synthesis from glucagon-treated (1.9 mg/kg) rat hepatocytes after 90 min of incubation, even inducing a glycogen breakdown at the highest concentrations (10^{-5}M and 10^{-4}M) (Fig.1). The glycogen increment from 0 to 90 min. in treated and untreated cells is 51.7 ± 2.8 ug equivalent glucose/mg prot.

1.b. Biochemical effects of oxytetracycline

Oxytetracycline did not affect LDH leakage, RNA synthesis and glycogen metabolism even at the highest concentration tested (10^{-3}M). The incorporation of ^{14}C-leucine into protein was slightly inhibited at this concentration, but 10^{-4}M oxytetracycline was without any effect (Fig.2).

1.c. Biochemical effects of the combination aflatoxin B_1 oxytetracycline

In order to detect a possible protective effect of oxytetracycline on the cytotoxicity induced by aflatoxin B_1, oxytetracycline was added to the incubation medium at the highest concentration without any effect on the evaluated criteria, i.e. 10^{-3}M for glycogen and RNA synthesis, and 10^{-4}M for protein synthesis.

The results presented in fig.2 show that there is no interaction between aflatoxin B_1 and oxytetracycline. Indeed, the association of the two chemicals produced the same effect on protein and RNA synthesis as the one observed for aflatoxin B_1 alone.

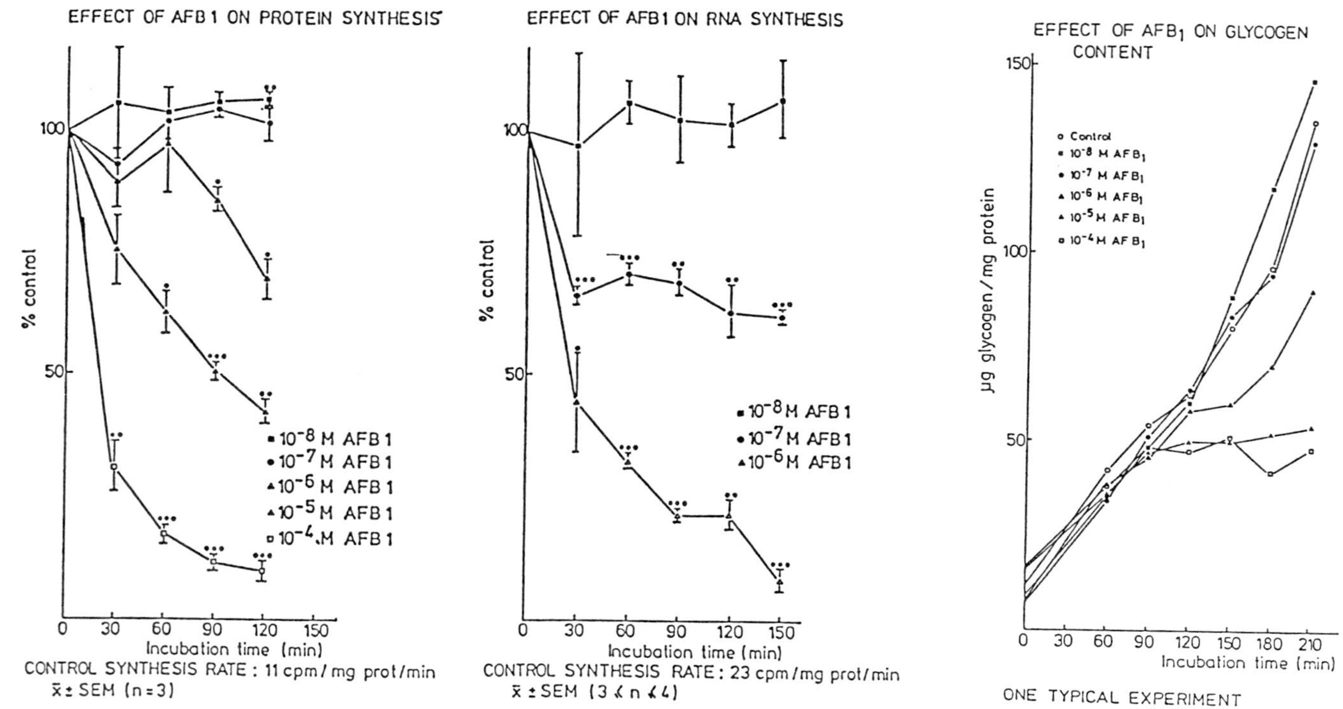

FIG.1 : EFFECTS OF AFLATOXIN B1 ON PROTEIN, RNA AND GLYCOGEN SYNTHESIS IN ISOLATED RAT HEPATOCYTES. *, ** and *** indicate a statistically significant difference from 100% ($p \leqslant 0.05$, $p \leqslant 0.01$ and $p \leqslant 0.001$ respectively).

TABLE 1

EFFECT OF OTC AND AFB1, ALONE OR IN COMBINATION, ON GLYCOGEN CONTENT IN RAT ISOLATED HEPATOCYTES FROM 90 TO 150 MINUTES.

CONDITIONS	GLYCOGEN INCREMENT g/mg prot[a]	n[b]
Control	49.5 ± 7.0	10
10^{-3}M OTC	49.1 ± 6.8	8
10^{-4}M AFB1	-2.0 ± 6.1[x]	9
10^{-3}M OTC + 10^{-4}M AFB1	27.8 ± 8.4[y]	9

a:Mean ± S.E.M.; x:$p \leq 0.001$ regarding to the control value; y:$p \leq 0.05$ regarding to AFB1-treated cells.
b:n:Number of independent experiments.

Aflatoxin B_1 reduced the increment of the glycogen level measured between 90 and 150 min.of incubation as compared to non-treated hepatocytes.

The glycogen increment in hepatocytes incubated in the presence of the mixture of drugs is not significantly different from that observed in untreated cells but it is significantly different from that observed in aflatoxin B1 treated cells. (Table 1).

1.d.Discussion.

The aim of this work was to investigate the possibility of an interaction between AFB_1 and OTC at a cellular level, in order to test the hypothesis put forward by Hatch and his collaborators (7,8), that OTC protects against AFB_1-induced necrosis. They postulated that OTC could interact directly with the toxic mechanisms of the mycotoxin.

Aflatoxin B_1 is known to inhibit RNA and protein synthesis. The

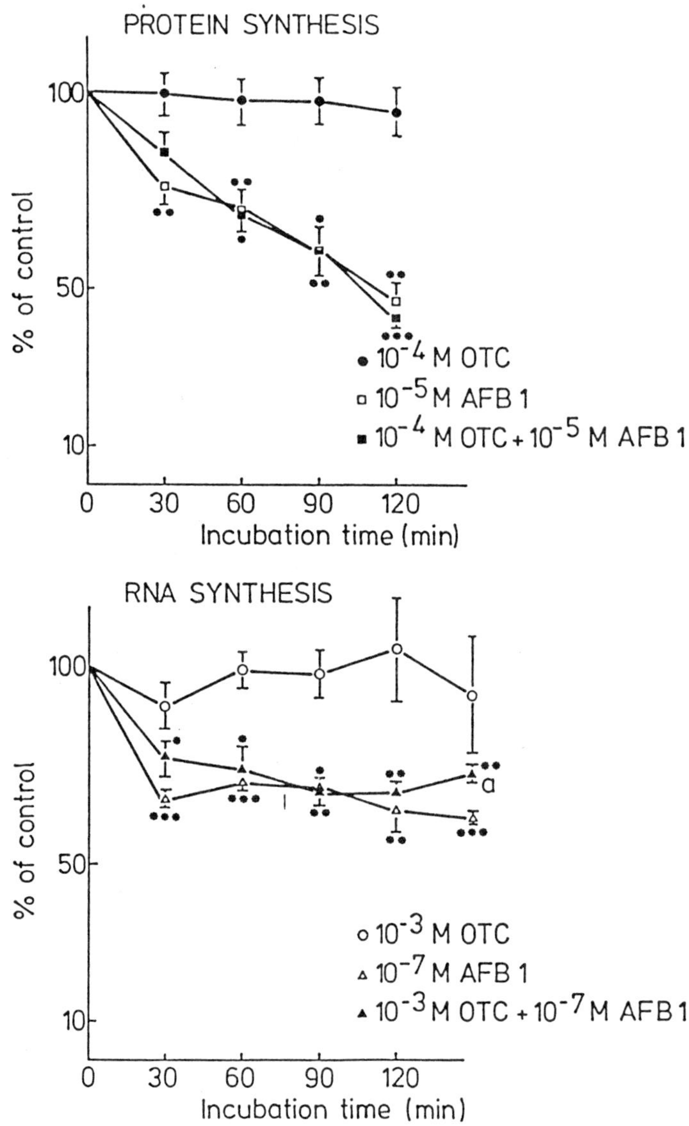

FIG.2 : EFFECTS OF AFLATOXIN B1 AND OXYTETRACYCLINE, ALONE OR IN COMBINATION, ON PROTEIN AND RNA SYNTHESIS IN RAT ISOLATED HEPATOCYTES.

x ± E.S.M. ($3 \leqslant n \leqslant 4$). *, ** and *** indicate a statistically significant difference from 100% ($p \leqslant 0.05$, $p \leqslant 0.01$ and $p \leqslant 0.001$ respectively). (a) indicates a statistically significant difference ($p \leqslant 0.05$) from the 10^{-7}M AFB1 value at the same incubation time.

effects were already observed in vivo in 1965 (9) and in vitro in 1966 (10) and they were further confirmed in vitro (11,12).

The mechanisms by which Aflatoxin B_1 exerts these inhibitions are complex. The inhibition of RNA synthesis seems to be dual. In 1977, Yu (13) presented evidences showing that the inhibition of RNA polymerase II would account for the inhibition of mRNA synthesis while impairment of DNA template function could be responsible for the inhibition of corresponding transfer and ribosomal RNA production.

The inhibition of protein synthesis is due, at least, to two mechanisms :inhibition of RNA synthesis (14) and direct impairment of translation (15,16,17).

In our study we confirm the inhibitory effect of AFB_1 on both RNA and protein synthesis (Fig.1).

In order to study the interaction between OTC and AFB_1 on these syntheses, the highest concentration of OTC which was without effect on the tested parameters was used. Nevertheless, we didn't observed any interaction between the two molecules neither on RNA nor on protein the two molecules on glycogen synthesis.

Concerning the evolution of glycogen content, the mechanism by which AFB_1 exerts its inhibition is not clearly understood. When AFB_1 and OTC are added simultaneously to the medium, an interaction is observed between the two molecules on glycogen synthesis.

Preliminary experiments conducted with a lower concentration of AFB_1 (10^{-5}M) seem to confirm these results.

2. Interaction between vitamin A and BHT/BHA

Retinol acetate (vitamin A) is often protected against oxidation by the addition of antioxydants such as butylated hydroxytoluene (BHT) and butylated hydroxyanisole (BHA). The hepatotoxicity of vitamin A is well known (18) and many reports have focussed on the biological effects of BHT and BHA (19).

Since those chemicals are often combined in pharmaceutical preparations, it was of interest to know if they do not mutually intensify their own effects. With the aim to search for such an interaction, LDH leakage, glycogen content and protein synthesis were monitored during the incubation of the isolated hepatocytes in the presence of mixtures of the 3 chemicals, i.e. retinol acetate, BHT and BHA combined according to their ratio (10/2.5/1) in a commercial preparation (20).

2.a. LDH leakage

Retinol acetate (10^{-3}M) induces an increase in LDH release which is statistically significant after 30 min of incubation. A similar rise in cellular lysis is observed if hepatocytes are incubated with the mixture BHT/BHA (2.5 10^{-4}M/ 10^{-4}M). When cells are incubated in the presence of the of the 3 chemicals at the same concentrations, the statistically significant increase in LDH leakage appears immediately (Fig.3)

A lower concentration of retinol acetate (10^{-4}M) either alone or in association with BHT/BHA (2.5 10^{-5}M/10^{-5}M) does not affect cell viability.

Due to its marked effect on LDH leakage at 10^{-3}M, a concentration which also produces an important impairment of cellular metabolic competence (data not shown), retinol acetate was tested for its effect on glycogen content and protein synthesis at lower concentrations (10^{-4}M and 5.10^{-5}M).

2.b. Glycogen metabolism and protein synthesis

At a concentration of 10^{-4}M, retinol acetate induces a loss of glycogen but no modification in protein synthesis. BHT/BHA (2.5 10^{-5}M/10^{-5}M) cause a decrease in the intracellular glycogen content but have no effect on protein synthesis. When the 3 drugs are added together to the culture medium at those concentrations, an increase of the effect on glycogen metabolism is observed and an inhibition of protein synthesis appears (Fig.4).

Retinol acetate, (5.10^{-5}M) and the mixture BHT/BHA, (1.25 10^{-5}M/5.10^{-6}M) have no significant effect on the biochemical parameters tested (Fig.4). However, when the 3 chemicals are added to the incubation medium, a significant

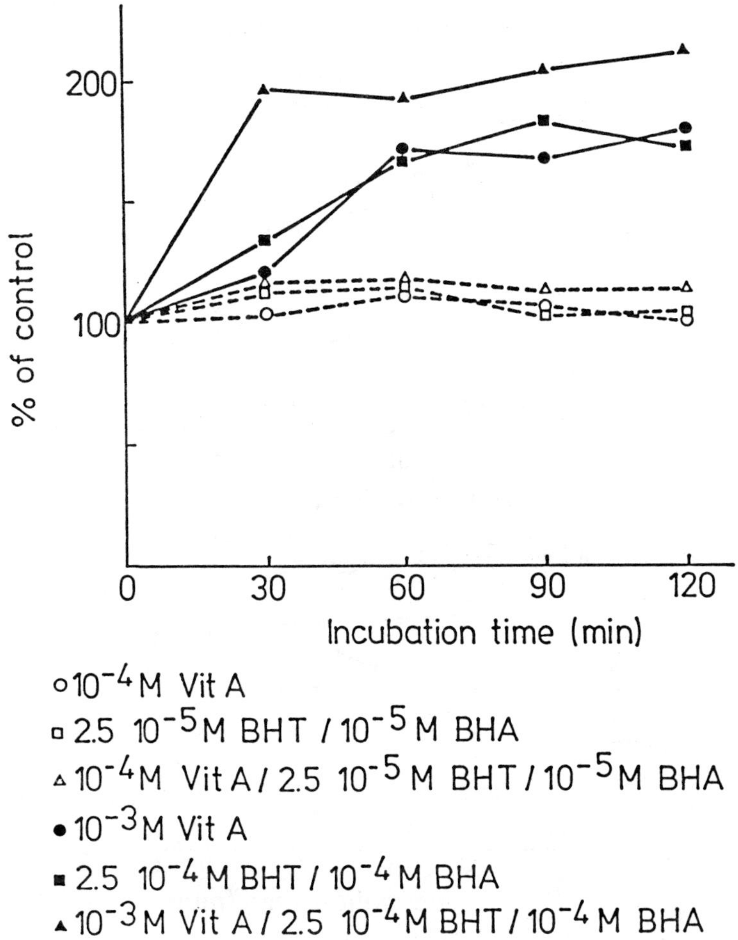

FIG.3 : EFFECT OF RETINOL ACETATE, BHT AND BHA, ALONE OR IN COMBINATION, ON LDH LEAKAGE FROM RAT ISOLATED HEPATOCYTES

decrease in both the glycogen content and the incorporation of ^{14}C-leucine into protein is observed as early as 30 min of incubation.

2.c Discussion

Retinol acetate is often associated with antioxidants like the mixture BHT/BHA. These substances have been widely

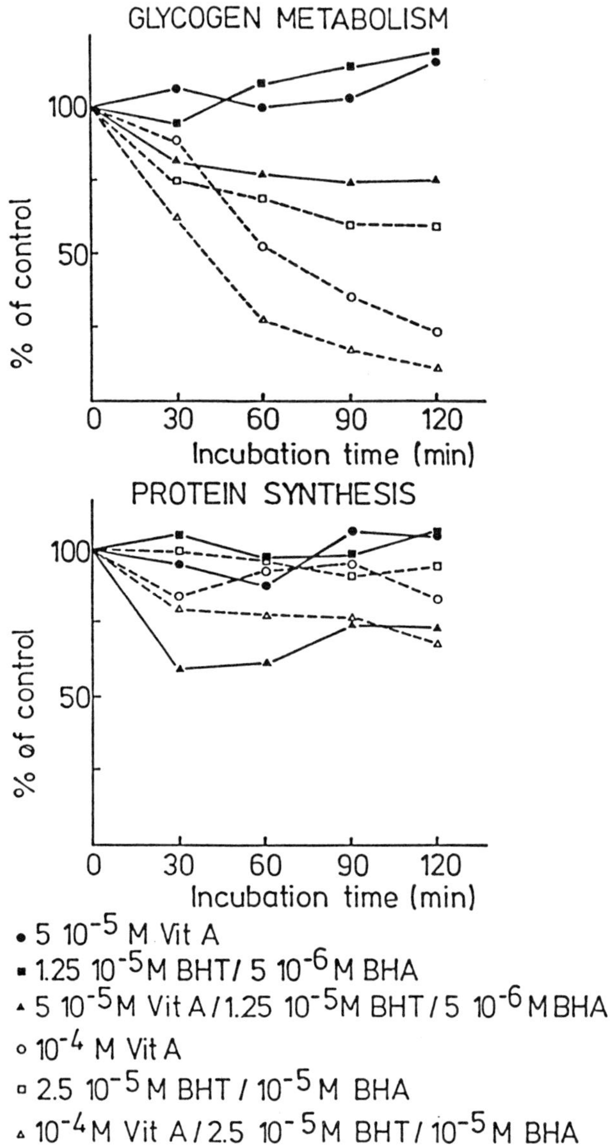

FIG.4 : EFFECTS OF RETINOL ACETATE, BHT AND BHA, ALONE OR IN COMBINATION, ON GLYCOGEN METABOLISM AND PROTEIN SYNTHESIS IN ISOLATED RAT HEPATOCYTES.

studied separately but their bio-toxicological effects remain partly controversial.

The liver is the major target of the vitamin A toxicity. The main pathology induced by hypervitaminosis A consists in perisinusoïdal fibrosis revealed by portal hypertension and leading in some cases to cirrhosis (21).
The effect of BHT on the liver is mainly described as a liver hypertrophy associated with a proliferation of smooth endoplasmic reticulum and an increase in the associated enzymatic activity. BHT also impairs protein synthesis as revealed by hemorrhages due to hypoprothrombinemia (for review:19).

Recently, McCormick and his collaborators (22,23) have demonstrated "in vivo" interactions between retinol acetate and BHT at the level of carcinogenic and hepatopathologic process. Their experiments showed that retinol acetate induces an hepatic fibrosis while BHT does not. However, when the two compounds are administred together, the incidence of fibrosis is much higher. From this, they conclude that BHT increases the retinol acetate induced toxicity.

From our results, it is not possible to confirm this hypothesis. As a matter of fact, as retinol acetate, at 5 10^{-5}M, has significant effect neither on glycogen metabolism nor on protein synthesis, it is not possible to conclude that the effects observed in a concommitant incubation with BHT/BHA - which are without any effect at this concentration - result from a potentiation of retinol acetate effects by BHT.

Whatever the exact nature of the interaction between retinol acetate and BHT is, their joint toxic actions may be of pharmaco-toxicological importance with regard to the use of vitamin A.

CONCLUSIONS

These studies support the feasibility of utilizing isolated hepatocytes as an in vitro model for investigating drug interactions. The effects of the different components either alone or in combination may be tested using cells prepared from the same animal. Biochemical processes such as glycogen and protein synthesis which are known to occur in our incubation conditions (2,3) are sensitive index of cellular alterations. Moreover, they appear as useful criteria to detect joint toxic actions.

Acknowledgements

This research was supported by the John Hopkins Center for Alternatives to Animal Testing (USA), Ana Laboratories (France) and Dr. Hens, president of the "Société Vétérinaire de Protection Animale (Belgium)". The "Union Belge pour l'Abolition de l'Experimentation sur l'Animal Vivant" is also gratefully acknowledged for providing a Bausch-Lomb spectrophotometer.

REFERENCES

1. KRACK, G., GRAVIER, O., ROBERFROID, M. and MERCIER, M. (1980 a). Subcellular fractionation of isolated rat hepatocyte. A comparison with liver homogenate. Biochim. Biophy. Acta, 632: 619-629.

2. GOETHALS, F., KRACK, G., DEBOYSER, D., VOSSEN, P. et ROBERFROID, M. (1984). Critical biochemical functions of isolated hepatocytes as sensitive indicators of chemical toxicity. Fund. Appl. Toxicol., 4: 441-450.

3. KRACK, G., GOETHALS, F., DEBOYSER, D. and ROBERFROID, M. (1980b). Interference of chemicals with glycogen metabolism in isolated hepatocytes. Toxicology, 18: 213-223.

4. SEGLEN, P.O. and SOLHEIM, A.E. (1978). Valine uptake and incorporation into protein in isolated rat hepatocytes. Eur. J. Biochem.85: 15-25.

5. POUNDS, J., MORRISON, D., WRIGHT, R., CASCIANO, D. and SHADDOCK, J. (1982). Effect of lead on calcium-mediated cell function in the isolated rat hepatocyte. Toxicol. Appl. Pharmacol., 63: 402-408.

6. LOWRY, O., ROSENBROUGH, N., FARR, L. and RANDALL, R. (1951). Protein measurement with the folin phenol reagent.
J. Biol. Chem., 183: 265-275.

7. CLARK, J. D., JAIN, A.V. and HATCH, R.C. (1982). Effect of various treatments on induced chronic aflatoxicosis in rabbits.
Am. J. Vet. Res., 43: 106-110

8. HATCH, R.C., CLARK, J.D., JAIN, A.V., MAHAFFEY, E.A. and WEISS, R. (1982). Effect of antibacterials, anabolic steroid and diethyldithiocarbamate on induced acute aflatoxicosis in goats.
Am. J. Vet. Res., 43: 639-643

9. LAFARGE, C., FRAYSINNET, C. and De RECONDO A.M. (1965) Inhibition par l'aflatoxine de la synthèse de RNA hépatique chez le rat.
Bull.Soc.Chim.Biol., 47: 1724-1725.

10. CLIFFORD, J.I. and REES, K.R. (1966). Aflatoxine : a site of action in the rat liver cell.
Nature, 209: 312-313.

11. McINTOSH, P.R., EVANS, I.M. and RABIN B.R. (1976) The effect of aflatoxin on the incorporation of RNA and protein precursors by isolated hepatocytes.
Br.J. Cancer,33: 440-449.

12. METCALFE, S.A. and NEAL, G.E. (1983).Some studies on the relationship between cytotoxicity of aflatoxin B_1 to rat hepatocytes and metabolism of the toxin.
Carcinogenesis, 4: 1013-1019 .

13. YU, F.L.(1977). Mechanisms of aflatoxin B_1 inhibition of rat hepatic nuclear RNA synthesis.
J.Biol.Chem. 252: 3245-3251.

14. PONG, R.S. and WOGAN, G.N. (1970). Time course and dose response characteristics of aflatoxin B_1 effects on rat liver RNA polymerase and ultrastructure. Cancer Res., 30: 294-304.

15. SARASIN, A. and MOULE, Y. (1975). Translational step inhibited in vivo by aflatoxin B_1 in rat liver polysomes. Europ.J.Biochem.,54: 329-340.

16. WHITE, J.S. and REES, K.R. (1980). The effect of aflatoxin B_1 on translation in cells in culture. Chem.Biol. Interactions.,32: 187-193.

17. LYMAN, B.A. DELVIN, T.M. and CH'IH J.J. (1986). Effect of aflatoxin B_1 on translation in isolated hepatocytes. Biochem.Phar.,34: 4184-4186.

18. JACQUES, E.A., BUSCHMANN, R.J. and LAYDEN, T.J. (1979). The histopathologic progression of vitamin A-induced hepatic injury. Gastroenterology, 76: 599.

19. BABICH, H. (1982). Butylated hydroxytoluene (BHT): a review. Environ. Res., 29: 1.

20. KRACK G., VOSSEN P., DEBOYSER D.,GOETHALS F. and ROBERFROID M. (1985). An in vitro model for acute Toxicity Screening using hepatocytes freshly isolated from adult mammals. In:Alternative methods in Toxicology, vol.3:In vitro Toxicology, 143-162.

21. GEUBEL, A.P., RAMIER, J. (1983). Hypervitaminose A: Physiopathologie et Toxicité Hépatique. Revue Médicale de Liège, 38: 679-684.

22. McCORMICK, D., MAY C., THOMAS, C. and DETRISAC, C. (1986). Anticarcinogenic and hepatotoxic interactions between retinyl acetate and butylated hydroxytoluene in rats.
Cancer Res., 46: 5264-5269.

23. McCORMICK D., MULTIN T., DETRISAC C. (1987). Potentiation of Vitamin A hepatotoxicity by Butylated Hydroxytoluene.
Toxicol.Appl.Pharmacol., 90: 1-9.

Poster A9

Comparative Hazard Assessment of Formaldehyde and Trioxane *In Vitro* Using Human Diploid Cell Strains

ROBERT A. KREIGER[1] and VINCENT F. GARRY[2]

[1]*Health Risk Assessment Section*
Minnesota Department of Health
Minneapolis, MN
[2]*Environmental Pathology Laboratory*
Department of Laboratory Medicine and Pathology
University of Minnesota
Minneapolis, MN

ABSTRACT

Formaldehyde toxicity was assessed at the cell and tissue level for long-term, low-dose exposure regimens. The experimental objective was to conduct a comparative hazard assessment in vitro for monomeric formaldehyde and trioxane. Trioxane is a possible process alternative for monomeric formaldehyde in resin manufacture and disinfection. Human diploid fibroblast strains were used as target cells. A skin cell strain (WS1) and a lung cell strain (WI-38) were both evaluated in these experiments. Indices of overt toxic effect included replication inhibition and cell death. Genotoxicity was evaluated by sister chromatid exchange (SCE) induction. Enhancement of virus infection in exposed cells was used as an index of sub-lethal damage. The results showed that monomeric formaldehyde was 6,000 to 13,000 times more toxic than trioxane, and that both test chemicals produced linear dose response patterns. Trioxane failed to induce SCE in either cell strain. SCE induction by formaldehyde monomer was directly proportional to toxic effects, and exhibited a linear dose response. Both toxicity and SCE induction by formaldehyde monomer operated over a very narrow dose range (0-3 ug/ml). Cells passaged at sub-lethal formaldehyde doses demonstrated cumulative SCE induction. Other findings indicated that virus infectivity and virulence were enhanced in cells exposed to formaldehyde or trioxane in vitro. The assay matrix demonstrated the capacity to measure the effects of main factors (cell strain, polymer form, exposure time) on indices of toxic response. The use of multiple toxicity indices permitted the measurement of strength and consistency of the cell and polymer effects within and between the various assay methods. Interaction of the main factors were shown to affect toxicity, SCE induction, and virus infection enhancement dose responses as much, or more than, single factor effects.

KEYWORDS: in vitro, formaldehyde, trioxane, SCE, virus enhancement

ABBREVIATIONS: HCHO, formaldehyde; SCE, sister chromatid exchange; PBS, phosphate buffered saline without calcium or magnesium; ug, microgram; FBS, fetal bovine serum; ED, effective dose; BrDU, 5-Bromo-2'-Deoxyuridine; DMEM, Dulbecco's Modified Eagle Medium; PFU, virus plaque forming unit; ppm, part per million by relative weights; ANOVA, analysis of variance.

INTRODUCTION

In vitro bioassay methods have been used for a number of specific applications in toxicology and human health risk assessments. One of the most useful and primitive levels of bioassay application is hazard assessment. This step identifies the biological effects resulting from exposure to a test chemical, describes comparative sensitivity for potential target tissues, and can provide essential data for resolving toxic mechanisms. A comparative in vitro hazard assessment for trioxane and formaldehyde was conducted to identify the pattern of toxic effects induced by these compounds. These chemicals were tested because they are potential process alternatives in resin manufacture and disinfection. Human lung and skin cells were selected as indicators of toxic effects for their relevance to inhalation and dermal exposure routes. Long-term, low-dose exposure regimens were applied to mimic potential human environmental and occupational exposures.

MATERIALS AND METHODS

Experimental Design

A correlative mathematical model was selected to describe the relationship between formaldehyde polymer type, cell strain, and dose responses. A diagram of the testing matrix is shown in Figure 1.

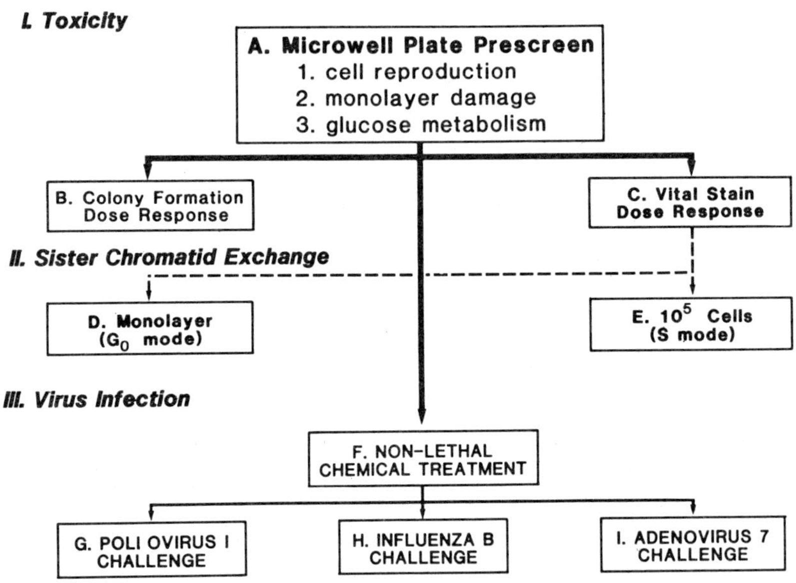

Figure 1. In vitro Toxicity Testing Schematic. Three levels of toxicity tests are shown in their hierarchical arrangement. Level I includes all cytotoxicity assays, Level II consists of genotoxicity assay variations, and Level III assesses sub-lethal damage as increased susceptibility to viral infection. The testing sequence begins at the microwell prescreen assay (A). Range-finding results from (A) are used to derive the doses for the more definitive assays of colony formation inhibition (B), vital stain toxicity (C), and chemical exposures preceeding virus challenge (F). Vital stain toxicity assay results (C) are used to set the doses in the SCE induction assays (D & E) in Level II.

Using this configuration of assays enhanced the ability to measure factor effects like cell strain and polymer type within and between different levels of the testing matrix. In this way, the strenth and consistency of factor effects could be evaluated and quantified.

Chemicals

The different attributes of the test chemicals are presented in Figure 2. Trioxane stocks were obtained as crystalline solids (Aldrich). Formaldehyde monomer was supplied as a 10% aqueous buffered solution not containing methanol (Mallinckrodt). Fresh stock solutions of each test compound were prepared immediately before use in cell culture medium plus 10% FBS. Ham's F-12 medium, Dulbecco's Modified Eagle Medium, PBS, colcemid (10 ug/ml) and trypsin solution (0.25%) were obtained from GIBCO laboratories. Fetal bovine serum was supplied by Hyclone Laboratories. DEAE dextran, crystal violet, Giemsa stain, and guinea pig red blood cells were obtained from the Sigma Chemical Company.

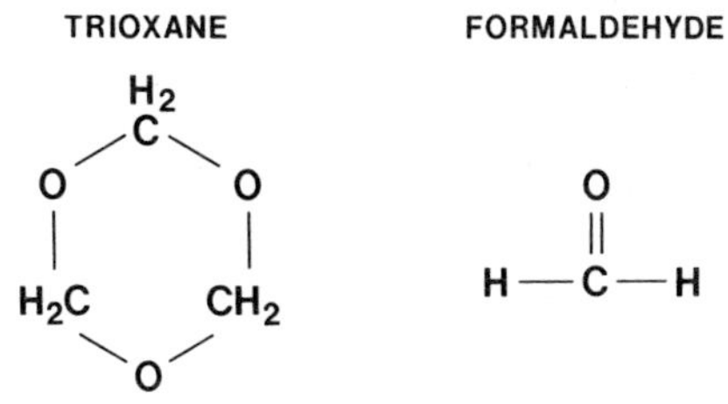

	TRIOXANE	FORMALDEHYDE
STRUCTURE	cyclic trimer (3n)	monomer
MW	90	30
BP	115°C	−20°C
MP	63°C	−92°C
SOLUBILITY	water, alcohol, ether	water
STABILITY	high	low
USES	solid fuel, waxes metal preservative petroleum additive acetyl resin disinfectant	urea and melamine resin fertilizer, dyes, reducing agent petroleum additive, textiles disinfectant drugs, cosmetics, dental work
MUTAGENICITY	No (AMES Test)	Yes
CARCINOGENICITY	unknown	animal carcinogen suspect human carcinogen

Figure 2. Test Chemical Attributes. Trioxane and formaldehyde properties are compared and contrasted. In the listing of physical parameters, MW is molecular weight, MP is melting point, and BP is boiling point.

Cells

Human diploid lung (WI-38) and skin fibroblast cultures were obtained from the American Type Culture Collection. Both strains were originally isolated from female embryonic tissue at the first trimester of gestation (1,2). Both strains were routinely cultured in DMEM plus 10% FBS. Normal chromosome number and doubling times were verified before using these target cell strains. Mycoplasma screening was periodically conducted for culture method quality control purposes (3). Working lots of each cell strain were mass cultured, sealed in ampules, and stored in liquid nitrogen using standard methods (4).

Microwell Plate Assay Methods

This prescreening method was based upon procedures developed for drug testing using HeLa cells (5,6,7). Modifications included using diploid human cells instead of HeLa cells, and measuring the additional toxicity indices of cell replication inhibition, monolayer damage and morphological cell changes, in addition to inhibition of glucose metabolism. Cultures of test cell strains were initiated by seeding 96 well culture plates with 1,000 cells per well. Test chemical dilutions prepared in DMEM plus 10% FBS were added to the plates 24 hours after seeding to assess effects on replication. Sterile paraffin oil (0.1 ml) was added to each well following chemical addition. Plates were then sealed with adhesive film and incubated for seven days at 37° C. Monolayer damage was assessed using the same basic method, but cells were incubated to reach confluency in the assay plates before chemical addition. Glucose metabolism was scored on the basis of color change in the medium. Yellow-orange color of the microwell medium was scored (+), indicating acid production from glucose. If the medium was pink-purple, glucose metabolism was scored (-). Replication, monolayer integrity, and cell morphology were scored as normal (+) or abnormal (-) after fixation and staining of the microwell plates. Fourty replicate wells were scored for each combination of cell strain, polymer type, and dose. Results were processed to yield probabilities for replication inhibition, monolayer damage, morphological change, and metabolic inhibition associated with the applied test chemical dose.

Colony Formation Methods

This index of toxic response measured the inhibition of cell replication resulting from test chemical exposure. Replication inhibition test methods have been adequately described by other investigators (8). For these experiments, 400 cells were plated in T-25 culture flasks, using Ham's F-12M medium. After 24 hours, test chemical aliquots prepared in culture medium were added to the flasks. Medium containing the test doses was removed after a 24 hour exposure. The cells were then washed with fresh medium, and a 5 ml volume of medium plus 10% FBS was added to each flask. These cultures were then incubated for 11 days to allow colony formation. Both cell strains were evaluated, as were both formaldehyde polymer types. Colonies were scored by decanting the medium, followed by fixation in methanol, and staining with crystal violet (0.5 % in water). Five replicate flasks were produced for each combination of cell strain, polymer type, and dose. Raw counts were tabulated using the SPSS statistical package (9), and dose response plots were generated. Linear regression was conducted by dividing raw colony counts by control mean counts, and graphing the results against dose. Residual analysis and analysis of variance were used to confirm the linearity of the assay results. Slopes of the dose response relationship were obtained for each combination of cell strain and formaldehyde polymer type.

Viable Count Methods

Culture flasks were seeded at 100,000 cells in DMEM plus 10% FBS, and incubated for 24 hours. A medium change was then conducted, including the addition of test chemical aliquots prepared in DMEM plus FBS. After a 24 hour exposure period, cells were harvested and assessed for viability by trypan blue dye exclusion methods (10). Hemocytometer counts were determined for live, dead, and total cells per sample. Five replicate flasks were counted for each combination of test conditions. Raw viable cell counts were transformed to survival probabilities by dividing them by unexposed control viable cell count means. Regression analysis methods for the viable count results also used SPSS statistical procedures.

Sister Chromatid Exchange Methods

The SCE induction test protocol was developed from a number of existing methods (11,12,13,14). Test flasks (T-75) were seeded with 10 ml of inoculum containing 10,000 cells/ml. SCE induction was tested in replicating cells, and in cell monolayers. In the replicating test mode, dilutions of formaldehyde or trioxane were added to the culture flasks with a fresh medium change 24 hours after the flasks were seeded. The medium containing the test doses was removed after 24 hours of exposure, flasks were washed with medium, and a fresh 10 ml volume of DMEM plus 10% FBS was added. The monolayer tests were conducted using similar methods, except the cells were cultured to confluency before adding test chemical doses. A third exposure mode was tested by culturing cells for 25 population doublings in sub-lethal doses of formaldehyde or trioxane. The final medium change contained 3 ug/ml BrDU. This addition was conducted in the dark, using photographic safe lights. Flasks were then foil wrapped, and incubated an additional 48 hours before harvesting. Colcemid solution was added to each flask after 44 hours, to produce a final concentration of 0.05 ug/ml of culture medium. Cell harvesting, slide preparation, and fixation of chromosomes followed existing procedures (14). SCEs were scored following the March of Dimes protocol (15). Results from the vital stain toxicity assay were used to calibrate the test chemical exposures. Effective doses (ED) representing lethality percentages were used to standardize trioxane and formaldehyde doses applied to the different cell strains. By equating the toxicity for each combination of cell strain and polymer, the SCE response was divorced from the confounding effects of differential toxicity. This means of setting dose levels produced an empirical index of genotoxicity that was more useful than doses expressed as molar concentrations or parts per million in culture medium.

Virus Infection Methods

Stock preparations of adenovirus 7, influenzavirus B, and poliovirus I were produced from pathological strains isolated by the Minnesota Department of Health. Virus isolates were cultured in primary monkey kidney cells, and identified by specific antibody neutralization tests. Plaque formation served as the endpoint for the selected viruses, with adenovirus and poliovirus producing zones of cell lysis. Influenza plaques were detected using hemadsorption, because red blood cells adhere to the infected cell membranes. Methods for conducting plaque forming unit assays have been described in a number of reviews (16,17). Cells were exposed to the test chemicals using two different protocols. In the acute exposure mode, cultures were incubated with the test dose for 24 hours. The concentrations used for acute exposure were 5 ug/ml for HCHO and 11,000 ug/ml for trioxane. The second exposure mode cloned cells for 25 population doublings in 1 ug/ml HCHO or 1000 ug/ml of trioxane. The dosages were determined by results from the microwell plate assay, using the highest doses not resulting in metabolic impairment. The dose was removed from the cultures, and a washing step removed residual chemical dose and FBS before virus inoculation of the exposed cultures. A small volume of virus inoculum (0.5 ml) in medium was then added to the washed monolayers to promote infection. The residual inoculum was then removed, the cultures overlaid with a DMEM - DEAE dextran agar medium, and incubated until plaques formed. Serial dilutions for each virus were assessed for each combination of cell strain, polymer type, and exposure mode. Adenovirus and poliovirus plaques were counted by gently decanting the agar overlay, fixing the cells in methanol, and staining the cells with crystal violet. Plaques were visualized as clear zones contrasting with the intact dark purple stained monolayer. Influenza plaques were developed by decanting the overlay, washing with PBS, and adding 0.4% guinea pig red blood cells at 4° C for 3 hours. Plaques were counted after 3 subsequent PBS washes using a phase microscope, appearing as zones of adherent red blood cells on the culture monolayers. Raw PFU counts were transformed to percentage of controls to allow comparison between cell strains and virus types, since the absolute PFU for any dilution was dependent upon cell strain, virus type, and virus dilution. This procedure also normalized the assay results, allowing analysis of variance (ANOVA) for the different experiment parameters. In addition, raw PFU counts were used in some instances to derive contrasts between control conditions and particular treatments of interest, but could not be used to compare results between cell strains or virus types.

RESULTS

Microwell Plate Results

A summary of the data collected for the microwell plate assay component of the test matrix is shown in Table 1. The results are expressed as dose ranges due to the variance inherent in binomial response assays.

Table 1

Microwell Plate Toxicity Assay Results For WI-38 and WS1 Cells Exposed To Formaldehyde or Trioxane

A. Mode 1 (Replicating Cell Damage)

CELL STRAIN	EFFECT*	HCHO DOSE RANGE (ug/ml)	TRIOXANE DOSE RANGE (ug/ml)
	NE	0 - 0.5	0 - 5,000
WI-38	MC	1.0 - 2.5	10,000 - 17,000
	MI	1.5 - 2.0	7,500 - 19,000
	CD	2.5 - 4.5	10,000 - 30,000
	NE	0 - 1.0	0 - 5,000
WS1	MC	2.0 - 5.0	7,000 - 23,000
	MI	3.0 - 8.0	7,000 - 30,000
	CD	4.0 - 8.0	9,000 - 30,000

A. Mode 2 (Monolayer Damage)

CELL STRAIN	EFFECT*	HCHO DOSE RANGE (ug/ml)	TRIOXANE DOSE RANGE (ug/ml)
	NE	0 - 2.0	0 - 7,500
WI-38	MI	3.0 - 6.0	9,000 - 40,000
	CD	5.0 - 7.0	15,000 - 40,000
	NE	0 - 3.0	0 - 11,000
WS1	MI	4.0 - 15.0	13,000 - 30,000
	CD	8.0 - 15.0	25,000 - 40,000

*EFFECT
NE = no effect
MC = morphological change
MI = glucose metabolic inhibition
CD = cell death

Results from these range-finding experiments demonstrated that trioxane was about 10,000 times less toxic than formaldehyde monomer, on a ppm basis. In addition, a differential response in the two target cell strains was indicated. WS1 cells seemed to tolerate higher doses of formaldehyde and trioxane than WI-38 cells. It also appeared that cell monolayers were more resistant to the toxic effects induced by the test chemicals than the replicating cell cultures. Test dose ranges for the colony formation and vital stain assays were derived from these test results. The test chemical doses to be used in the virus enhancement tier of the test matrix were also identified. Optimal doses allowing normal metabolism were selected, since virus reproduction depends on intact cell metabolic processes. A formaldehyde dose of 5 ug/ml and a trioxane dose of 11,000 ug/ml were chosen for 24 hour exposures preceding virus challenge. In addition, long-term doses applied for 25 population doublings were identified for trioxane (1,000 ug/ml) and formaldehyde (1 ug/ml).

Colony Formation and Vital Stain Results

Results from both the vital stain and colony formation assay methods produced plots of survival percentages vs. dose. Assessment of the regression data indicated that an unweighted least-squares linear regression model best described the relationship of dose and response, for both polymer types, and both cell strains. Slopes of the regression lines were used as a basis for comparison of toxic potency, since they describe the rate of change in survival depending upon dose. Results from the Colony Formation and Vital Stain assays conducted on replicating cultures are presented in Table 2.

Table 2

Cytotoxicity Results For WI-38 and WS1 Cells Exposed To Formaldehyde and Trioxane

A. Colony Formation - replication inhibition (24 hr exposure)

	slope	SE	m
1. WS1 Cells			
HCHO	-29.1	2.1	7,275
Trioxane	- 0.004	0.001	
2. WI-38 Cells			
HCHO	-50.3	3.8	12,575
Trioxane	- 0.004	0.0002	

B. Vital Stain - cytotoxicity (24 hr exposure)

	slope	SE	m
1. WS1 Cells			
HCHO	-18.7	1.5	4,665
Trioxane	- 0.004	0.0003	
2. WI-38 Cells			
HCHO	- 8.52	0.8	2,840
Trioxane	- 0.003	0.002	

Slope ratios have been used as a means of comparing the potencies of two compounds, provided the dose response lines converge at the Y-intercept (18). The slope numbers in Table 2 show the loss of viability percentage attributed to a unit dose of 1 ug/ml. The results show that formaldehyde is a far more potent cell toxicant than trioxane.

It is also evident that the relative potency of these compounds is different for WS1 cells compared to WI-38 cells. The data also demonstrate that vital stain assay results produce different results from replication inhibition assays. In addition, Tukey's test for non-additivity revealed that cell strain, polymer type, and dose exhibit strong interactions, over and above the additive effects attributed to each of these parameters singly (p=.05). These findings seem to show that even fairly simple in vitro bioassays can exhibit complexities related to the biological attributes of the target cells, and the particular chemicals being tested. Additional vital stain tests on cell monolayers were used in conjunction with results from the replicating cell cultures to set doses for the SCE induction assays. It was necessary to standardize SCE response to toxic effective dose (ED) to avoid confounding the SCE results with differential toxic effects caused by cell strain-polymer type interactions. A summary of the ED values is included in Figure 3.

Sister Chromatid Exchange Results

SCE induction for the test chemicals was evaluated in both replicating cultures and cell monolayers. The mean SCE count for unexposed cells ranged from 7 to 8 SCEs per cell. The control counts did not vary significantly with cell strain (p=.05). The most important finding was the inability of trioxane to induce SCE in either cell strain, in monolayers or replicating cultures. The SCE per cell remained unchanged from control values, even at trioxane doses producing 80% cell death. Conversely, formaldehyde was shown to induce SCE in both cell strains. Experiments using complete monolayers as target cultures produced positive SCE induction results. At higher doses (ED60-ED80), surviving cells exhibited significantly higher SCE means than untreated cultures (p=.05). The means for monolayer SCE at ED60 averaged 10.9 SCE per cell, and 15.4 SCE per cell at ED80. For cells exposed to 1 ug/ml of formaldehyde for long exposures (25 population doublings), only WI-38 demonstrated an SCE level elevated above controls (10.4 SCE/cell). For replicating cell cultures, SCE induction by formaldehyde was shown to be directly proportional to toxicity, following a linear response pattern. Trioxane did not induce SCE above the background counts. Slope estimates of SCE induction by formaldehyde indicated that WS1 cells accumulated SCE at about twice the rate as WI-38 cells. Graphs of the replicating cell results are shown in Figure 3, and the regression statisitics are also supplied.

A more detailed analysis of the SCE response is obtained from analysis of variance (ANOVA) applied to the SCE results. The main factors influencing SCE induction were identified as cell strain, polymer type, applied dose, and culture state (replicating or monolayer). In addition, the effects of factor interactions on SCE induction were also assessed and quantified. Interactions can be defined as the joint influence of the main factors on SCE induction over and above their separate effects. Of the single main factor effects, only cell strain was not significant (p=.13) with respect to effect on SCE induction. However, cell-polymer interaction was significant (p=.001), and even some 3-way interactions had significant effects on SCE induction, including cell-polymer-dose and polymer-state-dose. A model explaining SCE induction as a product of the main factors and their interactions accounted for 94% of the variance in SCE response, indicating a valid experimental method for describing SCE induction by formaldehyde in vitro. A summary of this data is shown in Table 3. Multiple classification analysis of the data indicated that cell strain differences accounted for only 6% of the SCE response. Cell state was responsible for 23% of the SCE response, and polymer type differences produced 49% of the SCE response variances. About 30% of the SCE response was attributed to factor interactions, demonstrating the importance of factor interactions in dose response observations.

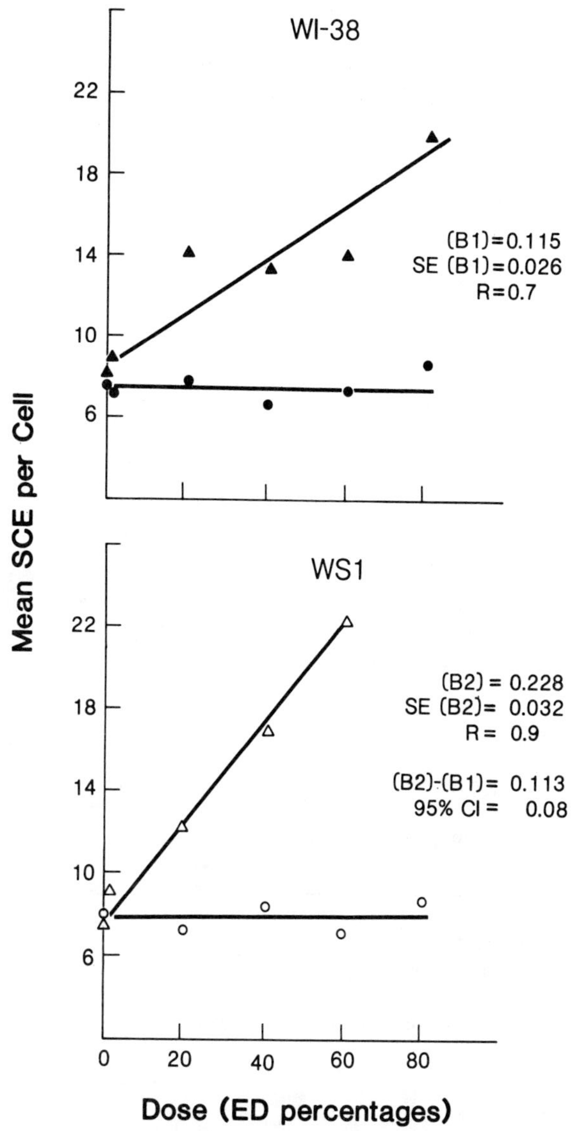

Figure 3. SCE Response in WI-38 and WS1 Cells Exposed to Formaldehyde or Trioxane As Replicating Cultures. Circles represent trioxane data points, triangles represent formaldehyde data points, and B represents the slope of regression lines. The slopes of WS1 and WI-38 SCE induction response demonstrate higher rates of SCE induction in WS1 cells. ED is the effective dose for a set toxicity percentage.

(ED) Values As ug/ml Doses

	WI-38 Cells				WS1 Cells			
(ED)	20	40	60	80	20	40	60	80
Formaldehyde	1.29	1.58	1.87	2.16	1.32	1.64	1.96	2.28
Trioxane	1300	2600	3900	5200	1200	2400	3600	4800

Table 3

Analysis Of Variance For SCE Results For Cells Exposed to Formaldehyde or Trioxane

Source of Variation	Sum of Squares	Degrees of Freedom	Mean Square	F	p
MAIN EFFECTS	1145.8	8	143.2	41.6	0.001
cell	8.8	1	8.8	2.5	0.133
polymer	559.1	1	559.1	162.5	0.001
state	114.9	1	114.9	33.4	0.001
dose	408.1	5	81.6	23.7	0.001
2-WAY INTERACTIONS	706.6	18	39.3	11.4	0.001
polymer cell	29.5	1	29.5	8.6	0.004
polymer state	71.8	1	71.8	20.9	0.001
polymer dose	324.8	5	65.0	18.9	0.001
cell state	0.7	1	0.7	0.2	0.646
cell dose	37.6	5	7.5	2.2	0.060
state dose	65.1	5	13.0	3.8	0.003
3-WAY INTERACTIONS	134.1	12	11.2	3.2	0.001
polymer cell state	0.5	1	0.5	0.2	0.697
polymer cell dose	52.7	4	13.2	3.8	0.006
polymer state dose	35.5	4	8.9	2.6	0.041
cell state dose	6.1	3	2.0	0.6	0.625
4-WAY INTERACTIONS	0.1	1	0.2	0.1	0.861
EXPLAINED	1906.6	39	50.9	14.8	0.001
RESIDUAL	413.6	120	3.4		
TOTAL	2399.6	159	15.1		

cell = cell strain effect
state = replicating culture or monolayer
dose = ED toxicity effect
polymer = polymer type effect independent of toxicity

Virus Infection Results

Unadjusted mean PFU counts for test conditions of interest were contrasted with control means to directly evaluate factor effects of interest. Results of these comparisons are presented in Table 4. The data demonstrate that WI-38 cells produced neither enhancement nor inhibition of polio or adenovirus infectivity resulting from previous exposure to formaldehyde or trioxane. Nor did 24 hour exposure to test chemicals alter responses to influenza virus challenge. However, WI-38 cells passaged in low doses of test chemicals did show significant enhancement of influenza infectivity (p=.05). WS1 cells produced a very different response pattern. Chronic low-dose formaldehyde exposure augmented poliovirus plaque formation. Also, test chemical exposure was very effective in producing adenovirus plaque formation enhancement. Lastly, influenza infectivity was greatly enhanced in WS1 cells exposed to trioxane over long culture periods, but no effect was seen with formaldehyde, or with short-term exposures to either test chemical.

Table 4

Contrasts Of Mean PFU Counts For Cells Exposed to Formaldehyde Or Trioxane Before Virus Challenge

Virus	Chemical	Dose Mode	PFU Contrast In WI-38 Cells	PFU Contrast In WS1 Cells
Polio I	HCHO	A	- 1.3	4.3
Polio I	HCHO	C	1.3	11.3*
Polio I	Trioxane	A	14.7	- 3.0
Polio I	Trioxane	C	- 8.4	- 8.0
Adeno 7	HCHO	A	15.7	28.0*
Adeno 7	HCHO	C	-60.4	24.0*
Adeno 7	Trioxane	A	3.3	- 7.3
Adeno 7	Trioxane	C	-22.0	25.0*
Flu B	HCHO	A	2.3	1.3
Flu B	HCHO	C	38.3*	- 1.3
Flu B	Trioxane	A	- 4.6	3.8
Flu B	Trioxane	C	43.0*	646.0*

A = 24 hour chemical dose before virus challenge
C = chronic chemical dose for 25 population doublings
* = contrast significant at p = .05
PFU = virus plaque forming unit
contrast = mean test PFU - mean control PFU from cells not exposed to test chemicals before virus challenge

Further data processing converting raw PFU counts to percentages of the concomitant control PFU values normalized the response variance, allowing ANOVA evaluation of cell strain, virus type, polymer type, and exposure time effects on PFU response. ANOVA tabulations for the virus enhancement experiments are shown in Table 5. The results showed that cell strain, virus type, polymer type and dose mode all significantly influence PFU (p =.001). The 2-way, 3-way, and 4-way factor interactions produced significant effects on PFU results as well, at times exceeding the main effects in their magnitude of influence on the PFU response. Analysis of the last portion of the ANOVA table reveals that the interactive factorial model fits the observed data very well, with 99% of the PFU response accounted for by the factor effects, and their interactions. Multiple classification analysis of the PFU results indicated that influenza virus was enhanced most by exposing the cells to the test chemicals, and that long exposure to low doses of test chemical enhanced virus infectivity more than short exposures at higher concentrations. WS1 cells were also identified as more susceptible to virus infection following exposure to the test chemicals than WI-38 cells. Other results not listed in Table 4 relate to induced changes in plaque size. Only cells exposed to the test chemicals for 25 population doublings were affected. Exposure to trioxane for 25 population doublings resulted in poliovirus plaques almost four times as large as those produced in control cultures, based upon surface area. Formaldehyde chronic exposure produced plaques approximately twice as large as control monolayers. No similar effects were produced by other viruses, or by the 24 hour exposure mode.

Table 5

ANOVA Analysis Of Virus PFU Enhancement By Exposure Of Cells To Formaldehyde or Trioxane

Source of Variation	Sum of Squares	Degrees of Freedom	Mean Square	F	p < .001
MAIN EFFECTS	351070.1	5	70214.0	55.2	yes
cell	59869.5	1	59869.5	47.0	yes
virus	169613.2	2	84806.6	66.6	yes
polymer	32038.8	1	32038.2	25.2	yes
dose	89549.1	1	89549.1	70.4	yes
2-WAY INTERACTIONS	593846.3	9	65982.9	51.8	yes
cell virus	38418.7	2	19209.3	15.1	yes
cell polymer	29459.8	1	29459.8	23.1	yes
cell dose	55778.7	1	55778.7	43.8	yes
virus polymer	158361.7	2	79180.9	62.2	yes
virus dose	224358.7	2	112184.3	88.1	yes
polymer dose	87459.6	1	87459.6	68.7	yes
3-WAY INTERACTIONS	359218.5	7	51316.9	40.3	yes
cell virus polymer	145689.6	2	72844.8	57.2	yes
cell virus dose	36424.3	2	18212.1	14.3	yes
cell dose polymer	63784.0	1	63784.0	50.1	yes
dose virus polymer	113320.6	2	56660.3	44.5	yes
4-WAY INTERACTIONS	107893.0	2	53946.5	42.4	yes
EXPLAINED	1412027.9	23	61392.5	48.2	yes
RESIDUAL	61089.3	48	1272.7		
TOTAL	1473117.2	71	20748.1		

cell = cell strain effect
virus = virus type effect
dose = acute or chronic chemical dose effect
polymer = polymer type effect independent of toxicity

CONCLUSIONS

Completion of a comparative hazard assessment for trioxane and formaldehyde <u>in vitro</u> using human target cells produced three basic conclusions. <u>First</u>, formaldehyde exposure did not exhibit the same toxicological effects as trioxane exposure. The cytotoxicity potencies for the two compounds were different, trioxane exposure did not induce SCE at any dose level, and both polymer forms showed different response patterns in the virus enhancement experiments. Secondly, lung and skin fibroblasts showed both qualitative and quantitative differences in response to exposure to formaldehyde and trioxane. Qualitative differences between cell strain response included SCE induction response patterns and dichotomy in virus enhancement results. Quantitative differences between the different cell strains were also evident, as illustrated by the response slopes in the cytotoxicty and SCE induction assays. Thirdly, some biological evidence was discovered regarding the mechanisms of action for the toxic effects produced by the test compounds. The cytotoxicity slope differences between formaldehyde and trioxane argue strongly against a common mechanism (18). Also the finding that trioxane does not induce SCE, even at doses inducing significant toxicity, indicates a different mechanism of action for the two compounds. The divergent biological effects produced by trioxane and formaldehyde also tend to refute the possibility that the toxic properties of trioxane result from formaldehyde monomer generated by metabolic processes, or present as a trace contaminant of trioxane. It is also unlikely that trioxane is metabolized by cells to form a more toxic intermediate. Ames tests of bacterial mutagenesis have been reported as negative for trioxane (19), even with metabolic activation by liver microsomes. In addition, micronucleus tests of trioxane in vivo using i.p. doses as high as 4250 mg/kg produced negative results (20). We also conducted some ancillary studies of colony formation and SCE effects of trioxane using microsomal S9 activation that demonstrated no evidence of metabolic activation of this compound.

The virus enhancement results showed that cells exposed to formaldehyde polymers differed in their resistance to virus infection. This finding is consistent, in general, with other studies documenting virus-chemical interaction (21,22,23). However, the in vitro results cannot be interpreted as indicating an increased infection risk for whole animals or man. Rather, they indicate only a potential for such action, that should be more fully investigated using in vivo methods.

A comparative hazard assessment for trioxane and formaldehyde indicated some promise for the possible use of trioxane as a formaldehyde substitute, based upon the measured indices of toxicity. Comparison of the test results also showed response trends consistent with existing information on formaldehyde and trioxane toxic effects. However, the magnitude of interaction effects found between the target cells, test chemicals, and dose application modes demonstrated a high degree of specificity related to hazard assessments conducted in vitro. The results imply that the biological-chemical attributes of the test system influence dose response measurements in vitro, and that the utility of resulting data depends directly upon the degree of concordance between the test hypothesis and the assay method.

REFERENCES

(1) Hayflick, L. and Moorhead, P. (1961). The serial cultivation of human diploid cell strains. Exp. Cell Res. 25:585-621.

(2) Cornfield, V. and R. Hay (1978). Effects of cysteine and glutamine restriction on human diploid fibroblasts in culture. In vitro 14(9):787-794.

(3) Chen, T. (1977). In situ detection of mycoplasma contamination in cell cultures by fluorescent Hoescht 33258 stain. Exp. Cell Res. 104:255-262.

(4) Hay, R. (1978). Preservation of cell culture stocks in liquid nitrogen. TCA Manual 5(2):787-790.

(5) Ekwall, B. and Sandstrom, B. (1978). Combined toxicity to HeLa cells of 30 drug pairs, studied by a two-dimensional microtitre method. Toxicol. Lett. 2:285-292.

(6) Ekwall, B. and Sandstrom, B. (1978). Improved use of the metabolic inhibition test to screen combined drug toxicity to HeLa cells - Preliminary study of 61 drug pairs. Toxicol. Lett. 2:293-298.

(7) Ekwall, B. (1983). Screening of compounds in mammalian cell cultures. pp 64-77. In: Cellular Systems For Toxicity Testing. G. Williams, V. Dunkel, and V. Ray (eds.). The New York Academy of Sciences, N. Y.

(8) Wininger, M., Kulik, F., and Ross, W. (1979). In vitro clonal cytotoxicity assay for chemicals using Chinese hamster ovary cells (CHO-K1). TCA Manual 5(2):1091-1093.

(9) Hull, C., and Nie, N. (1981). SPSS Update 7-9 - New Procedures and Facilities for Releases 7-9. McGraw-Hill Book Co., N.Y.

(10) Tolnai, S. (1975). A method for viable cell count. TCA Manual 1(1):37-38.

(11) Guerro, R., and Rounds, D. (1979). Use of sister chromatid exchange analysis as a bioassay for detecting mutagenic metabolites in urine. TCA Manual 5(2):1087-1089.

(12) Miller, R., Aronson, M., and Nichols, W. (1976). Effects of treatment on differential staining of BrDU labeled metaphase chromosomes. Chromosoma (Berl.) 55:1-11.

(13) Burkholder, G. (1982). The mechanisms responsible for reciprocal BrDU-Giemsa staining. Exp. Cell Res. 141:127-137.

(14) Lavappa, K. (1979). Sister chromatid exchange assay for the detection of chemical mutagens-carcinogens in cultured mammalian cells. TCA Manual 5(3):1121-1126.

(15) Bloom, A. and Paul, N. (eds.) (1981). Guidelines for studies of human populations exposed to mutagenic and reproductive hazards. Proceedings of a conference held Jan 26-27. Publ. March of Dimes Birth Defects Foundation, pp.3-35.

(16) Cooper, P. (1967). The plaque assay of viruses. In: Methods In Virology (K. Maramorsch and H. Koprowski, eds.) Vol. 3., Academic Press, N.Y.

(17) Dulbecco, R. and Vogt, M. (1954). Plaque formation and isolation of pure lines with poliomyelitis virus. J. Exp. Med. 99:167-182.

(18) Finney D. (1978). Statistical Method In Biological Assay. Third Edition, Charles Griffin and Company, Ltd., London.

(19) Kowalski, Z., Spiechowicz, E., and Baranski, B. (1984). Absence of mutagenicity of trioxane and dioxolane in Salmonella typhimurium. Mutat. Res. 136(3):169-171.

(20) Kowalski, Z. (1984). Genotoxic effects of dioxolane and trioxane in mice evaluated by the micronucleus test. Toxicol. Lett. 21(3):349-352.

(21) Schiff, L. (1977). Effect of nitrogen dioxide on influenza virus infection in hamster trachea organ culture. Proc. Soc. Exp. Biol. Med. 156:546-549.

(22) Staal, S., and Rowe, W. (1975). Enhancement of adenovirus infection in WI-38 and AGMK cells by pretreatment of cells with 5-iododeoxyuridine. Virology 64:513-519.

(23) Hatch, G., Conklin, P., Christensen, C., Casto, B., and Nesnow, S. (1983). Synergism in the transformation of hamster embryo cells treated with formaldehyde and adenovirus. Environ. Mutagen. 5:49-57.

Poster A10

High Performance Liquid Chromatography Analysis of the Novel Neutrophil Chemoattractants "Nourin" Released from Alkali-Burned Corneas

FATHIA METWALLY,[1] ANDREW COHEN,[1]
EDWARD F. ROSSOMANDO,[2] and SALWA A. ELGEBALY[1]

Departments of Surgery[1] and Biostructure and Function[2]
University of Connecticut School of Medicine
Farmington, CT 06032

ABSTRACT

We previously demonstrated the release of high levels of neutrophil chemotactic factors from alkali burned corneas isolated from bovine, rabbit, and human eyes. These cornea-derived neutrophil chemoattractants are referred to as Nourin. Initial biochemical characterization of Nourin suggested that they exhibit Mol wt value of greater than 300 KD. Our recent gel filtration HPLC analysis confirmed the high Mol wt nature of these factors. We also found that leukotriene B_4 (366 D), interleukin 1 (17 KD), and the complement split product C5a (15 KD) eluted from the column at fractions different from where Nourin were eluted. When these known low Mol wt chemoattractants were mixed with corneal supernatants containing Nourin prior to processing on the column, their elution position did not change, which indicates that the chemotactic activity of Nourin does not result from the binding of one of these factors to a high Mol wt protein. Radioimmunoassay confirmed the absence of leukotriene B_4. Further identification of Nourin will provide important information necessary to develop an Enzyme Linked Immuno Assay (ELISA) for rapid detection of the factors. It is our belief that the in-vitro generation of Nourin from corneas in response to injurious agents will provide a useful tool to predict the potential toxic effects of tested products considered for in-vivo use.

INTRODUCTION

Neutrophil chemotactic factors are important inflammatory mediators which activate and recruit leukocytes from the circulation into sites of tissue damage. Major sources of these factors are activated serum (e.g., the complement split product C5a and coagulation systems) [1,2] and immune cells (e.g., leukotriene B_4 and interleukin 1) [3,4]. Recently, we demonstrated the ability of corneal tissue to release high levels of the neutrophil chemoattractants Nourin in response to injury induced by chemical agents (e.g., hydrogen peroxide or sodium hydroxide) [5-7] or mechanical scraping [8]. Preliminary biochemical characterization of Nourin released from sodium hydroxide-injured corneas revealed that they are protease sensitive, heat unstable, extractable in organic solvents, and exhibit molecular weight value of greater than 300,000 daltons [7]. Using size exclusion high performance liquid chromatography (HPLC), we further investigated the molecular weight nature of these corneal factors. Our hypothesis is that Nourin released from alkali-burned corneas are different from previously known low molecular weight factors such as C5a (15,000 daltons), interleukin 1 (17,000 daltons), and leukotriene B_4 (366 daltons).

To test this hypothesis, the epithelial surface of corneas isolated from bovine eyes was exposed to 1N sodium hydroxide (NaOH) for 35 seconds at room temperature. The NaOH was then removed and the epithelial surfaces washed twice with buffer prior to incubation with culture medium (1 ml) for 1 hour at 37°C/5% CO_2 atmosphere. Supernatant solutions collected from five corneas were concentrated using Amicon membrane of cut-off 300,000 MW. Separation of various fractions was performed using gel filtration HPLC. Radiolabeled C5a, interleukin 1 (IL-1), and leukotriene B_4 (LTB_4) were also used to identify their elution position from the column and to investigate their binding capability to large molecular weight proteins.

MATERIAL AND METHODS

Corneal Cup Model

Corneas were isolated from fresh bovine eyes (1-2 hours post harvesting from slaughtered cows) and processed immediately for experiments [5-8]. To minimize damage to corneal epithelial cells, we carefully sectioned the eye 5-10 mm posterior to the limbus (Fig. 1). The attached lens and the iris were gently removed; the resulting "corneal cup" was then washed twice in saline and maintained in cold Minimal Essential Medium (MEM) (Flow Laboratories, Inc., McLean, VA) until used. The cup was then mounted in a paraffin well with the epithelial surface facing upwards and covered (above and below) by MEM. In all studies, serum-free MEM was used.

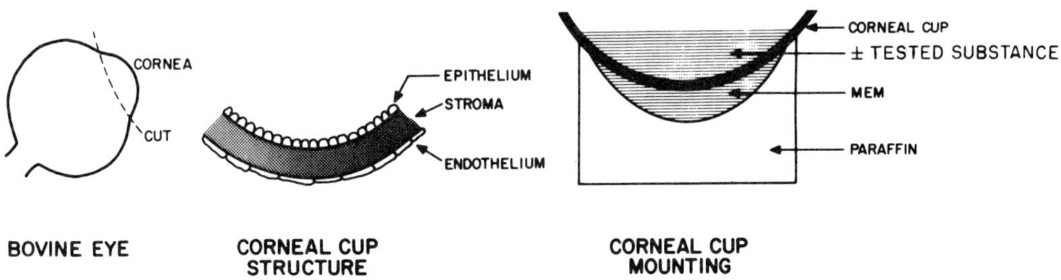

FIGURE 1. Isolation and Preparation of the Corneal Cup Model

NaOH Injury to Isolated Corneas

The epithelial surface of isolated bovine corneas was treated with 1N NaOH for 35 seconds at room temperature. The NaOH was then removed, and the epithelial surface was washed twice with buffer prior to incubation with serum-free MEM (1 ml) for 1 hour at 37°C/5% CO_2 atmosphere. Control corneas were treated with serum-free MEM for 1 hour under the same conditions. Supernatant solutions collected from 5 corneas were concentrated to 100 µl using Amicon membranes of cut-off 300,000 MW.

Size Exclusion High Performance Liquid Chromatography (HPLC)

HPLC analysis of supernatants collected from NaOH-treated corneas (fluids above and below the cornea) and control MEM-treated corneas (fluid above the cornea) were performed. The 100 µl Amicon concentrated materials (above the filter) were diluted 1:10 with mobile phase (0.1 M Na phosphate monobasic and 0.1 M Tris-pH to 6.5 with phosphoric acid) and then filtered through 0.45 µM millipore

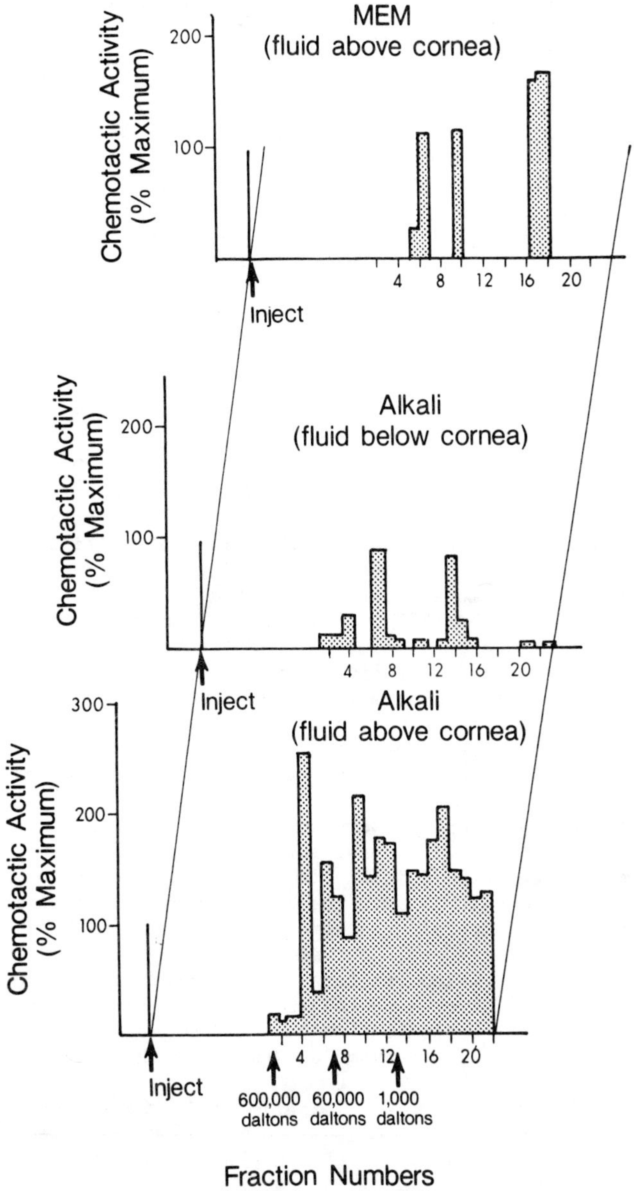

Figure 2: Neutrophil chemotactic activity detected in fractions collected from gel filtration HPLC of alkali burned and MEM-treated corneas.

filter type HA. A volume of 250 µl of the filtrate was injected to HPLC composed of two gel filtration columns, i.e., Bio-Rad TSK 50 (300,000 to greater than 1,500,000 daltons) and Bio-Rad TSK 250 (1,000 to 300,000 daltons). Fractions were collected from 10 minutes after injection to 30-35 minutes. Chart speed was 0.1 inches per minute. The flow rate was 1 ml/ minute/fraction. The detector (Waters-Lambda Max 480) was set at 280 nm wave length for protein and at 210 nm wave length for LTB_4 [9]. A volume of 20 µl radiolabeled I^{125}-C5a (3.5 µCi/8 ml) (Amersham, Arlington Heights, IL), I^{125}-IL-1 (200 µCi/µg) (New England Nuclear, Boston, MA), and ^3H-LTB_4 (178 Ci/nmol) (New England Nuclear, Boston, MA) were injected individually and after mixing well with supernatants obtained from NaOH-injured corneas in the gel filtration HPLC.

Neutrophil chemotactic activity was assayed in fractions 1 to 23 using modified Boyden chambers. The majority of the collected samples were tested for chemotactic activity within 1-7 days. Samples were stored at 4°C. Activity was significantly reduced following freezing.

Chemotaxis Assay

Rabbit peritoneal neutrophils were the indicator cells for these studies. Neutrophils were obtained from peritoneal washings 4-6 hours after glycogen injection (75 ml of 0.1% oyster glycogen in saline) of white New Zealand rabbits [10]. After collection, the leukocyte-rich exudate was strained through four layers of cheesecloth to remove large clumps of debris. The cells were then centrifuged down at low speed (250-500 xg) for 10 minutes at 4°C and resuspended in modified Hanks' Balanced Salt Solution (HBSS). Differential leukocyte counts were made using Wright's stained smears. The exudate usually yielded a highly homogenous population of neutrophils (90-95%).

Fractions collected from HPLC were assayed for neutrophil chemotactic activity using modified Boyden chambers [5,11,12]. F-Met-Leu-phe (10^{-9}M) was our positive control for 100% chemotactic response. HBSS was used as a negative control for random migration.

Rabbit peritoneal neutrophils were adjusted to a final density of 2.5 x 10^6 cells/ml in HBSS containing 0.1% bovine serum albumin (BSA). A 235 µl amount of neutrophil suspension was placed in the top compartment of each chamber containing micropore membrane of porosity 5 µM. The bottom compartment of the chamber contained 150 µl of experimental or control supernatants, F-Met-Leu-phe, or HBSS. Chambers were then incubated for 1 hour at 37°C/5% CO_2 atmosphere to permit cell migration. Following incubation, filters were removed, fixed (100% isopropyl alcohol), stained (hematoxylin), and mounted on glass slides for counting, using an Optomax image analyzer (Burlington, MA). Cell migration in response to the putative chemoattractants was expressed as % maximum chemotactic response.

$$\text{chemotactic activity} = \%\ \text{maximum} \quad \frac{CI_{\text{experimental}} - CI_{\text{HBSS}}}{CI_{\text{F-Met-Leu-phe}} - CI_{\text{HBSS}}} \times 100$$

CI: Chemotactic Index (distance traveled in the filter x cell number).

RESULTS

Neutrophil chemotactic activity detected in fractions collected from gel filtration HPLC of supernatants of NaOH (fluids above and below the cornea) and MEM-treated corneas (fluid above the cornea) is presented in Figure 2. Significant activity was detected in fluid above alkali-burned corneas as illustrated in fractions 2 to 22, which might suggest the heterogeneity of the factors. HPLC analysis, however, of fluid below alkali-burned corneas revealed markedly less chemotactic activity. Interestingly, although crude supernatants obtained from control MEM-treated corneas did not stimulate neutrophil migration [7], we found that upon fractionation, a number of fractions (e.g., 6-7, 9-10 and 16-18)

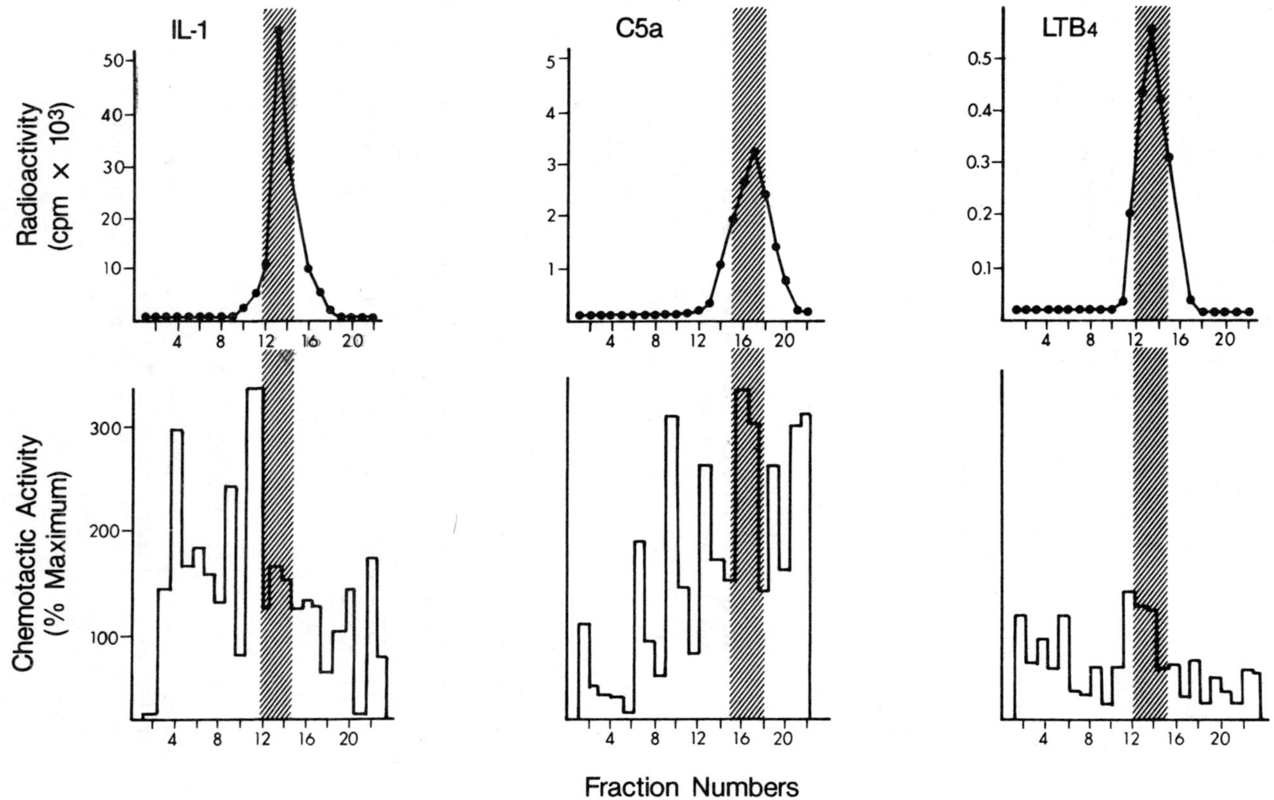

Figure 3: Radiolabeled chemoattractants (IL-1, C5a and LTB_4) and neutrophil chemotactic activity detected in fractions collected from gel filtration HPLC of alkali burned corneas (fluid above corneas).

exhibited activity. A possible explanation might be related to the elimination of chemotactic inhibitors in these fractions.

To determine whether activity detected in supernatants collected from alkali-burned corneas (fluid above the cornea) is related to LTB_4, IL-1 and C5a, radiolabeled isotopes of these factors were used. Chemoattractants injected individually to gel filtration HPLC were eluted at fractions 9 (IL-1), 11 (C5a), and 17 (LTB_4). Figure 3 illustrates elution of the three chemoattractants when mixed with 250 µl of concentrated supernatants obtained from NaOH-treated corneas. Chemotactic activity in the presence of these low molecular weight chemoattractants was also measured. Although we observed some shifts, the chemoattractants eluted at fractions 13 (IL-1), 17 (C5a), and 14 (LTB_4), which eliminates the possibility that activity detected in fractions 1 to 8 is the result of one or more of these chemoattractants bound to large molecular weight proteins. We also observed high chemotactic activity detected in fractions 10 to 18, where the low molecular weight factors were eluted, i.e., 12-15 (IL-1), 15-18 (C5a), and 12-16 (LTB_4).

DISCUSSION

Results of the present study indicate the detection of previously unidentified neutrophil chemotactic factors which, unlike other chemoattractants, are released from corneal tissue in response to alkali injury. For the purpose of discussion, these corneal factors are referred to as Nourin. Gel filtration HPLC analysis confirmed the high molecular weight (i.e., above 300,000 daltons) of these chemotactic factors. Furthermore, control studies showed that Nourin are different from IL-1 (17,000 daltons), C5a (15,000 daltons), and LTB_4 (366 daltons). Radioimmunoassay indicated the detection of very low levels of LTB_4 in supernatants of RPMI and NaOH-treated corneas (preliminary data). Using gel electrophoresis technique, ion exchange-HPLC, and reverse phase-HPLC, we are currently evaluating the chemical nature (i.e., lipoprotein vs. glycoprotein) and determining the molecular weight value of Nourin.

Further identification of the corneal Nourin will provide important information necessary to develop an ELISA for rapid detection of these factors. It is our belief that the in-vitro detection of Nourin in supernatants of corneas exposed to various tested agents will suggest the substance toxic effects on corneal tissue and predict their in-vivo toxicity, i.e., induction of corneal inflammation.

ACKNOWLEDGEMENTS

This work was supported in part by NIH grant EY 05495 and a grant from the Johns Hopkins Center for Alternatives to Animal Testing.

The authors would like to thank Mrs. Joanne D'Aprile for her help in the preparation of this manuscript.

REFERENCES

1. FERNANDEZ, H.N., HENSON, P.M., OTANI, A. and HUGLI, T.E. (1978), Chemotactic response to human C3a and C5a anaphylatoxins: I. Evaluation of C3a and C5a leukotaxis in vitro and under stimulated in vivo conditions. J. Immunol. 120:102-108.

2. KAY, A.B., PEPPER, D.S. and EWART, M.R. (1973), Generation of chemotactic activity for leukocytes by the action of thrombin on human fibrinogen. Nature New Biol. 243:56-57.

3. FORD-HUTCHINSON, A.W., BRAY, M.A., DOIY, M.U., SHIPLEY, M.E. and SMITH, M.J.H. (1980), Leukotriene B_4, potent chemokinetic and aggregating substance released from polymorphonuclear leukocyte. Nature 286:264-265.

4. CYBULSKY, M.I., COLDITZ, I.G. and MOVAT, H. (1986), The role of interleukin-1 in neutrophil leukocyte emigration induced by endotoxin. Am. J. Pathol. 124:367-372.

5. ELGEBALY, S.A., FOROUHAR F. and KREUTZER D.L. (1987), Characterization of neutrophil and monocyte-specific chemotactic factors derived from isolated corneas in response to hydrogen peroxide injury. Am. J. Pathol. 126:40-50.

6. ELGEBALY, S.A., FOROUHAR, F. and KREUTZER, D.L. (1987), In vitro detection of cornea-derived leukocytic chemotactic factors as indicators of corneal inflammation, Proceedings of the In Vitro Toxicology, Approach to Validation, A. Goldberg (Ed.) Mary Ann Liebert, Inc., New York, Vol. 5, 257-262.

7. ELGEBALY, S.A., DOWNES, R.T., BOHR, M., FOROUHAR, F., O'ROURKE, J. and KREUTZER, D.L. (1987), Inflammatory mediators in alkali-burned corneas: preliminary characterization. Curr. Eye Res. (in press).

8. ELGEBALY, S.A., SUNDER RAJ, N. and KREUTZER, D.L. (1986), Chemotactic factors released by mechanically injured corneal epithelial cells. Seventh International Eye Research 4:187 (abstract).

9. POUBELLE, P.E., BORGEAT, P. and ROLA-PLESZCZYNSKI, M. (1987), Assessment of leukotriene B_4 synthesis in human lymphocytes by using high performance liquid chromatography and radioimmunoassay methods. J. Immunol. 139:1273-1277.

10. TILL, G. and WARD, P.A. (1975), Two distinct chemotactic factor inactivators in human serum. J. Immunol. 114:843-845.

11. KREUTZER, D.L., O'FLAHERTY, J.T., ORR, W., SHOWELL, H.J., WARD, P.A. and BECKER, E.L. (1978), Quantitative comparisons of various biological responses of neutrophils to different active and inactive chemotactic factors. Immunopharmacology 1:39-49.

12. ELGEBALY SA. (1987), Inflammatory mediators in alkali-burned corneas: preliminary characterization. Curr. Eye Res. 6:1263-1274.

Poster A11

Acute and Protracted Injury to Corneal Epithelium as an Indication of the Biocompatibility of Various Pharmaceutical Vehicles

DALE R. MEYER and JAMES P. McCULLEY

Department of Ophthalmology
Southwestern Medical School
Dallas, TX 75235

ABSTRACT

Acute and protracted injury to terminally differentiated rabbit corneal epithelial cultures was evaluated after instillation of various ophthalmic vehicles in an effort to determine the biocompatibility of each of the different formulations, and the osmotic and pH tolerance of the tissue under experimental conditions designed to simulate acute and accumulative in vivo exposure. Acute damage was assessed by monitoring the release of radiolabeled nucleotides and corresponding changes in tissue morphology of the prelabeled cultures. Protracted damage was evaluated by reexamining the morphology of the same cultures after 24 hrs along with quantitative estimates of exfoliation, cell loss, and concomitant changes in protein synthesis.

Our testing results emphasize the importance of significant interactions which may be relevant to the assessment of more complex mixtures. The application of this type of strategy for the evaluation of ophthalmic drugs and commercial pharmaceutical preparations is discussed.

INTRODUCTION

The topical instillation of injurious drugs and pharmaceutical formulations onto the ocular surface primarily provokes a local cytolytic response which is generally accompanied by vasodilation and inflammatory cell infiltration. As a consequence of these events there is often a significant deterioration of the normal barrier function of the tissue which permits the rapid penetration of the agent through the corneal and conjunctival epithelium, resulting in internal damage to the eye.

While it may be difficult to examine the latter type of phenomenon with routine in vitro testing procedures, we thought it would be practical to develop a methodology to evaluate some of the immediate and delayed manifestations of damage by using an experimental preparation that possesses many of the cardinal features of its counterpart in vivo. Given the fact that Thelestam and Mollby (1–4) had previously shown that acute injury to the plasma membrane of cultured fibroblasts is often a more sensitive indication of cytotoxicity than changes in gross morphology, growth, and metabolism; we adopted there perspective to adopt an analytical protocol which enabled us to measure all these parameters in differentiated corneal epithelium cultures to establish an experimental model which was primarily designed to be eventually incorporated in an ophthalmic drug development program.

Our experience during the last six months has been very favorable, as we utilized this methodology to determine the biocompatibility of various pharmaceutical vehicles and the osmotic and pH tolerance of the tissues so we could gain a better understanding of the strengths and limitations of the individual assays.

We plan to discuss these considerations and describe some of the remarkable characteristic differences that we invariably found between the various formulations, since we think this type of information may provide some insight of the many salient factors that determine biological tolerance, which can be exploited in developing our knowledge of chemical interactions, and for establishing accurate guidelines for pharmaceutical specifications.

MATERIALS AND METHODS

Cell isolation and cultures. We now routinely harvest corneal epithelium from enucleated rabbit eyes that we purchase from Pel Freez Biologicals, which alleviates the need to sacrifice animals, and gives us an unlimited supply of donor tissue.

The cells are harvested by a modification of the methods described by Johnson–Muller and Gross (5). After the endothelium has been removed, the excised corneal buttons are incubated overnight in a 0.25% trypsin/Hanks balanced salt solution (HBSS) at 4°C. The following morning the corneas are placed in serum-free MEM containing hyaluronidase and bacterial collagenase and reincubated at 35°C for about 45 min. After this treatment, the cells are gently removed from the stromal surface with a scalpel blade, the cell clumps are collected, and resuspended in fresh medium for rinsing. The sedimented cells are resuspended and inoculated into 24–well dishes at approximately 1 x 10^4 cells/16 mm well. The cultures are grown in the nutrient formulation (SHEM) described by Jumblatt and Neufeld (6) except for the deletion of epidermal growth factor. Under these conditions, the cells rapidly proliferate until a confluent monolayer is reached, then differentiate to eventually form a multilayered (3 to 5 cells thick) tissue which possesses most of the cardinal attributes of native epithelium in situ (6). Terminal development is generally completed by 10 to 14 days which is highlighted by the onset of a stable rate of tissue remodeling and exfoliation that is characteristic of the tissue. Differentiated tissue can be easily maintained for at least several more weeks provided the cultures are refed 3 or 4 times per week since metabolic activity is extremely high.

Pharmaceutical vehicles. Three intraocular and two topical vehicles were evaluated with our testing methodology. The isotonic intraocular vehicles included unbuffered saline, 1.5 mM phosphate buffered saline (PBS), and a balanced salt solution (BSS) that was formulated with high strength potassium, calcium and magnesium, and buffered with 25.8 mM sodium acetate and 5.8 mM sodium citrate, which is identical in composition to an intraocular irrigating solution that is commercially available. The isotonic topical vehicles include a saline buffered with acetate/citrate at the same concentration, and a more complex formulation (CBA) that was buffered with 50 mM sodium borate, 12.5 mM citric acid, and 25 mM trisodium phosphate which we considered to be representative of some of the types of vehicles that are used for commercial pharmaceutical preparations.

Osmotic values of the pharmaceutical vehicles were also adjusted in 100 mOsm increments usually between 100 to 800 mOsm by changing the concentration of sodium chloride used in the formulation, to determine the osmotic tolerance of the tissue. Hypotonic solutions were formulated by reducing NaCl or omitting it entirely. Additional NaCl was added to adjust the tonicity of the hypertonic solutions.

All the solutions were freshly prepared with USP grade reagents in double glass distilled water, and adjusted to a final pH of 7.4 $\pm$ 0.2 with dilute HCl or NaOH before sterilization. The solutions were sterilized by filtration through a 0.2 mu membrane filter and stored in sealed borosilicate glass bottles. Aliquots of each of the experimental solutions were measured in triplicate by vapor pressure osmometry to confirm tonicity. The pHs were also checked immediately before testing and readjusted as necessary to maintain these specifications.

The pH values of the same vehicles were also adjusted in 1.0 unit increments from 1 to 12 to determine the pH tolerance of the tissue after instillation of the various formulations. In some of these experiments, we substituted 20 mM glycine for the phosphate and acetate/citrate buffers in formulating the alkaline solutions, since the buffering capacity of the constituents was generally unstable above pH values of 8.0 to 8.5.

Time–dependent toxicity. Acute and protracted damage to the differentiated epithelium was always evaluated after the instillation of the various formulations by using a half log series of exposure intervals (e.g., 4 to 128 min) as described by Takahashi (7), which we utilized to determine the shortest exposure that was damaging and whether or not the manifestations of injury were gradual or sharply delineated. Acute damage was assessed by measuring the release of radiolabeled cytosolic markers and corresponding changes in tissue morphology. Protracted damage was ascertained by reexamining the morphology of the same cultures at 24 hrs, along with quantitative estimates of exfoliation, cell loss and concomitant changes in protein synthesis as described below.

Acute damage. Cultures were rinsed with HBSS and prelabeled with 2.5 uCi/ml of ^{3}H–uridine for 2 hrs in SHEM containing 58 nM of uridine carrier to preferentially label intermediate molecular weight nucleotides as demonstrated by Thelestam and Mollby (2–4). After labeling, the radiotracer solution was removed, the culture was rinsed again with HBSS, and the test formulation was instilled on top of the tissue. All the cultures were then reincubated at 35°C under ambient atmospheric conditions, which permitted us to maintain an extracellular pH coincident with the value of the test formulations. Each of the experimental solutions was removed after a predetermined time and the cultures were refed with an equal volume of nutrient (SHEM) for a maximum total of 256 min. At that time, the medium was removed and pooled with the test solutions for assay of released radioactivity by liquid scintillation spectrometry. The latter procedure was initiated to maintain a constant collection time for assay. Each experimental exposure was assayed in duplicate and compared to negative controls (n = 4 to 6) maintained during the same interval with nutrient medium under the same conditions. Equivalent aliquots of medium were then collected from the control cultures for determination of the spontaneous efflux of the cytosolic markers during the interval measured. Released radioactivity was expressed as a percentage of maximum release:

$$\frac{[(\text{Exp Release}) - (\text{Spontaneous Release})]}{[(\text{Maximal Release} - (\text{Spontaneous Release})]} \times 100$$

as determined by lysing additional controls in a 67 mM sodium borate buffer immediately after prelabeling. After the release samples were finally collected, the cultures were again refed and placed under the usual incubation (5% CO_2 in air) conditions to be evaluated the next day.

Corresponding changes in the morphology of the cultures were also evaluated by phase contrast microscopy immediately after instillation of the vehicles, and at 256 min after the final refeeding. The general status of the tissue was graded by using a semi–quantitative scale from 0 to 5 to indicate whether their appearance was normal or marginal, or whether there was evidence of surface, penetrating, or perforating damage. Penetrating damage, for example, was easily detected because of the stratified characteristics of the cultures, and the minimal criterion for perforation was the appearance of at least focal areas of denuded substratum. Morphologic evidence of injury was fairly consistent by 256 min, and the changes we saw were almost invariably more severe after longer exposures. Because of its consistency, we felt that our final assessment was a good frame of reference for evaluating the sensitivity of our release assay.

Protracted damage. Delayed or residual damage was initially evaluated at 24 hrs by reexamining the cultures by phase contrast microscopy. The cellular material that had been sloughed during the intervening period was subsequently collected, washed to removed residual serum, and assayed for total protein content by the method described by Lowry et al (8) to determine the amount of exfoliation. After the nutrient medium was removed, the cultures were then rinsed with HBSS, and reincubated with either 1.25 uCi or 2.5 uCi/ml or ^{14}C–leucine in SHEM containing 100 uM leucine carrier for 4 hrs to determine the amount of the precursor incorporated in tissue protein. The incubations were terminated by aspiration, the cells rinsed with physiologic saline, and harvested with a buffered 0.2% trypsin/EDTA solution. The tissue was pelleted by centrifuging and rinsed with saline before hydrolysis in alkali. The tissue pellet was then dissolved in 0.1N NaOH. An aliquot of each sample was assayed for protein by the method of Lowry, et al. The remaining solution was assayed for radioactivity by liquid scintillation spectrometry after correction of residual tritium spillover. Protein synthesis values were normalized (CPM/mg protein) and expressed as a percentage of control.

Statistical analysis. A general description of acute damage was accomplished by employing a modification of the analysis described by Takahashi (7,9) to calculate CDT_{50} values which indicated the time of exposure that was necessary to injure 50% of the tissue. We modified his procedures

by only including the values between 16% to 84% of maximal release in our computations because of the asymptotic characteristics of most of our time–response curves which we think is a consequence of the complex cytoarchitecture of the cultures. Moreover, we often extended the exposure to 256 min in some of the experiments when ^{3}H–nucleotide release was not high enough after 128 min to permit us to calculate accurate values.

The statistical significance of the other quantitative measurements was ascertained by calculating 99% confidence intervals in the corresponding control data by using the X ± 3 SD to determine whether experimental values were derived from the same population.

RESULTS AND DISCUSSION

Osmotic Tolerance

Intraocular Vehicles

The remarkable differences in acute tolerance of the three intraocular vehicles that we examined are illustrated in Fig. 1, which shows release of ^{3}H–nucleotides after instillation of the various formulations. In these particular experiments, the first two groups of hypertonic vehicles were clearly more damaging than the corresponding hypertonics balanced salt solutions, which are differences that should be taken into consideration when this methodology is utilized for pharmaceutical screening and formulation development.

Generally speaking, appreciable (or rapid change) release of the tritiated markers usually corresponded with the development of penetrating injury, with the exception of the two most hypertonic (800 mOsm and 1000 mOsm) balance salt solutions where overall efflux remained very low even though these formulations were very injurious after 64 to 128 min exposures (refer to Fig. 1 and Table 1). In view of this finding, we don't always consider this to be the most

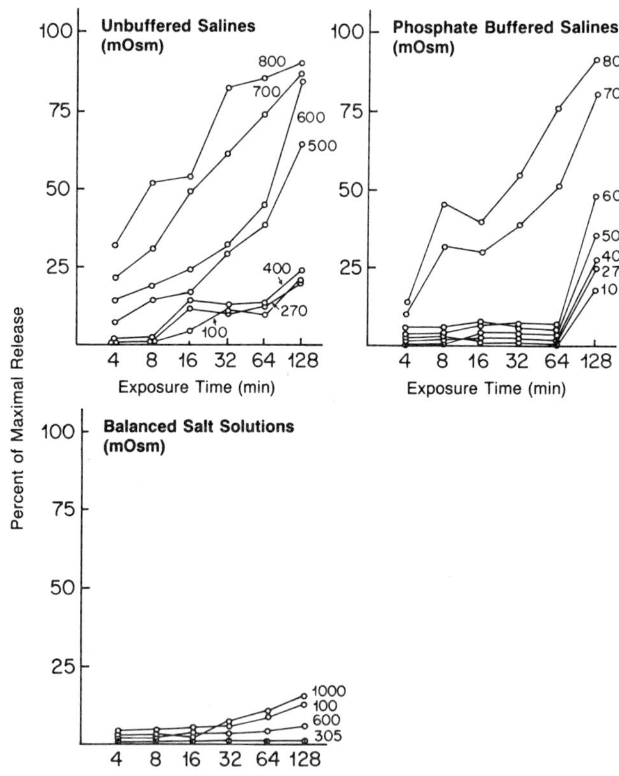

Fig. 1. Acute Osmotic Tolerance of Corneal Epithelium after Instillation of Various Intraocular Vehicles

sensitive feature of our testing methodology, since other criteria were frequently more effective in detecting more subtle differences between the prototype vehicles.

The onset of significant ^3H release, for example, typically coincided with the development of surface damage after the instillation of the unbuffered salines, but this wasn't so apparent after contact with the buffered solutions where it mainly corresponded with changes in the osmotic value of the vehicle. It was clearly evident that changing the tonicity of the solutions in varying degrees from an isotonic value generally resulted in quicker initial release of the cytosolic markers. A gradual change in these values was particularly apparent after instillation of the balanced salt formulations, which we think is a consequence of its chelating properties which may have subtle impact on the permissive tolerance of the tissue even when citrate is formulated in an otherwise compatible vehicle. This type of acuity suggests that latency measurements may be a very sensitive indication of low grade osmotic damage which may not always be discernible by any other criterion. This type of measurement may also be suitable for evaluating the additive (a possibly synergistic) interaction of individual components in more complex mixtures where it might be possible to detect a gradual response that might have some predictive value for identifying potential biological and chemical incompatibilities. We certainly plan to investigate this application in the future.

Table 1: Different Features of Acute Damage after Instillation of Intraocular Vehicles

Formulation (mOsm)	Onset (min) [1]Signif. ^3H Release	Surface Injury	Penetrating Injury	CDT_{50}
Unbuffered Salines				
100-300	8-16	4	ND	>256
400	16	4	ND	195.4
500	4	-	4	74.6
600	4	-	4	38.7
700	4	-	4	17.4
800	4	-	4	8.7
PBSs				
100-300	16-128	4	ND	>256
400	128	4	ND	206.5
500	16	4	ND	168.9
600	16	4	ND	130.6
700	4	-	4	36.7
800	4	-	4	21.1
BSSs				
100	4	[2]ND	ND	>256
200	32	ND	ND	>256
305	128	ND	ND	>256
400	32	ND	ND	>256
600	16	128	ND	>256
800	8	-	128	>256
1000	4	-	64	>256

[1]Compared to control ($p < .01$); [2]Not detectable after a 128 min exposure.

Using the less rigorous criteria described in the table enabled us to compare and contrast each of the different vehicles on the basis of penetrating injury and median damage scores. We typically found that 100 to 400 mOsm unbuffered salines, for example, were tolerated for up to 128 min, causing only low grade focal damage to the superficial cell layers. More extreme hypertonic solutions (500 to 800 mOsm) proved to be much more damaging by causing penetrating injury and pronounced release of ^3H–nucleotides after exposures of 4 to 16 min. Damage was very progressive after the instillation of these vehicles, which was clearly evident by the series of decreasing CDT_{50} values.

Most of the hypertonic phosphate buffered vehicles were much better tolerated, but striking damage was observed after the instillation of the 700 to 800 mOsm formulations which indicated that 600 mOsm was approximately the upper limit of tolerance.

The same corresponding hypertonic balance salt solutions were by far the least toxic, since we didn't even find any discernible change in the morphology of the tissue until after 128 min exposures to the 600 mOsm formulation. Instillation of the 800 mOsm and 1000 mOsm solutions were more injurious, but we were never able to determine any CDT_{50} values since there wasn't enough damage even after extending exposure to 256 min. Under these circumstances, hypertonic balanced salt solutions were clearly better tolerated than the other vehicles, which is a finding that could be exploited in development projects where hypertonicity may be unavoidable.

Table 2: Evidence of Persistent Damage at Twenty-Four Hours after Exposure

Formulation (mOsm)	Minimum Previous Exposure (min)			
	[1]Signif. Exfol.	[2]CD	Residual injury: Surface	Residual injury: Penetrating
Unbuffered Salines				
100-400	4-16	128	128	ND
500	4	4	4	ND
600	4	4	4	ND
700	4	4	4	128
800	4	4	4	16
PBSs				
100-600	128	128	128	ND
700	4	4	4	128
800	4	4	4	16
BSSs				
100-600	4	ND	ND	ND
800	4	128	4	128
1000	4	128	4	32

[1]Significant exfoliation compared to control ($p < .01$).

[2]Cell desquamation was empirically defined as a 3 to 8 fold increase in exfoliation.

Major differences between the intraocular vehicles were even more striking when we reexamined the cultures the next day at approximately 24 hrs after the initial exposure. Protracted damage was clearly evident in all the cultures that had previous contact with the unbuffered salines, since exfoliation was consistently elevated ($p < .01$) and protein synthesis was invariably reduced ($p < .01$) to about 60% to 80% of total values, even in the cultures that exhibited only residual surface damage (Tables 2 & 3). Residual penetrating damage was still evident after exposure to the 700 to 800 mOsm solutions, but there was generally no particular correspondence between the type of exposure and the magnitude of change that we observed in the quantitative assay. The absence of any consistent experimental differences indicated that the reduction in macromolecular synthesis that we invariably observed was probably the consequence of a pervasive perturbation of extracellular pH, since none of the vehicles were buffered. There could have also been a minor problem with the stability of the pH values of the solutions during the original exposure, since the vehicles may have become mildly acidic while in contact with the tissue because of the absorption of atmospheric carbon dioxide. As a consequence of our observations, we don't even think isotonic vehicles should be used for most pharmaceutical formulations.

Protracted damage after instillation of 100 to 600 mOsm phosphate buffered vehicles was not nearly as striking since exfoliation was only affected by 128 min exposures, even though there was some evidence of heightened tissue remodeling after 32 to 64 min exposures because of the elevated protein synthesis values (Tables 2 & 4). Exfoliation and residual morphologic damage

Table 3: Protracted Injury as Demonstrated by Changes in Protein Synthesis after Exposure to Unbuffered Salines

Formulation (mOsm)	[1]Previous Exposure (min) 4	8	16	32	64	128
100	89	[b]84	[b]60	[b]67	[b]65	[b]60
200	[b]81	[b]84	[b]60	[b]64	[b]69	[b]64
270	93	85	[b]66	[b]79	[b]81	[b]79
400	91	[b]82	[b]63	[b]72	[b]65	[b]74
500	[b]66	[b]60	[b]62	[b]78	[b]76	[b]75
600	[b]67	[b]61	[b]56	[b]57	[b]69	[b]81
700	[b]63	[b]62	[b]60	[b]66	[b]65	[b]67
800	[b]59	[b]54	[b]80	[b]40	[b]70	[b]82

[1]Normalized (CPM/mg protein) values are expressed as a percentage of control
[b]Significant reduction of protein synthesis compared to control ($p < .01$).

Table 4: Protracted Injury as Demonstrated by Changes in Protein Synthesis after Exposure to Phosphate Buffered Salines

Formulation (mOsm)	[1]Previous Exposure (min) 4	8	16	32	64	128
100	[b]82	87	90	[a]129	[a]150	105
200	[b]83	[b]76	92	[a]120	[a]124	94
280	89	[b]88	101	[a]121	112	102
400	96	84	104	109	[a]129	108
500	104	104	94	[a]125	[a]135	114
600	92	[b]80	110	117	[a]156	106
700	[a]143	[a]132	[a]119	[a]120	103	102
800	118	105	91	115	[a]121	92

[1]Normalized values (% control).
[a,b]Significant elevation or reduction, respectively ($p < .01$).

were more pronounced after previous contact with the 700 to 800 mOsm solutions even though protein synthesis wasn't particularly affected by the 800 mOsm vehicle, and neither of the two groups exhibited any consistent terminal cell loss.

Protracted damage after previous exposure to the balanced salt solution was generally the least remarkable, except for the fact that there was inevitably significant exfoliation ($p < .01$) in all of the cultures, which we again attribute to its chelating properties (Tables 2 & 5). There was some evidence of reduced protein synthesis (and cell loss) after 64 to 128 min exposures to the two hypotonic vehicles, but we failed to find any abnormal morphology, so we think it is questionable whether this is toxicologically important. The two most hypertonic vehicles, on the other hand, were unequivocally damaging after 64 to 128 min exposures since moderate to extensive residual penetrating injuries of these cultures, along with significant reductions ($p < .01$) in protein synthesis and cell loss. But we don't think this is of any practical consequence, since it is unlikely that this type of extreme exposure would ever be duplicated in vivo, even after repeated instillation of ophthalmic drugs.

Table 5: Protracted Injury as Demonstrated by Residual Tissue Loss and Changes in Protein Synthesis after Exposure to Balanced Salt Solutions

Formulation (mOsm)	[1]Previous Exposure (min) 4	8	16	32	64	128
100	91	85	92	94	[b]81	97
200	91	86	99	104	95	[bd]78
305	93	88	88	95	99	101
400	84	95	84	87	93	83
600	111	110	89	89	93	96
800	89	87	83	83	[d]95	[bd]53
1000	83	86	86	96	[bd]25	[bd]7

[1]Normalized synthesis values (% control).

[b]Significant reduction ($p < .01$).

[d]Decreased tissue protein values ($p < .01$).

Most of our observations from the first series of experiments support the view that formulating many topical preparations of balanced salt vehicles might certainly reduce their potential toxicity which could increase their margin of safety, particularly when the final formulations are not isotonic. This particular conclusion was also supported by more recent studies when we evaluated two other types of buffered vehicles which were more frequently used for these types of medications.

Topical vehicles

Hypotonic topical formulations generally caused much more ^3H release than the corresponding intraocular type vehicles which confirmed our hypothesis that tonicity was a much more critical

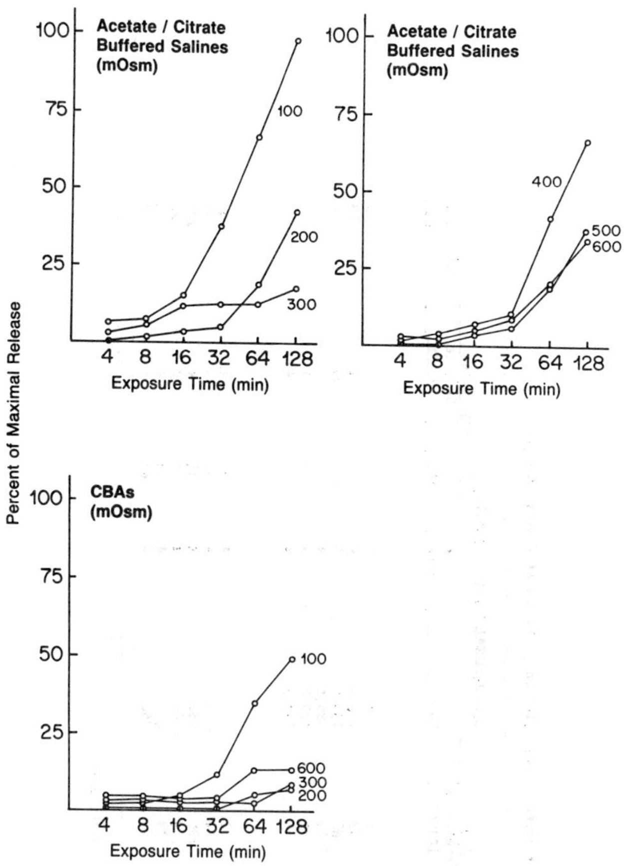

Fig. 2. Acute Osmotic Tolerance of Corneal Epithelium after Instillation of Various Topical Vehicles

factor for these types of vehicles (see fig. 2). On the other hand, the correspondence between ^3H release and osmotic damage was very peculiar, since it was quite apparent that release of the cytosolic marker gradually decreased as we increased the tonicity of the hypertonic solutions, even though there was usually striking cellular retraction and evidence of some penetration almost immediately after we instilled these vehicles on top of the tissue. We think this phenomenon may be characteristic of incomplete vehicles with chelating properties since we found the same general relationship at the after the instillation of the CBA vehicles. As a matter of fact, in this particular experiment, the onset of appreciable release was greatly delayed and its overall magnitude was not nearly as striking, which we don't think was coincidental since these particular formulations contained about twice as much citrate.

It is certainly defensible to suggest that there may be a direct quantitative relationship between the concentration of the chelating agents and the degree of antagonism or suppression of the ^3H release; since in the final analysis, citrate's affinity for Ca^{2+} could have a significant impact on the permeability and integrity of the plasma membrane of the cells. This conjecture is particularly exciting since it is well understood that Ca^{2+} is a necessary factor for phospholipase A_2 activity which is the rate limiting step in the activation of the arachidonic acid cascade (10), which is ultimately responsible for the hydrolysis of membrane lipids and the consequential production and release of prostonoids and other inflammatory mediators (11). Because of the

Table 6: Manifestations of Acute and Protracted Damage after Instillation of Topical Vehicles

	Minimal Exposure (min)						
	Acute			Protracted			
Formulation (mOsm)	Sign. ^3H Release	Penetrating Injury	CDT_{50}	[1]Sign Exfol	[2]CD	Surface Injury	Penetrating Injury
Acetate/citrate							
100	4	32	41.7	4	--	4	32
200	4	32	118.8	4	--	4	128
300	4	ND	159.8	4	--	ND	ND
400	4	64	86.4	4	--	4	32
500	16	32	120.2	4	--	4	16
600	8	16	120.2	4	--	4	16
CBAs							
100	16	32	125.0	4	32	4	ND
200	64	64	>256	4	16	4	ND
270	128	128	>256	4	16	4	128
400	64	128	>256	4	4	4	ND
500	64	128	>256	4	64	4	128
600	64	64	>256	4	64	4	64

[1]Compared to control ($p < .01$); [2]3 to 8 fold increase

critical role of calcium in this entire chain of events, chelation may have a modest indirect antiinflammatory effect by binding free Ca^{2+} in the cytoplasm of the cells and thereby reducing membrane hydrolysis and permeability which may also be reflected by the decreased release of the soluble ^3H–nucleotides. This is a proposition that would be worthwhile to investigate in the future experiments, particularly since corneal and conjunctival epithelium are capable of synthesizing and releasing cyclooxygenase (12–15) and lipooxygenase products (12–16) which have potent inflammatory and chemotactic properties.

Nevertheless, we shouldn't assume that these particular vehicles were generally tolerated even though ^3H release was much lower, since many other features of the experiments indicated that the correlation between ^3H release and morphologic evidence of injury was fairly low, so that the quantitative measurements actually underestimated the degree of damage induced by most formulations.

The data shown in Table 6 clearly demonstrated that the acetate/citrate buffered vehicles were more rapidly damaging than the corresponding CBA vehicles as documented by the quicker development of penetrating injury and the markedly lower CDT_{50} values. Acute damage resulting from the first set of vehicles with the exception of the isotonic solutions was much more persistent since residual morphologic damage was still relatively unchanged at 24 hrs, whereas there was quite a bit of indirect evidence to indicate that appreciable wound healing took place during the intervening period after the initial contact with the various CBA formulations. In these particular groups residual damage was much less severe and often confined to only the superficial layers of the tissue. Significant exfoliation was apparent after the instillation of all of the vehicles but the CD values couldn't be determined for the first set of experiments because of the large amount of tissue that was lost in the acute phase of the experiment. The exfoliation that occurred within 2 to 4 hrs after placing the vehicles on the cultures was documented by microscopy, but we didn't collect the debris for pooling with the samples that we collected the next day. As a consequence, our exfoliation assays in this particular experiments probably underestimated the magnitude of tissue loss by at least 1 to 2–fold.

We think that this general finding indicates that the osmotic tolerance of the epithelium is remarkably restricted after the instillation of the topical vehicles, since only the isotonic acetate/citrate buffered vehicle was very tolerated, even though the relative CDT_{50} values of the hypertonic solutions were not particularly low. We don't think the CBA formations were very compatible either, but the manifestations of injury were such that most of our indices seemed to suggest that the damage was much less pervasive.

Chelation generally appears to increase the probability of penetrating damage, which is exacerbated by high tonicities. This is not very surprising. Extensive exfoliation is typically the norm, but the degree of persistent damage that is evident by 24 hrs may be entirely explained by the concentration of the chelating constituents in the formulations. Low to moderate concentrations of citrate, for example, may be much more damaging in some respects than higher concentrations (e.g., the 12.5 mM found in the CBAs) which may be more effecting in inhibiting phospholipase A_2 activity. This factor could limit penetrating injury and thereby promote subsequent tissue remodeling which could account for the relative differences that we found between the two different basic prototype formulations.

Support of this point of view can also be demonstrated from the data shown in Table 7, which depicts one particular aspect of the metabolic status of the tissue. Reduced protein synthesis and cell loss is frequently observed in the cultures in the first series of experiments after 32 to 128 min of prior exposure to the acetate/citrate buffered salines, which is in distinct contrast to the pronounced hyperplasia that was almost invariably observed after prior exposure to the CBA formulations. This is a very interesting distinction, per se, but it also demonstrates that statistically significant increases in protein synthesis should also be considered to be toxicologically significant even when striking indications of morphologic damage are no longer apparent.

Table 7: Protracted Injury as Indicated by Residual Tissue Loss and Changes in Protein Synthesis

Topical Formul. (mOsm)	[1]Previous Exposure (min) 4	8	16	32	64	128
Acetate/citrate						
100	113	99	86	[b]84	[bd]64	[bd]42
200	100	98	91	86	[d]84	[bd]79
300	98	94	94	89	93	[d]97
400	104	106	97	94	[bd]81	[bd]83
500	[a]119	[a]132	[ad]128	[ad]121	[d]108	[bd]82
600	[a]119	116	108	91	[b]71	[bd]57
CBAs						
100	118	[a]139	[a]140	[a]137	[a]144	116
200	[ad]148	[ad]206	[ad]175	[a]147	[a]154	[a]162
270	101	113	[ad]154	[a]143	[ad]154	[a]162
400	[ad]158	[ad]142	[ad]135	[ad]158	[a]163	[a]131
500	[ad]165	[a]125	[a]154	[ad]144	[ad]199	[a]142
600	[ad]127	[ad]117	[ad]127	[d]122	[d]124	[d]118

[1]Normalized values (% control).

[a,b]Significant elevation or reduction, respectively ($p < .01$).

[d]Decreased tissue protein ($p < .01$).

pH Tolerance

Intraocular vehicles

The range of permissive pH values that were tolerated by the epithelium was much more sharply delineated than osmolality (Fig. 3), which implies that this particular characteristic may be a more critical factor in determining the toxicity of most pharmaceutical formulations. Buffered intraocular vehicles between the pH values of 4 to 9 caused very little ^{3}H release, but the very acidic and alkaline solutions were extremely destructive and caused very rapid release of the radiolabeled cytosolic markers.

These tolerance limits were not invariant, however, since the acidic balanced salt formulations proved to be much more damaging than the corresponding phosphate buffered vehicles. This seemed to be a rather curious phenomenon which certainly suggests that its chelating properties may accentuate the toxicity of acidic solutions.

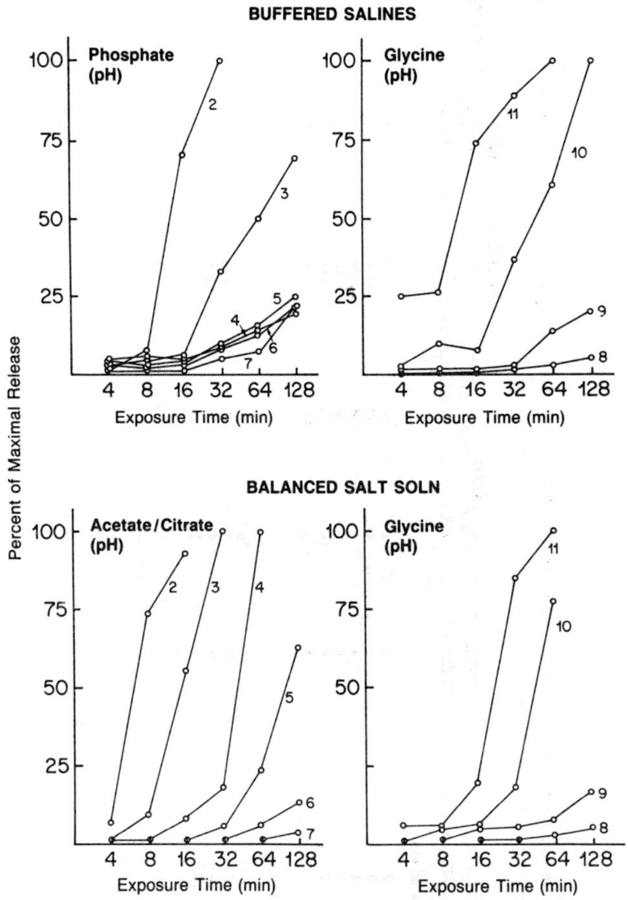

Fig. 3: **Acute pH tolerance of corneal endothelium after the instillation of various intraocular vehicles.**

Table 8: Manifestations of Acute and Protracted Damage after Instillation of Acidic and Alkaline Intraocular Vehicles

Formulation (pH)	Minimal Exposure (min)					
	Acute				Protracted	
	Sign. ^{3}H Release	Surface Injury	Penetrating Injury	CDT_{50}	Surface Injury	Penetrating Injury
Phosphate						
2	8	4	16	6.9	4	8
3	4	4	32	62.5	4	32
4	4	4	128	>128	4	ND
5	4	4	128	>128	32	ND
6	4	16	ND	>128	ND	ND
7	4	128	ND	>128	ND	ND
Glycine						
7.5	32	128	ND	>128	ND	ND
8	32	4	ND	>128	ND	ND
9	4	4	128	>128	8	128
10	1	1	32	22.9	1	4
11	1	1	8	8.5	1	4
12	0.5	--	0.5	<0.5	--	--

The information shown in Table 8 indicates that the buffered vehicles adjusted to pH values between 6 to 8 were acutely tolerated. Acidic and alkaline vehicles were typically injurious, but the alkaline solutions were much more destructive as indicated by the more rapid onset of penetrating injury and corresponding decrease in the CDT_{50} values. An alkaline solution at a pH of 12 wasn't tolerated at all, since the tissue was completely hydrolyzed within 30 seconds of contact, which was the shortest exposure we examined. Protracted damage was also not nearly as striking after previous contact with the mildly acidic solutions (e.g. pHs 4 to 5) since most of the cultures appears to, at least, partially recover from the initial damage. These observations were very contrasting to the persistent effects that were observed after prior exposure to the mildly alkaline solutions that were adjusted to pH values between 10 to 11.

Exfoliation determinations weren't tabulated for any of the pH experiments since we typically found that most of our experimental values were significantly reduced below the controls. We think this peculiar relative consistency was a consequence of the type of tissue damage that we invariably saw. In these particular studies, mostly debris rather than intact cells were typically sloughed, which apparently contained very little protein. As a consequence, we couldn't appropriately compare these values to the control group unless we used an accurate correction factor. Since we really didn't know what this value might be, we simply decided to delete this information from our final analysis.

Table 9: Protracted Injury as Indicated by Residual Tissue Loss and Changes in Protein Synthesis

Intraocular Formul. (pH)	[1]Previous Exposure (min)					
	4	8	16	32	64	128
Phosphate						
2	89	[bd]50	[bd]0	--	--	--
3	[bd]70	[bd]74	[bd]73	[bd]75	[bd]62	[bd]41
4	106	[b]78	[b]66	114	[d]107	[d]96
5	[a]126	91	[a]123	109	[ad]156	[d]117
6	[a]121	94	116	115	110	116
7	104	111	97	88	118	112
Glycine						
7.5	108	112	103	96	94	98
8	[ad]131	[ad]125	[ad]117	[d]109	[d]106	[d]115
9	[ad]130	[ad]118	[d]106	[d]104	[d]102	[d]110
10	[d]102	[d]94	[d]96	[bd]71	[bd]0	--
11	[d]108	[bd]86	[bd]57	[bd]39	[bd]0	--
12	0	--	--	--	--	--

[1]Normalized values (% control).

[a,b]Significant elevation or reduction, respectively ($p < .01$).

[d]Decreased tissue protein values ($p < .01$).

Table 10: Manifestations of Acute and Protracted Damage after Instillation of Modified Balanced Salt Solutions

	Minimal Exposure (min)					
	Acute				Protracted	
Formulation (pH)	Sign. ^3H Release	Surface Injury	Penetrating Injury	CDT_{50}	Surface Injury	Penetrating Injury
Acetate/citrate						
2	0.5	0.5	2	6.8	0.5	2
3	8	4	8	15.4	4	8
4	16	4	8	39.9	4	16
5	32	4	16	101.1	16	128
6	64	4	ND	>128	128	ND
7	128	16	ND	>128	128	ND
Glycine						
8	64	128	ND	>128	ND	ND
9	16	16	64	>128	64	128
10	16	4	16	46.8	--	64
11	4	4	16	19.8	16	32
12	0.5	0.5	0.5	10.5	--	--

The experimental data shown in Table 9 were fairly complementary although it was a little surprising that even the slightly alkaline solutions proved to be so toxic. Acidic solutions at pH values of 5 or less affected protein synthesis to varying degrees, which was usually accompanied by significant tissue loss. Persistent damage was much more pervasive, however, after exposure to the alkaline solution since tissue loss was invariable observed in all of the groups with the exception of pH 7.5. We think that this is probably the consequence of surface tissue loss, since we did observe a transient induction of protein synthesis after 4 to 16 min exposures to vehicles at pHs of 8 and 9, which probably represented some minor tissue remodeling.

The experimental data shown in Table 10 demonstrate that the effective range of tolerance, (e.g., pH 6 to 8) for the balanced salt solutions was essentially no different from the buffered salines when the formulations were adjusted to within normal physiologic values. Alkaline solutions were slightly better tolerated than the saline vehicles but the acidic solutions below pH 6 were much more damaging as we previously mentioned. The increased toxicity of the acidic formulations was clearly reflected by quicker development of penetrating damage and the large decrease in the corresponding CDT_{50} values. There weren't much evidence to indicate recovery from the initial damage since penetrating injury was quite persistent. And, this overall view was generally supported by our assessment of protein synthesis and cell loss at 24 hrs, which is shown in Table 11.

Table 11: Protracted Injury as Indicated by Residual Tissue Loss and Changes in Protein Synthesis

BSS Formul. (pH)	[1]Previous Exposure (min) 4	8	16	32	64	128
Acetate/citrate						
2	$^{bd}7$	$^{bd}1$	--	--	--	--
3	$^{a}121$	$^{bd}16$	$^{bd}0$	--	--	--
4	112	92	$^{bd}17$	$^{bd}0$	--	--
5	90	95	97	97	116	$^{bd}7$
6	99	87	88	88	102	101
7	97	95	102	94	105	89
Glycine						
8	98	99	98	115	99	112
9	103	116	96	95	117	111
10	107	104	98	95	$^{d}113$	$^{d}111$
11	88	90	$^{d}98$	$^{bd}74$	$^{bd}52$	$^{bd}18$
12	0	--	--	--	--	--

[1]Normalized values (% control).

[a,b]Significant elevation or reduction, respectively ($p < .01$).

[d]Decreased tissue protein values ($p < .01$).

Table 12: Manifestations of Acute and Protracted Damage after Instillation of Acidic and Alkaline Topical Vehicles

Formulation (pH)	Minimal Exposure (min)					
	Acute				Protracted	
	Sign. ^3H Release	Surface Injury	Penetrating Injury	CDT_{50}	Surface Injury	Penetrating Injury
Acetate/citrate						
2	1	1	4	--	1	4
3	1	--	1	8.6	--	1
4	1	1	4	17.5	1	8
5	2	2	16	33.8	2	32
6	4	4	128	>128	4	128
7	4	4	128	>128	4	128
7.5	4	4	ND	>128	ND	ND
CBAs						
2	4	--	4	6.8	--	4
3	4	--	4	67.7	--	4
4	4	--	4	111.4	--	4
5	4	--	4	>128	--	4
6	4	--	4	>128	--	4
7	4	--	4	>128	--	4
7.5	128	4	128	>128	4	128
8	4	4	64	41.6	4	64
9	4	4	32	28.2	4	32
10	4	4	32	22.0	4	32
11	4	4	8	5.6	4	8
12	0.5	--	4	<0.5	--	<0.5

Topical vehicles

It wasn't very surprising that the modified topical vehicles were generally more toxic than the intraocular vehicles. The acidic acetate/citrate buffered vehicles were typically more rapidly damaging than most of the corresponding balanced salt formulations (see Table 12). We examined some of the acidic solutions (pHs 2 to 4) from exposures as short as 1 min which didn't seem to make much difference in their toxicity. The corresponding acidic CBA solutions were a bit slower acting, although penetrating damage was invariably observed even after 4 min exposures. The initial damage was fairly pronounced and there was little evidence of a recovery by 24 hrs when we reexamined the cultures. It was interesting that the formulation of a pH of 7 was about as acutely toxic as some of the acidic solutions, since the formulation at pH 7.5 was distinctly better tolerated. This particular difference certainly indicates that slightly alkaline solutions may be least toxic even though the permissive range seems to be remarkably narrow for this particular vehicle. Alkaline solutions were certainly better tolerated for at least 16 min until we increased the pH value above 10.

Table 13: Protracted Injury as Indicated by Residual Tissue Loss and Changes in Protein Synthesis

Acetate/citrate	[1]Previous Exposure (min)							
(pH)	1	2	4	8	16	32	64	128
2	$^{ad}121$	$^{d}106$	$^{bd}62$	$^{bd}8$	$^{bd}0$	--	--	--
3	$^{bd}72$	$^{bd}16$	$^{bd}6$	$^{bd}0$	--	--	--	--
4	$^{d}110$	$^{bd}87$	$^{bd}84$	$^{bd}31$	$^{bd}0$	--	--	--
5	--	$^{d}98$	$^{d}88$	$^{d}101$	$^{bd}63$	$^{bd}47$	$^{bd}0$	--
6	--	--	$^{ad}117$	$^{ad}113$	$^{ad}120$	$^{ad}120$	$^{ad}120$	$^{d}94$
7	--	--	$^{ad}124$	$^{ad}116$	$^{ad}115$	$^{ad}127$	$^{d}96$	$^{d}101$
7.5	--	--	98	$^{c}94$	$^{c}94$	89	93	$^{d}97$

[1]Normalized values (% control).

[a,b]Significant elevation or reduction, respectively.

[c,d]Increased or decreased tissue protein ($p < .01$).

Significant consequences of the previous exposures to acetate/citrate buffered vehicles were also clearly evident the next day after we evaluated the metabolic status of the tissue, since we invariably found reduced protein synthesis and/or cell loss in all the groups except for the cultures that were tested with the formulation at pH 7.5. Damage was apparently the least severe after exposure to pHs 6 and 7 since we consistently saw a modest induction of protein synthesis even though tissue protein values were lower than the controls. There was probably a modest amount of tissue remodeling in most of these cultures as differentiated corneal epithelium generally have a fairly large capacity to regenerate as long as the basal cells aren't irreparably damaged (see Table 13).

Our final assessment of the cultures that were previously exposed to the CBA formulations was very similar (Table 14). Reduced protein synthesis, which was often accompanied by significant cell loss, was frequently observed in most of the groups, indicating that most of the damage was fairly persistent. We didn't find any evidence of consistent hyperplasia, which is in marked contrast to our previous experience from the osmotic tolerance studies as highlighted by inclusion of the isotonic formulation at a pH of 7.5. This striking difference again reemphasizes the fact that modestly alkaline formulations are generally tolerated better for short periods of contact.

Table 14: Protracted Injury as Indicated by Residual Tissue Loss and Changes in Protein Synthesis

CBA	[1]Previous Exposure (min)					
(pH)	4	8	16	32	64	128
2	95	[bd]68	[bd]23	[bd]5	--	--
3	84	86	[d]89	[bd]49	[bd]1	--
4	[b]69	[b]73	[bd]78	[bd]67	[bd]15	--
5	[b]66	[b]68	[b]76	[b]65	[b]65	[bd]61
6	85	[b]79	[b]71	[b]78	[b]84	[bd]78
7	88	86	[b]72	[b]76	[bd]69	[bd]32
7.5	101	113	[ad]154	[a]143	[ad]154	[a]162
8	97	114	95	[d]91	[bd]40	[bd]26
9	112	89	96	[bd]70	[bd]40	[bd]7
10	90	107	84	[bd]49	[bd]4	--
11	100	[bd]26	[bd]0	--	--	--
12	[bd]0	--	--	--	--	--

[1]Normalized values (% control).

[a,b]Significant elevation or reduction, respectively ($p < .01$).

[d]Decreased tissue protein values ($p < .01$).

CONCLUSIONS

There are clearly a number of conclusions that we think we can formulate from the basis of these experiments which can have some practical value as we apply this information to further investigation:

1. Remarkable differences were apparent in the biocompatibility of the various pharmaceutical vehicles that we examined.
2. There was generally a good correspondence between ^3H release and acute damage except for the type of injury caused by the osmotically modified topical formulations with chelating properties.
3. Protracted injury was often more apparent (or striking) than acute damage which can probably be attributed to the cytoarchitecture of the tissue.
4. Statistically significant changes in protein synthesis in either direction are considered to be toxicologically important even in the absence of striking changes in tissue morphology.
5. The relative rank order of toxicity of the various formulations that we examined was : A/Cs > CBAs > unbuffered salines > PBSs > BSSs.
6. Permissible osmotic values of biocompatible vehicles were approximately 100 to 600 mOsm.
7. The range of permissible pH values of the same vehicles was approximately 6.0 to 7.5.
8. Osmotic and pH tolerance limits of the typical vehicles were much more restrictive.
9. This type of methodology should be an effective tool in drug development, and for establishing accurate guidelines for various pharmaceutical formulations.

ACKNOWLEDGEMENTS

Supported in part by a grant from the Center for Alternatives to Animal Testing; and unrestricted research grant from Cilco, Inc.; and an unrestricted development grant from Research to Prevent Blindness, Inc., New York, New York. The excellent technical assistance of Ms. V. Shine and Mr. R. Pisana is greatly appreciated. The manuscript was carefully prepared by Ms. Pat Clarke.

REFERENCES

1. Thelestam, M. and Mollby, R. (1975a), Sensitive assay for the detection of toxin-induced damage to the cytoplasmic membrane of human diploid fibroblasts. Infection and Immunity, 12:225.
2. Thelestam, M. and Mollby, R. (1975b), Determination of toxin-induced leakage of different-size nucleotides through the plasma membrane of human diploid fibroblasts. Infection and Immunity, 11:640.
3. Thelestam, M. and Mollby, R. (1976), Cytotoxic effects in the plasma membrane of human diploid fibroblasts - a comparative study of leakage tests. Med. Biol. 54:39.
4. Thelestam, M. and Mollby, R. (1979), Classification of microbial, plant and animal cytolysins based on their membrane-damaging effects on human fibroblasts. Biochim. Biophys. Acta. 557:156.
5. Johnson-Muller, B.J. and Gross, J. (1978), Regulation of corneal collagenase production: epithelial-strand cell interactions. Proc. natl. Acad. Sci. U.S.A., 75:4417.
6. Jumblatt, M.M. and Neufeld, A. (1983), B-adrenergic and serotonergic responsiveness of rabbit corneal epithelial cells in culture. Invest. Ophthalmol. Vis. Sci. 24:1139.

7. Takahashi, N. (1982), Quantitative cytotoxicity of preservatives evaluated in cell culture with Chang's human conjunctival cells - effect of temperature on cytotoxicity. Jpn. J. Ophthalmol., 26:234.
8. Lowry, O.H., Rosenbrough, N.J., Farr, A.L., and Randall, R.J. (1951), Protein measurement with the folin phenol reagent. J. Biol. Chem., 193:265.
9. Takahashi, N. (1983), A new method evaluating quantitative time-dependent cytotoxicity of ophthalmic solutions in cell culture. Beta-adrenergic blocking agents. Graefe's Arch. Clin. Exp. Ophthalmol. 220:264.
10. Meyer, D.R. (1987), Potential approaches for the development of in vitro alternatives to eye irritancy tests. In: A Critical Evaluation of Alternatives to Acute Ocular Irritation Testing, J.M. Frazier, et al. Alternative Methods in Toxicology Series, Vol 4, A.M. Goldberg (ed.), Mary Ann Liebert Inc., New York, 31–44.
11. Dubin, N.H. (1985), Prostaglandin production as an index of in vitro cytotoxicity. In, In Vitro Toxicology, A.M. Goldberg (Ed.), Alternatives Methods in Toxicology, Vol. 3, Mary Ann Lieberg, Inc., New York, 43–52.
12. Bazan, H.E.P, Bickle, D.L., Beuerman, R., Bazan, N.G. (1985), Cryogenic lesion alters the metabolism of arachidonic acid in rabbit cornea layers. Invest. Ophthalmol. Vis. Sci. 26:474.
13. Leopold, I.H. (1982), Pharmacology of cellular elements of inflammation. In, Biomedical Foundations of Ophthalmology, I.H. Leopold (Ed.), Vol. 3, Harper and Row Publ. Inc., New york, Ch 33.
14. Weissman, G. (1980), Prostaglandins in acute inflammation. Current Concepts, The Upjohn Co.
15. Kulkarni, P.S. and Srivivasin, B.D. (1981), The effect of topical and intraperitoneal indomethacin on the generation of PGE 2-like activity in rabbit conjunctiva and iris ciliary body. Exp. Eye Res., 33:121.
16. Bazan, E.P., Bickle, D.L., et al (1985), Inflammation-induced stimulation of the synthesis of prostaglandins and lipooxygenase-reaction products in rabbit cornea. Current Eye Res. 4:175.

Poster A12

In Vitro Toxicology Data on Respirable Particles and Fibres and Its Evaluation for Statistical Significance

D. NADEAU,[1] D. PARADIS,[1] L. FOUQUETTE,[1] and J. DUNNIGAN[2]

[1]*Laboratoire de Caractérisation de l'Amiante*
Département de Biologie
Université de Sherbrooke
Sherbrooke, Québec
Canada, J1K 2R1
[2]*L'Institut de l'Amiante*
Division Santé et Environnement
Université de Sherbrooke
Sherbrooke, Québec
Canada, J1K 2R1

ABSTRACT

We investigated the impact of the use of nonparametric methods on the interpretation of the biological significance of cytotoxicity data. In our in vitro assay, we use rat pulmonary alveolar macrophages to determine the cytotoxic potential of natural or man-made respirable particles. The cytotoxicity parameters include the extracellular release of the cytoplasmic enzyme LDH (membrane permeability), the ATP cell contents (viability index) and the lactic acid production (metabolism). To evaluate the performance of the two statistical methods, we used a nonparametric Kruskal-Wallis one-way analysis of variance (ANOVA) coupled to a multiple comparisons test (Conover's t test) on rank and, a parametric one-way ANOVA coupled to a multiple comparisons test (Scheffe's test, Duncan's test and/or Dunnett's t test). The analysis were performed on three to eight sets of independent experiments. Overall, it was found that with the nonparametric tests, a statistical significance could be established with less data sets. Moreover, both statistical methods were in almost complete agreement when the results of the eight experiments were pooled. It is therefore concluded that, in our assay, the use of selected nonparametric analyses does not lead to any statistical bias in the interpretation of experimental data. They also provided useful information when trends are needed to step up a biological evaluation (screening), using a very small number of experiments (e.g. triplicate).

INTRODUCTION

In order to substantiate an interpretation of experimental data, it is a common practice to perform some kinds of statistical analysis. In fact, almost every published data are supported by a confidence limit derived from one type or another of analysis for comparing two arithmetic means (e.g. the Student's t test). However, in practice, it is quite frequently required that the results of more than two treatments have to be compared. The procedures for such comparisons include an analysis of variance (ANOVA) and a multiple comparisons procedure such as the Dunnett's t test (1). Those statistical analyses are parametric methods and require calculations to be performed on the current data values. They are available in many computer-compatible statistical packages and the descriptive statistics (mean, standard deviation, etc.) can even be implemented on a pocket calculator.

Recently, Theodorsson-Norheim (2) suggested that the use of nonparametric methods for the analysis of experimental data could be a valuable tool in the comparisons of many small groups of data. As he pointed out, biomedical data are quite frequently not normally distributed; they also contain outlier values and the size of the experimental groups for comparison are often relatively small. Consequently, he suggested that nonparametric statistical methods of analysis «may outperform their parametric analogues in the practical research situation».

Many nonparametric tests are based on a ranking procedure of the data rather than on the value of the data itself (e.g. Mann-Whitney). Because this ranking process can be tedious if performed manually, this approach has been somewhat disregarded by the investigators. However, with the spreading of personal computers, it is no longer a disadvantage. A BASIC program was proposed by Theodorsson-Norheim (2) to perform the Kruskal-Wallis test, which was described by the author as a nonparametric ANOVA for multiple comparisons. In this paper, we wish to report our experience in the evaluation of *in vitro* cytotoxicity data with respirable particles based on both parametric and nonparametric statistical methods.

MATERIALS AND METHODS

Particles and fibres

For the comparisons of the *in vitro* effects of fibres, we used the UICC B (Canadian chrysotile) asbestos standard (3) and, a «short» fraction of the fibrous polyacrylonitrile DOLAN 10® (Hoechst AG). The latter was isolated by flotation in water (4), after a 10 min opening in a blender. This synthetic fibre is used as a reinforcing material for cement and, possibly, for friction material.

For the study of the particulate materials, we used titanium dioxide (TiO_2) and the quartz DQ12 (5) as our reference particles for comparing the effects of the amorphous calcium silicate insulating material KAYLO 10® (Fiberglass Canada/ Owens-Corning, USA). After crushing, the calcium silicate particles passing through a 20 mesh screen were separated at 15,000 rpm on an Multi-Plex selector (Alpine AG; model 100 MZR laboratory type).

The TiO_2 and the DQ12-quartz particles were selected respectively for their relative innocuousness (6) or their strong cytotoxic effects on pulmonary alveolar macrophages (PAM) (7). The labels F1, F2, P1, P2 on the figures will be referring respectively to the UICC chrysotile fibres, the DOLAN 10® fibres, the -15,000 rpm and the +15,000 rpm Alpine fractions of KAYLO 10®.

Cell culture

Our *in vitro* model for studying the toxic effects of natural or man-made respirable fibres and particles on PAM in culture has been described elsewhere (1). Briefly, PAM are obtained from the lungs of healthy black hooded Long-Evans male rats by *in situ* bronchoalveolar lavages. The free airways cells (⩾ 95% viable PAM) are washed, numbered and allowed to form a cell monolayer in multiwell plates. The adherence medium is then replaced with fresh culture medium containing a suspension of the particles to be tested. This procedure corresponds to our fresh monolayer assay. However, in this study we used 1×10^5 cells/well (micro-assay), that is four times less cells than our regular cytotoxicity assay (1). Consequently, to have a better basis of comparison with previous data, the dose indicated on the figures and in the tables show the total (μg) tested when we use 4 x 10^5 PAM. The total amount of particles actually incubated in presence of 1 x 10^5 cells should be divided by four, that is ranging from 6.25 to 125 μg.

After a contact period of 18 hrs, the medium and the cells are collected to measure various cytotoxicity parameters such as the extracellular leakage of the cytoplasmic lactate dehydrogenase (LDH), the cellular ATP levels and the lactic acid (lactate) production by the cells. With varying sensitivities, those parameters are indicative of cellular damage induced by the substance assayed.

Statistical analyses

The results from replicate experiments, at least three and with different cells populations, were collected and compared with the ANOVA and the multiple comparison tests. For the purpose of comparing the two statistical approaches, in the first set of experiments (fibres), the results of eight separate dose-response assays were accumulated and analysed in groups of three, five and eight experiments. These three sets of data were generated at random from the pool of eight experiments. In the second series of experiments (particles), a set of three assays was performed and analysed.

The experimental results were subjected first to an ANOVA, Dunnett's Scheffe's and Duncan's tests. The BASIC programs from Tallarida and Murray (8) were used for the ANOVA and the Dunnett's t test. The parametric tests (ANOVA, Scheffe's and Duncan's tests) were also checked on the SAS system (9) to verify the exactitude of the calculations of our BASIC programs. The BASIC program described by Theordosson-Norheim (2) was used for the nonparametric Kruskal-Wallis test. In all cases, the level of statistical significance was set at $p \leq 0.05$.

RESULTS AND DISCUSSIONS

Fibres

As seen in tables 1 to 3, the selected fibres are cytotoxic to PAM. In a dose-dependant fashion, both the chrysotile asbestos (F1) and the DOLAN 10® polyacrylonitrile (F2) fibres induced significant extracellular releases of LDH (Fig. 1 to 3; a and b), significant decreases in cellular ATP (Fig. 1 to 3; c and d) and significant reductions in the production of lactic acid (Fig. 1 to 3; e and f).

When the fibre-exposed cell monolayers are compared to the control PAM (dose 0), one can observe that with the parametric analyses, the frequency of statistically significant differences seen with the LDH parameter progressively increases with the number of experiments (Fig. 1 to 3; a). This progression of the statistical significance was not observed with the nonparametric analysis since all the data points were already significant with a triplicate set of experiments (Fig. 1 to 3; b).

As for the other parameters, the same observations apply. However, one can notice that for the ATP levels (Fig. 1 to 3; c vs d), and especially for the lactic acid productions (Fig. 1 to 3; e vs f), the sensitivities of these parameters are such that more experiments are needed to reveal a statistical significance with both methods of analysis. Also, with the parametric analyses, the Scheffe's test consistently appears to require more data points than the Duncan's or Dunnett's tests. Despite the strong difference in reactivity between the two types of fibres, they were not compared between each other because factors such as the size (length and diameter) distributions have not been evaluated.

Particles

Our experimental *in vitro* design was extended further to evaluate intra-groups differences in cytotoxicity between mineral samples of fairly

TABLE 1. Dose-responses for the extracellular LDH release from PAM monolayers exposed to natural or man-made fibres

Experimental groups	Dose[a] (μg)	Number of experiments n=3	n=5	n=8
		Percentages of liberation[b]		
Controls	0	5.6 ± 1.2[c]	6.2 ± 1.2	5.8 ± 0.9
Chrysotile asbestos (F1)	25	17.0 ± 1.3	18.3 ± 1.3	17.4 ± 1.2
	50	14.7 ± 1.3	16.3 ± 1.5	15.0 ± 1.5
	100	13.1 ± 2.0	15.2 ± 1.8	14.9 ± 1.3
	250	21.6 ± 2.5	23.0 ± 1.9	22.4 ± 1.4
	500	36.1 ± 4.0	35.3 ± 3.2	32.0 ± 3.0
DOLAN 10 (F2)	25	18.2 ± 2.9	20.1 ± 2.0	18.5 ± 1.8
	50	24.1 ± 2.5	24.8 ± 1.8	24.5 ± 1.1
	100	32.2 ± 5.4	32.7 ± 3.6	31.0 ± 3.0
	250	36.5 ± 2.8	36.4 ± 2.6	33.5 ± 3.3
	500	54.4 ± 6.3	53.7 ± 4.8	51.5 ± 4.2

a The actual total amounts assayed ranged from 6.25 to 125 μg (see MATERIALS AND METHODS for more details).

b The values are expressed as a percentage of the total cell activity of each respective group (1).

c Mean values ± standard error (S.E.).

TABLE 2. Dose-response for the cellular ATP levels from PAM monolayers exposed to natural or man-made fibres

Experimental groups	Dose[a] (μg)	Number of experiments n=3	n=5	n=8
		Percentages of control[b]		
Controls	0	100.0 ± 1.9[c]	100.0 ± 1.8	100.0 ± 1.9
Chrysotile asbestos (F1)	25	88.7 ± 1.5	88.8 ± 8.7	83.2 ± 7.0
	50	93.5 ± 8.6	90.5 ± 5.8	85.9 ± 5.1
	100	81.3 ± 2.7	85.7 ± 4.2	82.8 ± 3.7
	250	69.2 ± 3.3	71.3 ± 2.9	67.9 ± 3.3
	500	48.1 ± 1.4	51.6 ± 9.6	48.1 ± 7.0
DOLAN 10 (F2)	25	77.2 ± 9.1	83.6 ± 8.5	78.6 ± 6.7
	50	61.9 ± 8.2	67.6 ± 7.4	64.7 ± 5.5
	100	59.6 ± 9.7	62.1 ± 7.0	61.7 ± 4.8
	250	51.1 ± 4.4	53.6 ± 4.6	48.4 ± 4.7
	500	28.1 ± 1.4	29.1 ± 1.3	28.5 ± 1.2

a The actual total amounts assayed ranged from 6.25 to 125 μg (see MATERIALS AND METHODS for more details).

b The values are expressed as a percentage relative to the cell contents of control PAM monolayers (~150 ng) (1).

c Mean values ± S.E.

TABLE 3. Dose-responses for the lactic acid production from PAM monolayers exposed to natural or man-made fibres

Experimental groups	Dose[a] (μg)	n=3	n=5	n=8
		Number of experiments		
		Percentages of control[b]		
Controls	0	100.0 ± 2.4[c]	100.0 ± 1.5	100.0 ± 1.1
Chrysotile asbestos (F1)	25	89.6 ± 5.6	91.5 ± 4.5	89.9 ± 3.3
	50	98.2 ± 2.5	95.7 ± 4.2	93.4 ± 3.2
	100	93.9 ± 4.3	94.8 ± 3.7	96.5 ± 2.5
	250	83.7 ± 1.2	88.7 ± 8.7	88.4 ± 5.4
	500	77.8 ± 2.2	80.7 ± 1.6	78.1 ± 9.7
DOLAN 10 (F2)	25	104.1 ± 1.1	107.1 ± 8.0	107.1 ± 5.1
	50	113.7 ± 1.5	114.0 ± 1.1	112.5 ± 7.5
	100	105.1 ± 2.1	111.2 ± 1.3	109.1 ± 8.1
	250	102.6 ± 1.2	107.1 ± 9.0	103.0 ± 5.9
	500	59.7 ± 6.3	68.0 ± 6.2	64.7 ± 4.1

a The actual total amounts assayed ranged from 6.25 to 125 μg (see MATERIALS AND METHODS for more details).

b The values are expressed as a percentage relative to the production of control PAM monolayers (~30 μg) (1).

c Mean values ± S.E.

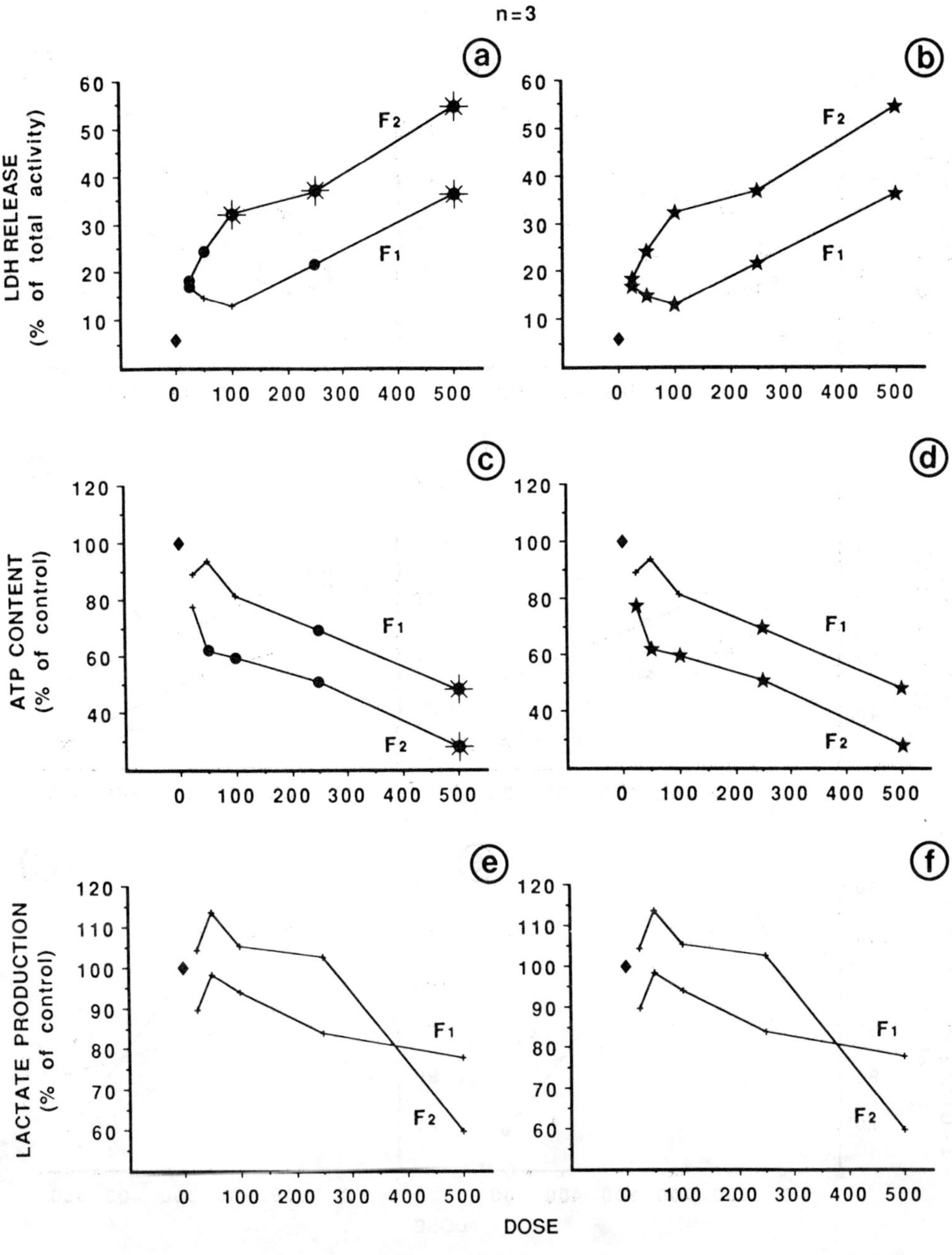

FIG 1. Statistical significance of the cytotoxicity parameters according to parametric (a,c,e) and nonparametric (b,d,f) approaches (n=3). F1: UICC B Chrysotile asbestos fibres; F2: DOLAN 10 polyacrylonitrile fibres.

(◆) Controls values.
(+) No difference with the control values.
(●) Difference with the control values according to Dunnett's and Duncan's tests.
(☼) Difference with the control values according to Scheffe's test.
(★) Difference with the control values according to Kruskal-Wallis' test.

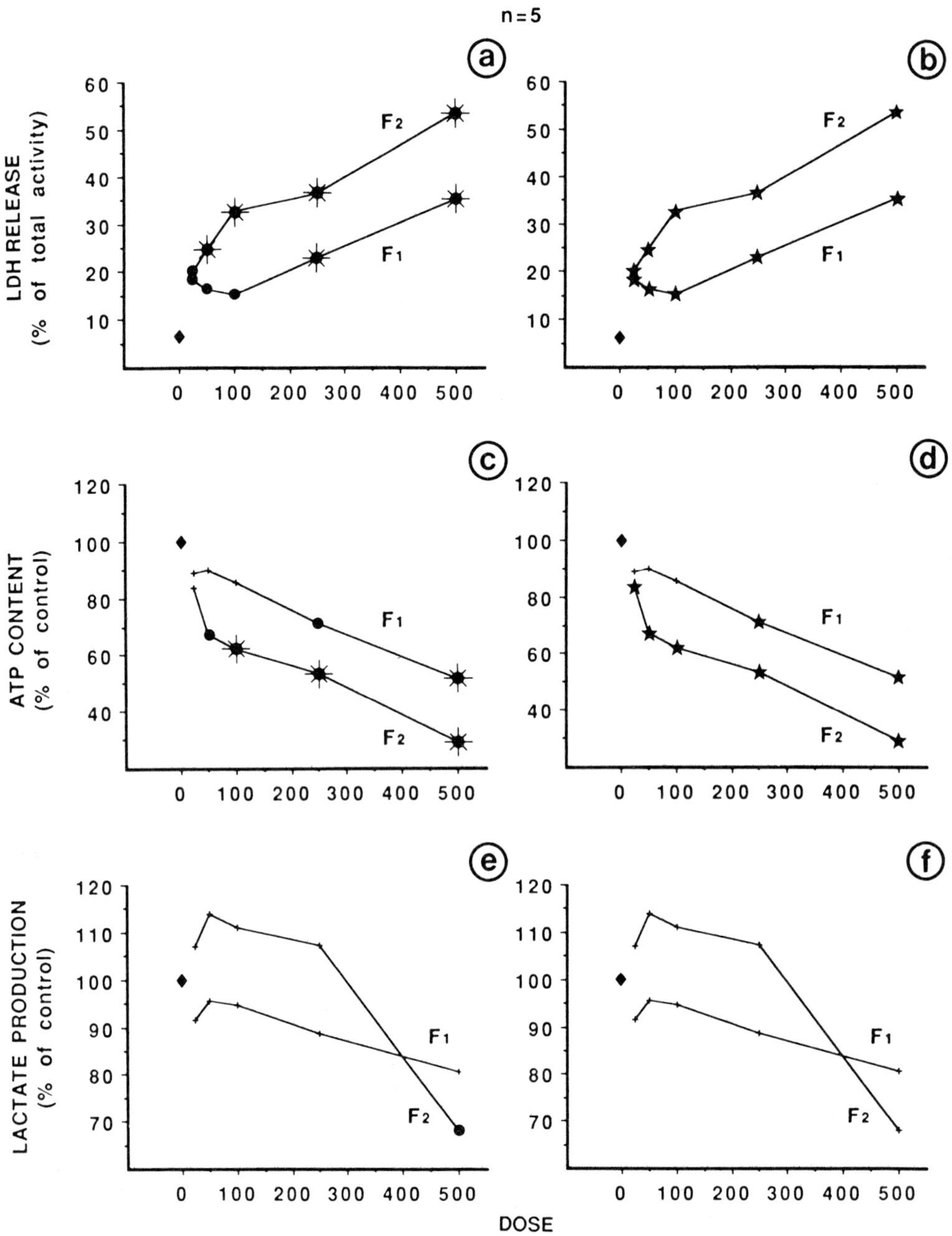

FIG 2. Statistical significance of the cytotoxicity parameters according to parametric (a,c,e) and nonparametric (b,d,f) approaches (n=5). F1: UICC B Chrysotile asbestos fibres; F2: DOLAN 10 polyacrylonitrile fibres.

(◆) Controls values.
(+) No difference with the control values.
(●) Difference with the control values according to Dunnett's and Duncan's tests.
(☼) Difference with the control values according to Scheffe's test.
(★) Difference with the control values according to Kruskal-Wallis' test.

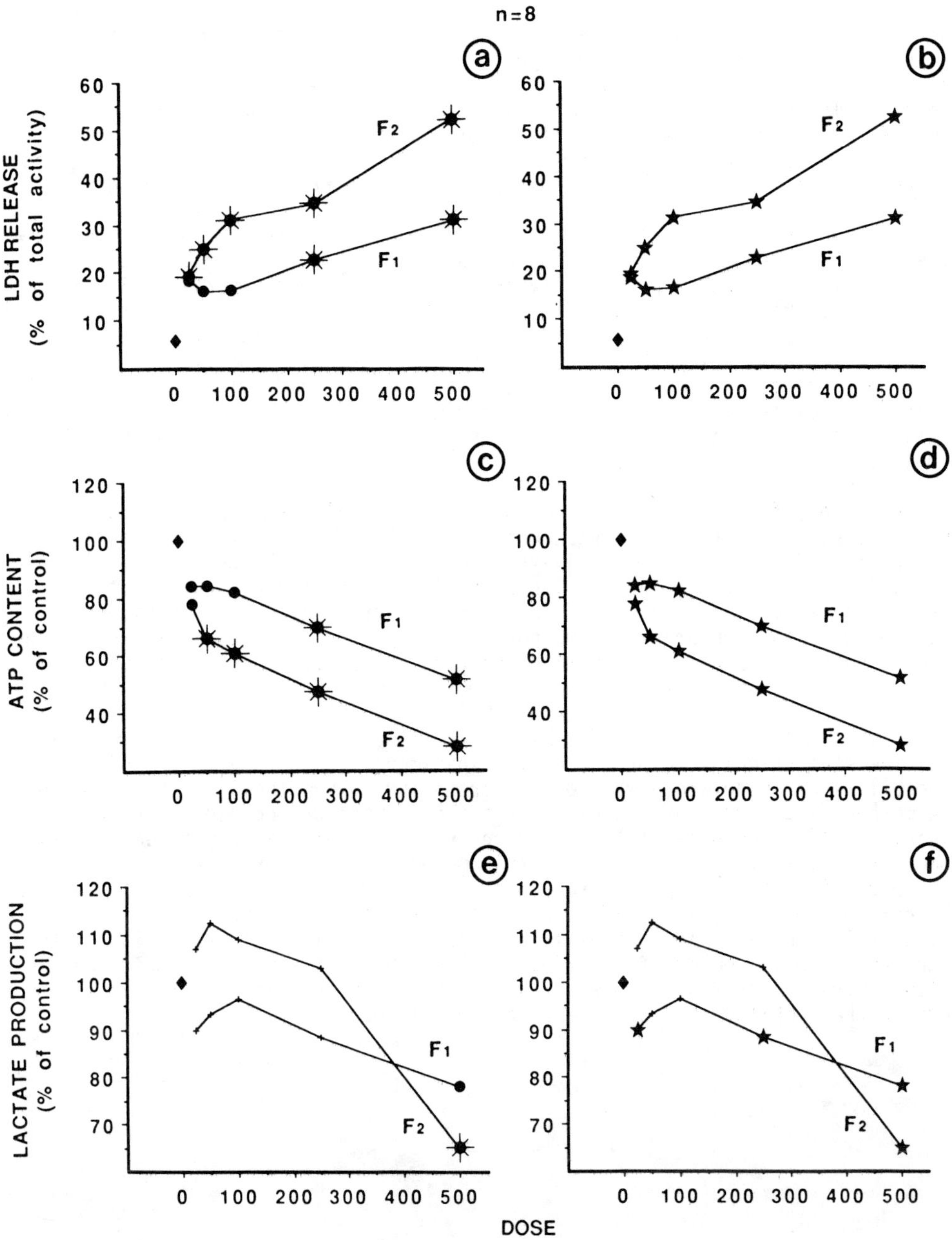

FIG 3. Statistical significance of the cytotoxicity parameters according to parametric (a,c,e) and nonparametric (b,d,f) approaches (n=8). F1: UICC B Chrysotile asbestos fibres; F2: DOLAN 10 polyacrylonitrile fibres.

(◆) Controls values.
(+) No difference with the control values.
(●) Difference with the control values according to Dunnett's and Duncan's tests.
(☼) Difference with the control values according to Scheffe's test.
(★) Difference with the control values according to Kruskal-Wallis' test.

homogenous sizes, with only a triplicate set of experiments. For that purpose, only two doses of particles were evaluated. As mentioned before, the references materials (TiO_2 and quartz DQ12) were selected because they are at each end of the spectrum of biological reactivity. In our culture conditions, the respectively low and high cytotoxicities of the TiO_2 and quartz particles towards PAM were confirmed (Table 4). For the calcium silicate fractions of KAYLO 10® (P1 and P2), there seems to be a difference in the biological response of each particle. This could be related to small differences in dimensions.

As seen in Figure 4, the calcium silicate samples are moderately cytotoxic to PAM when compared to the non-exposed cell monolayers (controls). With the LDH parameter, the nonparametric method show a slight edge in discrimination (Fig. 4; a vs b). As for the ATP levels, both types of statistical analysis are more or less equivalent; moreover, the parametric methods do not test equal as it was observed with the LDH parameter (Fig. 4; c vs d). For the third parameter, the production of lactic acid, only the highly cytotoxic DQ12-quartz particles present a statistical difference when compared to control PAM. Either statistical method was ineffective in revealing an effect for the KAYLO 10® samples.

With very few exceptions, the Table 5 shows that the nonparametric analysis is equivalent or better than those obtained with the parametric methods for showing the differences in reactivity between each and everyone of the particles tested. This observation appears to be valid for the three cytotoxicity parameters measured. Finally, a summary of the trend of each comparison obtained with the nonparametric method, that is if the biological effect of the mineral particles are lower, equal or higher, is presented in Table 6.

CONCLUSION

The statistical interpretation of experimental data is a matter of probability of being wrong when one is proposing an hypothesis. The choice of one method of analysis over another is not easy when one considers the risk of misinterpreting the data (10). As demonstrated in this study, it seems that, in some cases, parametric and nonparametric methods can support the same interpretation of the experimental data. We found that the approach proposed by Theodorsson-Norheim (2) is relatively simple to implement on a small computer and that it can be quite a valuable tool for the statistical evaluation of the data from a small number of experiments. Moreover, this nonparametric approach allows overall comparisons between experimental groups that normally would require the combined uses of several parametric methods (1).

TABLE 4. Dose-related cytotoxic effects of mineral particles on PAM monolayers

Experimental groups	Dose[b] (μg)	Cytotoxicity parameters[a] LDH (%)	ATP (%)	LACTATE (%)
Controls	0	5.3 ± 1.4[c]	100.0 ± 3.9	100.0 ± 5.0
Quartz DQ12	50	59.7 ± 3.4	20.0 ± 1.9	43.7 ± 13.8
	250	74.5 ± 4.1	7.5 ± 1.5	49.5 ± 13.7
TiO_2	50	7.9 ± 2.1	90.1 ± 9.7	101.0 ± 6.6
	250	7.8 ± 0.8	87.4 ± 8.2	99.3 ± 7.8
KAYLO 10 (P1)	50	8.9 ± 0.3	108.9 ± 14.6	117.5 ± 18.0
	250	43.3 ± 3.1	56.0 ± 6.5	98.1 ± 9.6
KAYLO 10 (P2)	50	20.6 ± 3.0	84.4 ± 13.7	108.9 ± 7.3
	250	59.5 ± 5.6	42.3 ± 6.8	88.7 ± 10.5

a See the legends of TABLES 1 to 3 for more details.

b The actual total amounts assayed are 12.5 and 62.5 μg (See MATERIALS AND METHODS for more details).

c Mean values ± S.E.

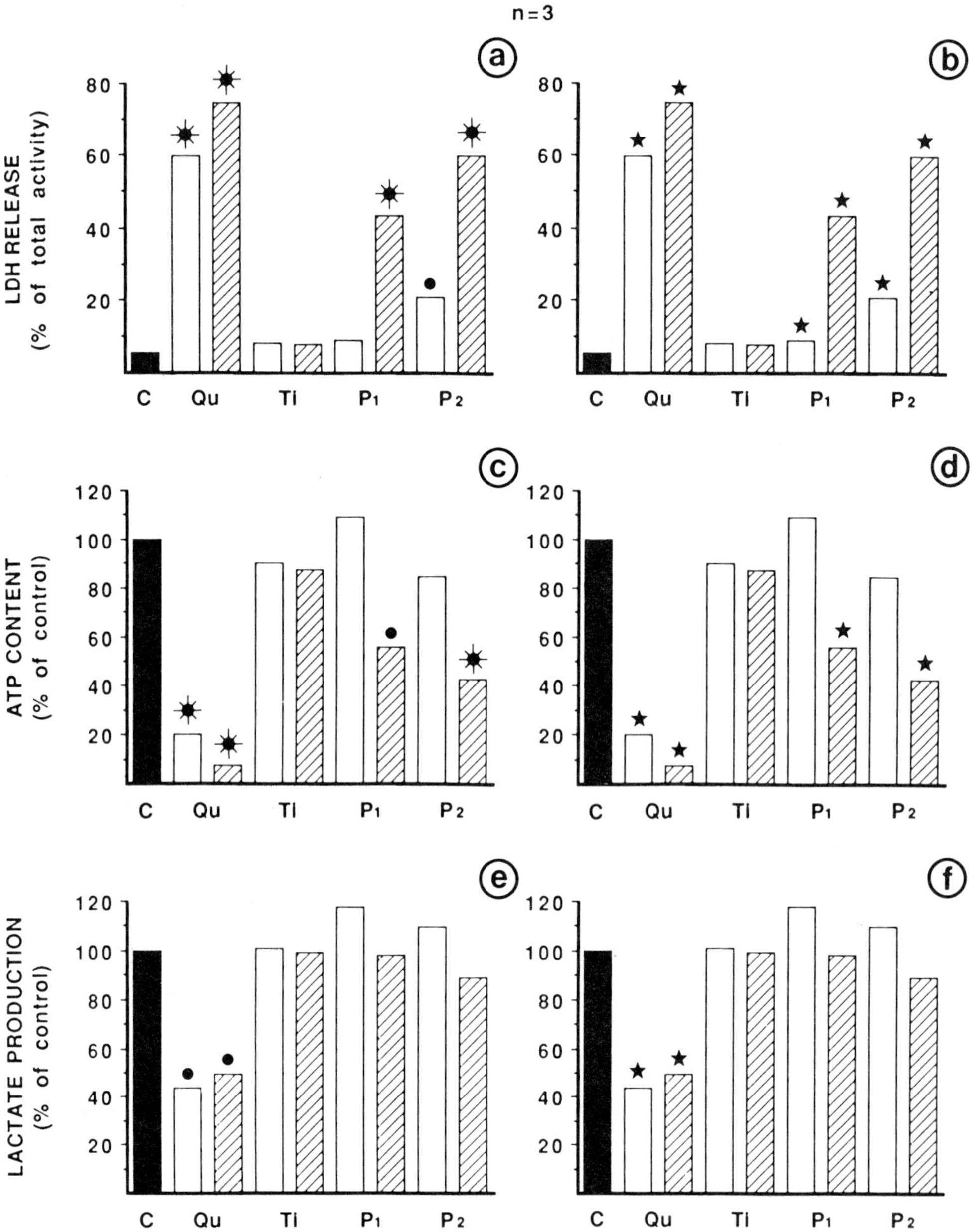

FIG 4. Statistical significance of the cytotoxicity parameters according to parametric (a,c,e) and nonparametric (b,d,f) approaches (n=3), for low (□) and high (▨) doses of different mineral particles. Quartz DQ12 (Qu); Titanium dioxide (Ti); KAYLO 10, fraction 1 (P1); and KAYLO 10, fraction 2 (P2); Control values (c).

(●) Difference with the control values according to Dunnett's and Duncan's tests.
(☼) Difference with the control values according to Scheffe's test.
(★) Difference with the control values according to Kruskal-Wallis' test.

TABLE 5. Multiple comparisons of the biological effects of different mineral particles on PAM and statistical significance of each cytotoxicity parameter according to parametric and nonparametric approaches.

LDH releases

	A	B	C	D	E	F	G	H	I
A	X	abc	abc	---	---	a	abc	a c	abc
B		X	c	abc	abc	abc	c	abc	---
C			X	abc	abc	abc	abc	abc	c
D				X	---	---	abc	a c	abc
E					X	---	abc	a c	abc
F						X	abc	c	abc
G							X	b c	c
H								X	abc
I									X

ATP levels

	A	B	C	D	E	F	G	H	I
A	X	abc	abc	---	---	---	a c	---	abc
B		X	---	abc	abc	abc	c	abc	---
C			X	abc	abc	abc	a c	abc	c
D				X	---	---	a c	---	abc
E					X	---	a c	---	a c
F						X	abc	---	abc
G							X	a c	---
H								X	a c
I									X

Lactate productions

	A	B	C	D	E	F	G	H	I
A	X	a c	a c	---	---	---	---	---	---
B		X	---	a c	a c	abc	a c	abc	c
C			X	a c	a c	abc	a c	abc	c
D				X	---	---	---	---	---
E					X	---	---	---	---
F						X	---	---	---
G							X	---	---
H								X	---
I									X

A Controls (n=3)
B Quartz DQ12 low dose (50 µg)*
C Quartz DQ12 high dose (250 µg)**
D TiO_2 low dose
E TiO_2 high dose
F P1 particle of KAYLO 10 low dose
G P1 particle of KAYLO 10 high dose
H P2 particle of KAYLO 10 low dose
I P2 particle of KAYLO 10 high dose

--- Not statiscally different
a Significant difference according to Kruskal-Wallis' test (2)
b Significant difference according to Scheffe's test (8)
c Significant difference according to Duncan's test (9)

* Actual amount tested: 12.5 µg
** Actual amount tested: 62.5 µg
(See MATERIALS AND METHODS for more details)

TABLE 6. Comparisons of the biological effects of different mineral particles on PAM and statistical significance of each cytotoxicity parameter according to a nonparametric approach.

	LDH releases									ATP levels									Lactate productions								
	A	B	C	D	E	F	G	H	I	A	B	C	D	E	F	G	H	I	A	B	C	D	E	F	G	H	I
A	X	<	<	=	=	<	<	<	<	X	>	>	=	=	=	>	=	>	X	<	<	=	=	=	=	=	=
B		X	=	>	>	>	=	>	=		X	=	<	<	<	=	<	=		X	=	<	<	<	<	<	<
C			X	>	>	>	>	>	=			X	<	<	<	<	<	=			X	<	<	<	<	<	<
D				X	=	=	<	<	<				X	=	=	>	=	>				X	=	=	=	=	=
E					X	=	<	<	<					X	=	>	=	>					X	=	=	=	=
F						X	>	=	<						X	>	=	>						X	=	=	=
G							X	=	=							X	<	=							X	=	=
H								X	<								X	>								X	=
I									X									X									X

A Controls (n=3)
B Quartz DQ12 low dose (50 μg)*
C Quartz DQ12 high dose (250 μg)**
D TiO_2 low dose
E TiO_2 high dose
F P1 particle of KAYLO 10 low dose
G P1 particle of KAYLO 10 high dose
H P2 particle of KAYLO 10 low dose
I P2 particle of KAYLO 10 high dose

= Not statiscally different
> Significantly higher according to Kruskal-Wallis' test (2)
< Significantly lower according to Kruskal-Wallis' test (2)

* Actual amount tested: 12.5 μg
** Actual amount tested: 62.5 μg
(See MATERIALS AND METHODS for more details)

REFERENCES

1. NADEAU, D., FOUQUETTE-COUTURE, L., PARADIS, D., KHORAMI, J., LANE, D. and DUNNIGAN, J. (1987), Cytotoxicity of respirable dusts from industrial minerals: comparison of two naturally occurring and two man-made silicates. Drug Chem. Toxicol. 10(1&2):49-86.

2. THEODORSSON-NORHEIM, E. (1986), Kruskal-Wallis test: BASIC computer program to perform nonparametric one-way analysis of variance and multiple comparisons on rank of several independent samples. Comput. Method. Program. Biomed. 23:57-62.

3. TIMBRELL, V. (1970), Characteristics of the International Union Against Cancer standard reference samples of asbestos. Proceedings of an International Conference on Pneumoconiosis, Johannesburg, 1969, H.A. Shapiro (Ed.) Oxford University Press, London, 28-36.

4. JOLICOEUR, C., ROBERGE, P. and FORTIER, J.L. (1981), Separation of short fibers from bulk chrysotile abestos fiber materials: analysis and physico-chemical characterization. Can. J. Chem. 59:1140-1148.

5. ROBOCK, K. (1973), Standard quartz DQ12 < 5 μm for experimental pneumoconiosis research projects in the Federal Republic of Germany. Ann. Occup. Hyg. 16:63-66.

6. ALLISON, A.C. (1978), Inflammatory and fibrogenic effects of toxic particles. Europ. J. Rheumat. Inflam. 1:130-134.

7. HILL, J.O. and HOBBS, C.H. (1982), Comparative cytotoxicity of DQ12-quartz and fly ash particles from coal combustion. Toxicol. Lett. 10:399-403.

8. TALLARIDA, R.J. and MURRAY, R.B. (1981), Manual of pharmacologic calculations with computer programs. Springer-Verlag New York Inc., 150 pages.

9. SAS Institute Inc. (1982), SAS User's Guide, 1982 Edition.

10. GORE, S.M., JONES, J.G. and RYTTER, E.C. (1977), Misuse of statistical methods: critical assessment of articles in BMJ from January to March 1976. Br. Med. J. 1:85-87.

FOOTNOTES

Send all correspondance and reprint requests to: Denis Nadeau, Ph.D.
This work was supported by L'Institut de l'amiante, Division de la Recherche, Montréal, Québec, Canada H3A 2M8 (Grant #19, Project LCA). The authors wish also to thank Mr. Bruno Gagné for the art work, Ms Réjeanne Laplante and Ms Linda Dawson for typing the manuscript, and Dr. Klauss Robock for kindly providing the DQ12-quartz sample.

Poster A13

In Vitro Ocular Irritancy Prediction: Assays in Serum-Free Media Correlate Better with *In Vivo* Data

CHARLES SHOPSIS[1] and BEN ENG[2]

[1]*Department of Chemistry*
Adelphi University
Garden City, NY 11530
[2]*Laboratory Animal Research Center*
The Rockefeller University
New York, NY 10021

ABSTRACT

To evaluate potential in vitro alternatives to the Draize test for ocular irritancy, several toxicity assay systems, culture conditions and target cells have been compared. A uridine uptake inhibition (UUI) assay, (Shopsis & Sathe, Toxicology 29:195, 1984, and a computer-coupled cell growth/protein accumulation (CGP) assay (Shopsis & Eng, Toxicol. Lett. 26:1-8, 1985) have been employed with 3T3 cells, NS-LMTK$^-$ cells (LMTK$^-$ cells adapted to growth in defined, serum-free medium) and tertiary normal human epidermal keratinocytes (NHEK cells, Clonetics Corp.). Seven surfactants and eight surfactant-based substances supplied by the Soap and Detergent Association, Inc. (SDA) for an interlaboratory validation study were used as test agents. With the pure surfactants, all assays and conditions ranked the test agents identically and correctly distinguished between the irritating cationic surfactants and the less toxic anionic and non-ionic compounds. With the SDA agents, for which detailed Draize scores were provided, correlation coefficients of comparisons of standardized scores for the in vivo and in vitro data were: for the UUI assay with 3T3 cells, serum-free, r = 0.77, in media with 10% fetal calf serum (FCS), r = 0.60. With the CGP assay, for 3T3 cells in media with 10% FCS, r = 0.58; for NS-LMTK$^-$ cells in serum-free medium, r = 0.79; for NHEK cells (serum-free) r = 0.87. Rank correlation coefficients of these analyses were patterned similarly. These data suggest that: 1) for the surfactant-based substances studied here, serum-free culture conditions are preferable for ocular irritancy prediction; 2) NHEK cells may be useful as substrates for in vitro toxicity tests.

INTRODUCTION

The development of *in vitro* toxicity testing procedures has received a great deal of attention in recent years. Concerns for animal welfare, for the reduction in cost of toxicity tests, and for the potential hazard of the large numbers of inadequately tested chemicals and mixtures in our environment have motivated this work. One major focus of interest has been the development of *in vitro* alternatives to the Draize test for ocular irritancy (1). The subjective endpoint and documented interlaboratory variability (2) of this test have made it a prime target for replacement.

A number of potential *in vitro* Draize test alternatives have been reviewed recently (3), but assessment of the relative merits and validity of these assays has been difficult, because few of the proposed tests have been applied to a large number of substrates, and no standard set of in vivo data against which these alternatives can be compared has been published. Many assay systems have been used to assess the toxicity of a few surfactants, and there has generally been good qualitative agreement, both among the various *in vitro* assay systems and in comparisons of *in vitro* data with *in vivo* descriptions of irritancy. However, these data are insufficient to determine the relative merits of the assay systems.

Our laboratory has developed several *in vitro* toxicity tests, on the assumption that a battery of such tests may be required to serve as pre-screening or replacement assays for *in vivo* tests (4). Two of these procedures are utilized in this study. One measures the effects of xenobiotics on the uptake of ^{3}H-uridine by cultured cells (5). This sub-lethal, reversible (6,7) toxic endpoint detects perturbations in the transport and accumulation of uridine, and thus detects damage to cell membrane function and reduction in activity of uridine kinase (UK), the rate-limiting metabolic event in uridine uptake. The activity of UK is high in actively growing cultures and low in quiescent cultures, and thus serves as an indicator of the growth status of cells (8). We have reported that this assay correlated well with the ocular irritancy with a large number of test agents (4,5,6,9,11,12), but the *in vivo* data used for these comparisons unavoidably consisted largely of qualitative, verbal descriptions of irritancy. The second assay system employed in this study is an automated cell growth assay in which growth is monitored as the accumulation of total cell protein (10). It's development was predicated on the idea that cell growth inhibition is an early and common manifestation of almost all toxic action. This assay system has also been applied to a large number of test agents (4,10,11,12), but as described above, assessment of its validity is compromised by the quality of the available *in vivo* data.

A recent interlaboratory study, sponsored by the Soap and Detergent Association, Inc.,(unpublished), provides a useful model for procedures that may help validate candidates for *in vitro* alternative assays. In this study eight coded surfactant-based test agents were supplied to a number of laboratories engaged in *in vitro* assay development. The agents were tested for ocular irritancy to rabbits by a contract laboratory, using standard Draize test procedures. Our laboratory analyzed these eight test substances with three different assay protocols during the "blind" phase of this study; the cell growth/protein assay applied to Balb/c 3T3 cells, and the uridine uptake inhibition procedure applied to these 3T3 cells in the presence and absence of serum in the "treatment" media. After the release of the in vivo data from this study, we applied two additional variations of the cell growth/protein assay to these test agents; the assay was applied to normal human epidermal keratinocytes (supplied by Clonetics Corp.) and mouse fibroblasts capable of growth in serum-free medium. In this report we compare the results of the application of these five *in vitro* toxicity testing protocols to surfactants and to the 8 SDA test agents.

MATERIALS AND METHODS

Cells and culture conditions

Balb/c 3T3, a mouse fibroblast cell line, was maintained as described previously (6). NS-LMTK⁻ cells were derived in our laboratory from LMTK cells (obtained from the American Type Culture Collection). LMTK are a derivative of mouse L929 cells that lack thymidine kinase and have minimal nutritional requirements. NS-LMTK⁻ cells were derived by serial passage of LMTK in DME/F12 media (comprised of a 1:1 mixture of Ham's F12 and Dulbecco's modified Eagle's medium (DMEM) and antibiotics as described previously, (6)), supplemented with successively lower concentrations of serum. Cells capable of growth in this defined, serum-free media were cloned and a colony picked for use in toxicity experiments. These cells grew well in suspension in DME/F12 media without any supplementation, and as adherent cells in DME/F12 media supplemented with 40 ug/ml recrystallized bovine serum albumin (Sigma Chemical Co., St. Louis, MO). They were used as adherent cultures in the experiments described here. For subculture, dishes were treated with trypsin and the cell suspensions obtained were treated with trypsin inhibitor prior to replating.

NHEK cells are normal human epidermal keratinocytes, obtained in their second passage from Clonetics, Corp., San Diego, CA. These cells, derived from patients undergoing elective surgical procedures, are cultured in KGM medium supplied by Clonetics, a serum-free low protein medium supplemented with growth factors. The cells were passaged by trypsinization and trypsin inhibitor treatment, using the protocols and reagents supplied by Clonetics, and were utilized for assay of toxicants in their third passage.

Assay Systems

Cell growth/protein assay

The growth inhibitory potencies of test agents were measured with an automated assay that detects their abilities to reduce the accumulation of total cell protein (10). Cells were plated at low density in 96 well tissue culture plates (3×10^3 per well for 3T3 cells, and 5×10^3 per well for NHEK and NS-LMTK⁻ cells). After 24 hrs, for 3T3 cells, or 48 hrs for the other cells, medium was removed and replaced with either the cells' normal growth medium, for control wells, or normal growth media containing various concentrations of test agents. Eight replicate wells served as controls, and each experimental treatment was applied to four replicate wells. After an additional 24 hrs (3T3 cells) or 48 hrs (NHEK or NS-LMTK⁻ cells), cultures were examined with phase microscopy to obtain a qualitative indication of toxic effects, media were again removed, and cells were washed twice in Tris-buffered saline pH 7.4 (TBS, (6)). At this point, plates can be stored indefinitely at -20°C. For analysis, cell protein was solubilized by adding 50 ul of 0.1N NaOH to each well. 200 ul of a 1:3 dilution of a Coomassie blue protein reagent (Bio-Rad, Richmond, CA) in distilled water was then added. A standard curve was prepared in row 1 of each plate using a stock solution of bovine serum albumin (BSA, 200 ug/ml in 0.1 N NaOH) by placing 0 to 10 ug of BSA in the wells, adding 0.1 N NaOH to a final volume of 50 ul, and then adding the Coomassie blue reagent as described above. The well with 0 ug BSA served as a blank. The plates were scanned in a Dynatech MR600 microplate reader, using a reference wavelength of 410 mu and an absorption wavelength of 630 mu. The data was sent to a microcomputer programmed to plot the standard curve and calculate the cell protein/well and the percent change in cell protein/well relative to mock-treated control wells. Control wells typically contain about 3.5 ug of cell protein at the end of the experiments, corresponding to an optical density of about 0.6. The concentration of test agent inducing a 50% decrease in cell protein (designated the P-50), determined as described in Data Analysis, below, was used to compare the potency of test agents.

Uridine uptake inhibition assay

The uridine uptake inhibition assay was performed as described previously (5,6). Briefly, 3T3 cells plated in 35 mm dishes at 5 X 10^4 per dish were incubated for 48 hrs in normal growth medium. Medium was then removed and triplicate cultures were treated with test media, consisting of either normal growth medium (DMEM supplemented with 10% fetal calf serum (FCS)) or DMEM (for serum-free experiments) containing various concentrations of test agents. After 4 hrs, test media were removed, cells were washed 2X with TBS, 1.0 ml of TBS and ^{3}H-uridine (33 uM, 1.67uCi/ml) were added to each dish, and cells were incubated for 15 min at 37^0. Cultures were then washed 3X with cold TBS and lysed with 0.1 N NaOH. One aliquot of the lysate was transferred to liquid scintillation vials and counted to determine uridine taken up, and another was analyzed for protein content. The concentration of test agent inducing a 50% decrease in uridine uptake (designated the UI-50), determined as described in data analysis, below, was used to compare the potency of test agents.

Determination of cell growth rates

Growth rates for the cells used in this study were determined by measuring the rate of accumulation of total cell protein. Cells were plated into 96 well culture plates at a density of 2 X 10^3 cells per well in the appropriate medium for each cell type as described in "Cells and Culture Conditions" above. At 24 hr intervals, 8 replicate wells were washed twice with TBS and drained, and the plate was then returned to the incubator. Cultures received fresh medium on the third and fifth days. After 7 days, the wells were analyzed for cell protein content as described for the cell growth/protein assay above. Doubling time was determined from the linear portion of plots of the log of cell protein vs. duration of incubation

Supplies

Antibiotics, media and serum were purchased from Gibco, Grand Island, NY. Other chemicals were purchased from Sigma Chemical Co., St. Louis, MO, and tissue culture dishes were obtained from Becton-Dickinson, Oxnard, CA. Eight test agents described in Table 2 were supplied by the Soap and Detergent Association, N.Y., NY, in the context of a blind interlaboratory study on the prediction of ocular irritancy.

Data Analysis

The toxic potencies of test agents in vitro were quantified by linear regression analysis of the relationship between log of test agent concentration and uridine uptake or cell protein per well relative to untreated control cultures. The concentration of test agent, in ug/ml, required to induce a 50% decrease in uridine uptake rate or total cell protein, designated the UI-50 and P-50 respectively, were interpolated from these analyses and used to quantify cytotoxicity. In vitro and in vivo data were then compared 1) by ranking the test agents and calculating Spearman rank correlation coefficients, and 2) by converting both sets of data to standard scores (so that both sets of data have a mean of 0 and and standard deviation of 1, and calculating correlation coefficients between the sets of standard scores. Because of the much broader numerical range of the in vitro data relative to the in vivo data (Table 3), in vitro data were transformed to their logarithms prior to the calculation of standard scores. Raw data and standard scores for the in vivo effects of the 8 SDA test agents were supplied by Arthur D. Little, Inc. on behalf of the Soap and Detergent Association.

RESULTS

Derivation of NS-LMTK⁻ Cells and Determination of Cell Growth Rates

One goal of this study was to determine the effects of serum in the test media on the results of in vitro toxicity assays. In the uridine uptake assay protocol, the period of exposure of cells to test media is relatively brief, enabling the use of serum-free media even with cells that require serum for growth. The longer exposure to test media in the cell growth/protein assay requires cells capable of growth in serum-free media for these comparisons. Therefore we adapted $LMTK^-$ cells to growth in defined, serum-free medium as described in Methods. These cells (called $NS\text{-}LMTK^-$), when plated at a density of 2×10^3 in 96 well plates, grow with a doubling time of 25 hrs. NHEK cells cultured in serum-free KGM medium have a similar growth rate, doubling every 24 hrs. The doubling time for 3T3 cells cultured in DMEM and supplemented with 10% FCS was 14 hrs. The initial cell densities and incubation times for the cell growth/protein assay, described in Methods, were based on these determinations.

Table I compares the cytotoxicities of seven surfactants, using the uridine uptake assay on Balb/c 3T3 cells treated in the presence and absence of serum, and the cell growth/protein assay on: 3T3 cells tested in the presence of 10% serum, and, in serum-free medium, $NS\text{-}LMTK^-$ cells and NHEK cells. The relative rank of toxicity of the surfactants is identical with all protocols. However, the absolute values of the UI-50's and P-50's for anionic and non-ionic surfactants are lower in the three serum-free protocols. The relative ranking of cytotoxicity of these seven agents are in accord with their ocular irritancies; the cationic surfactants cetyl pyridinium bromide and benzalkonium chloride are strongly irritating, anionic surfactants (Na lauryl SO_4 and triethanolamine lauryl SO_4) are less irritating and the non-ionic Tween 40, 60, and 80 are least irritating (13,14). It is noteworthy that the UI-50 and P-50 values are similar for 3T3 cells treated with test agents in 10% FCS, despite the differences in duration of the test agent treatment in those assay procedures (4 hrs vs. 24 hrs).

Table 1

Cytotoxicity of Surfactants in Various Assay Conditions

Test Agent	Uridine Uptake Assay[1] 3T3 Cells No Serum	Uridine Uptake Assay[1] 3T3 Cells 10 % Serum	Cell Growth/Protein Assay[2] 3T3 10 % Serum	Cell Growth/Protein Assay[2] NS-LMTK⁻ No Serum	Cell Growth/Protein Assay[2] NHEK No Serum
Cetyl pyridinium Br	0.01	0.01	0.2	0.1	0.2
Benzalkonium Cl	0.5	0.7	0.3	3.0	0.35
Sodium lauryl SO_4	29	80	74	6	6
Triethanolamine lauryl SO_4	89	180	160	9	15
Tween 40	100	225	165	45	30
Tween 60	111	230	180	55	35
Tween 80	ND	400	380	70	40

1. Uridine uptake inhibition assay as described in Methods. Data are the UI-50 values, the concentrations of test agents, in ug/ml, that reduce uridine uptake by 50%.
2. Cell growth/protein assay as described in Methods. Data are the P-50 values, the concentrations of test agents, in ug/ml, that reduce total cell protein by 50%.

Table 2 lists the eight agents received in the Soap and Detergent Association (SDA) sponsored interlaboratory in vitro assay validation study, and indicates their compositions, pH's, and ocular irritancies. In contrast to the single component substances whose in vitro toxicities are listed in Table 1, 6 of these substances are complex mixtures typical of the final product formulations that are tested for ocular irritancy by commercial enterprises.

Table 3 lists the average maximum Draize scores and in vitro cytotoxicities (using the 5 assay protocols employed in the experiment described in Table 1) of the eight SDA agents. In contrast to the results obtained with "pure" surfactants (Table 1), the relative ranking of cytotoxicity of the SDA agents differed in the various assay protocols. Although the maximum Draize score data would suggest that the in vivo ranking of agents 1, 2 and 5 are indistinguishable, differences in other aspects of the Draize test results (days required for ocular damage to clear, median Draize score, etc.) yielded clear distinctions between these agents (see Table 4).

The scoring scales of the Draize test and the in vitro tests differ markedly. The former is scored on a non-parametric scale with a minimum of 0 and a maximum of 110, representing the sum of 3 distinct components of ocular injury, subjectively determined after treatment with a single concentration of test agent. The in vitro endpoints in this study, determined from an analysis of dose-response data, are the concentrations of test agent in ug/ml that produce a 50% effect in the indicated parameter. For the 8 SDA test agents, these values ranged from 0.01 to almost 8000 ug/ml. In order to make quantitative comparisons between the two sets of data, the raw data was converted to standard or "Z" scores as described in Methods. Table 4 presents such standard scores for the five sets of in vitro toxicity determinations performed on the 8 SDA agents, along with the standard scores provided by the SDA for the ocular irritancies of these materials. The standard scores for the ocular irritancies of the SDA agents are based a composite of the scores for the average maximum Draize score of the animals tested, the median score, the days required for clearance of ocular damage, and the scores for damage to the cornea, iris, and conjunctiva. These data were provided by the Soap and Detergent Association.

Table 5 provides correlation coefficients that compare the in vitro effects of the eight SDA agents, as determined with the 5 assay protocols, to the ocular irritancies of these materials. Part A makes comparisons between the standard scores for the in vitro assays and the standard scores of both the various components of the Draize test and the composite standard score of the Draize test. The serum-free in vitro protocols provide higher correlation coefficients than the assays carried out in serum-containing media, with the cell growth/protein assay applied to NHEK cells yielding the highest correlations. Part B of Table 5 indicates the results of analogous comparisons between the rankings of toxicity of the 8 SDA agents in the 5 in vitro assays and the Draize test. As with the standard score correlation coefficients, these Spearman rank correlation coefficients are higher when serum-free in vitro assays are compared to the in vivo data, and highest for the cell growth/protein assay applied to NHEK cells.

Table 2

Composition of Soap and Detergent Association Test Samples[1]

Code #	Component	Weight Percent	pH, 1% solution	Ocular[2] Irritancy
1.	Na lauryl SO_4	92.9	7.6	moderate
2.	Liquid laundry detergent		7.0	moderate
	water	50-74		
	alkyl ethoxylate	10-24		
	ethanol	5-9		
	ditallow dimethyl ammonium chloride	1-4		
3.	Liquid laundry detergent		7.0	extreme
	water	50-74		
	linear alkylbenzene sulfonate	25-49		
	alkyl ethoxylate	10-24		
	ethanol	5-9		
	triethanolamine	1-4		
	coconut fatty acid	1-4		
	magnesium hydroxide	1-4		
4.	Light duty liquid household cleaner		9.1	mild
	water	75-99		
	2-butoxyethanol	1-4		
	trisodium phosphate	1-4		
	linear alkylbenzene sulfonate	1-4		
5.	Light duty liquid detergent		7.1	moderate
	water	50-74		
	magnesium alkyl ethoxylate SO_4	25-49		
	magnesium alkyl SO_4	5-9		
	ethanol	5-9		
	ammonium chloride	1-4		
	ammonium xylene sulfonate	1-4		
	alkylamine oxide	1-4		
6.	Granular laundry detergent		10.3	severe
	complex Na phosphates	25-49		
	Na SO_4	25-49		
	Na carbonate	10-24		
	water	5-9		
	Na alkyl SO_4	5-9		
	Na alkyl ethoxylate SO_4	5-9		
	Na linear alkylbenzene sulfonate	1-4		
	Na silicate	1-4		
7.	Granular laundry detergent		8.9	moderate
	Na SO_4	40-50		
	Na carbonate	25-35		
	Na linear alkylbenzene sulfonate	10-15		
	water	3-5		
8.	Tween 20	100	5.8	non-irritating

1. Information on composition and irritancy provided by the Soap and Detergent Association.
2. Ocular irritancy classification based on Draize test scores according to the scale of Kay and Calandra (15).

Table 3

Draize Scores and Cytotoxicity of SDA Test Agents

SDA Agent[1]	Average Maximum Draize Score[2]	Uridine Uptake Assay[3] 3T3 Cells No Serum	Uridine Uptake Assay[3] 3T3 Cells 10 % FCS	Cell Growth/Protein Assay[4] NHEK Cells	Cell Growth/Protein Assay[4] NS-LMTK⁻ Cells	Cell Growth/Protein Assay[4] 3T3 Cells 10 % FCS
1	23.2	26	90	9.2	5.3	84
2	24.2	9	17	22	2.6	19
3	52.2	5	21	6	3.8	22
4	3.0	1153	7700	222	367	6750
5	24.3	61	297	31	13	214
6	33.7	91	548	16	16	436
7	30.0	48	318	12	18	331
8	0	107	186	92	50	152

1. Soap and Detergent Association code number. See Table 2.
2. Data supplied by the Soap and Detergent Association.
3. Uridine uptake inhibition assay as described in Methods. Data are the UI-50 values, the concentrations of test agents, in ug/ml, that reduce uridine uptake by 50%.
4. Cell growth/protein assay as described in Methods. Data are the P-50 values, the concentrations of test agents, in ug/ml, that reduce total cell protein by 50%.

Table 4

Standard Scores of SDA Test Agents In Vitro and In Vivo[1]

SDA Agent[2]	Draize	Uridine Uptake Assay[3] 3T3 Cells No Serum	Uridine Uptake Assay[3] 3T3 Cells 10 % FCS	Cell Growth/Protein Assay[4] NHEK Cells	Cell Growth/Protein Assay[4] NS-LMTK⁻ Cells	Cell Growth/Protein Assay[4] 3T3 Cells 10% FCS
1	-0.04	0.39	0.41	0.83	0.68	0.45
2	0.30	1.03	1.26	0.12	1.12	1.27
3	1.32	1.38	1.15	1.16	0.88	0.98
4	-1.24	-1.88	-1.88	-1.80	-1.99	-1.98
5	0.36	-0.12	-0.21	-0.19	0.12	-0.07
6	0.48	-0.36	-0.52	0.34	-0.01	-0.46
7	0.22	0.02	-0.24	0.62	-0.07	-0.31
8	-1.39	-0.46	0.03	-1.08	-0.73	0.11

1. Standard scores for Draize data, provided by the SDA, were computed from a composite of maximum, median, conjunctival, corneal and iridal scores and "days to clear" (15). Standard scores for in vitro data were computed from the UI-50 and P-50 data in Table 3 as described in Methods.
2. Soap and Detergent Association code number. See Table 2.
3. Concentration of test agent that reduces uridine uptake by 50%, as described in Methods.
4. Concentration of test agent that reduces total cell protein by 50%, as described in Methods.

Table 5

Correlation Coefficients
Components of Draize Test Scores vs. In Vitro Toxicity Data

A. Standard Score[1] Correlation Coefficients
Draize Test Standard Scores vs. *In Vitro* Assay Standard Scores

In Vivo	In Vitro Assays				
Draize Test Component	Uridine Uptake Assay		Cell Growth/Protein Assay		
	3T3 No Serum	3T3 10% FCS	3T3 10% FCS	NHEK No Serum	NS-LMTK⁻ No Serum
Maximum Draize	0.74	0.55	0.51	0.88	0.71
Corneal Score	0.72	0.59	0.53	0.70	0.60
Iridal Score	0.68	0.51	0.51	0.88	0.78
Days to Clear	0.75	0.63	0.62	0.70	0.79
Conjunctival Score	0.54	0.36	0.36	0.81	0.68
Median Score	0.76	0.63	0.59	0.76	0.71
Composite Score[2]	0.77	0.60	0.58	0.87	0.79

B. Spearman Rank Correlation Coefficients
Draize Test Rank vs. *In Vitro* Assay Ranks

In Vivo	In Vitro Assays				
Draize Test Component	Uridine Uptake Assay		Cell Growth/Protein Assay		
	3T3 No Serum	3T3 10% FCS	3T3 10% FCS	NHEK No Serum	NS-LMTK⁻ No Serum
Maximum Draize	0.55	0.07	0.07	0.69	0.45
Corneal Score	0.66	0.36	0.36	0.61	0.71
Iridal Score	0.46	0.00	0.00	0.62	0.39
Days to Clear	0.76	0.47	0.47	0.53	0.77
Conjunctival Score	0.22	-0.28	-0.28	0.51	0.18
Median Score	0.68	0.43	0.43	0.63	0.78
Composite Score[2]	0.52	0.10	0.10	0.62	0.50

1. Standard scores were derived as described in the text.
2. Composite standard scores, provided by the SDA, are the averages of standardized scores for the six Draize test components listed.
3. Composite rank is based on the sum of the ranks of scores of these six Draize test components. These *in vivo* data were provided by the Soap and Detergent Association.

DISCUSSION

The great interest in the development of alternative *in vitro* toxicity assays has resulted in a large number of prospective alternatives to the Draize test for ocular irritancy (3). A major impediment to the application of these systems to toxicity testing in regulatory, industrial and research laboratories is the lack of data available to enable their validation. Interlaboratory studies, such as the Soap and Detergent Association sponsored effort described in part here, provide a very valuable means for obtaining the needed validation data.

The 5 assay conditions applied here provided identical rankings for pure surfactants (Table 1), suggesting that such "simple" test agents may be of limited use in distinguishing between various proposed *in vitro* assay systems. It is of interest in this regard that major differences in duration of test agent treatment (4 hrs vs. 24 hrs) had little effect on cytotoxicity. This is probably attributable to the rapid lytic action of these substances on cell membranes. Analogous studies using divalent metal salts as test agents resulted in similar rankings of toxicity but different sensitivities of cells in assays of differing durations (Shopsis, unpublished data).

In contrast, significant differences in ranking of toxicity was observed when the eight SDA agents were analyzed *in vitro* (Tables 3-5). Use of serum-free medium during treatment of the cells with test agents provided results that agreed better with *in vivo* data than the use of media containing 10% fetal calf serum. Of the 15 test substances examined in this report, 12 were substantially more cytotoxic in serum-free conditions, and the other three agents were similarly cytotoxic in the presence and absence of serum. This suggests that serum may interact with test agents to mitigate their cytotoxicities to varying extents. Serum has been shown to significantly alter the growth inhibitory potency (16) and genotoxicity (17) of test agents in other assay systems.

In this study three different cell systems were tested in serum-free conditions, and of these, results obtained with normal human epidermal keratinocytes (NHEK) correlated best with ocular irritancy. In contrast to the 3T3 and NS-LMTK⁻ cells, NHEK cells in their 3rd passage in KGM media retain many of the properties of differentiated cells. This feature may enable them to respond to chemical insult in a manner more closely akin to the cells of an living animal than do the cells of relatively undifferentiated cell lines. Continuing validation studies with substances representative of those used in toxicological assessments will be useful in determining the importance of culture conditions and the differentiated status of cells in *in vitro* toxicity assays.

ACKNOWLEDGMENTS

We thank the Soap and Detergent Association, Inc., for their development and support of the interlaboratory validation study, Revlon, Inc. for funding of the early stages of this work, and Clonetics, Corp. for supplying NHEK cells.

REFERENCES

1. DRAIZE, J.H., WOODWARD, G., and CALVERY, H.O., (1944), Methods for the study of irritation and toxicity of substances applied topically to the skin and mucous membranes. J. Pharmacol. Exp. Ther. 82:377.

2. WEIL, C.S. & SCALA, R.A., (1971), Study of intra- and inter-laboratory variability in the results of rabbit eye and skin irritation tests. Toxicol. Appl. Pharmacol., 19:276.

3. FRAZIER, J.M., GAD, S.C., GOLDBERG, A.M., McCULLEY, J.P., (1987), eds., A Critical Evaluation of Alternatives to Acute Ocular Irritation Testing, Mary Ann Liebert, Inc. NY.

4. SHOPSIS, C.S., BORENFREUND, E., STARK, D.M., (1987), Validation studies on a battery of potential in vitro alternatives to the Draize test, in Alternative Methods in Toxicology, vol. 5, A.M. Goldberg (Ed.), Mary Ann Liebert, Inc. NY., 31-44.

5. SHOPSIS, C.S., (1984), Inhibition of uridine uptake by cultured cells: a rapid, sub-lethal cytotoxicity test. J. Tiss. Cult. Meth. 9:19.

6. SHOPSIS, C.S., SATHE, S., (1984), Uridine uptake as a cytotoxicity test: correlations with the Draize test. Toxicology 29:195.

7. HYSMITH, R.H., WELCH, T.K., BOOR, P.J. (1987), The comparative study of cardiovascular toxins utilizing a sensitive indicator of sublethal toxic injury. In Vitro 23:129

8. KOREN, R., (1980), The relevance of the state of growth and transformation of cells to their patterns of metabolic uptake. Int. Rev. Cytol. 68:127.

9. SHOPSIS, C.S., BORENFREUND, E., WALBERG, J., STARK, D.M., (1985), A battery of potential alternatives to the Draize test: uridine uptake inhibition, morpholgical cytotoxicity, macrophage chemotaxis and exfoliative cytology. Fd. Chem. Toxic. 23:259.

10. SHOPSIS, C.S., ENG, B., (1985), Rapid cytotoxicity testing using a semi-automated protein determination on cultured cells. Toxicol. Lett. 26:1.

11. STARK, D.M., SHOPSIS, C.S., BORENFREUND, E., BABICH, H., (1986), Progress and problems in evaluating alternative assays in toxicology. Fd. Chem. Toxic. 24:449.

12. STARK, D.M., BORENFREUND, E., WALBERG, J., SHOPSIS, C.S., (1985), Comparison of several alternative assays for measuring potential toxicants. in Alternative Methods in Toxicology, vol. 3, A.M. Goldberg (Ed.), Mary Ann Liebert, Inc. NY., 371-390.

13. NORTH-ROOT H., YACKOVICH, F., DEMETRULIAS, J., GACULA, M., Jr., HEINZE, J. E., (1982), Evaluation of an in vitro cell toxicity test using rabbit corneal cells to predict the eye irritation potential of surfactants. Toxicol. Lett. 14:207.

14. GRANT, M.E., (1974), Toxicology of the Eye, 2nd edition, Charles C. Thomas, Springfield, IL.

15. KAY, J.H., CALANDRA, J.C., (1962), Interpretation of eye irritancy tests. J. Soc. Cosmet. Chem. 13:281.

16. MUMMERY, C.L., VAN DEN BRINK, S., VAN DER SAAG, P.T., DE LAAT, S.W., (1983), Screening for cytotoxicity in neuroblastoma cells 1. Dependence of growth inhibition on the presence of serum. Toxicol. Lett. 18:201.

17. COULOMB, H.M., GU, Z.W., LOIREAU, M., CHOUROULINKOV, I., (1984), Effect of serum concentration on cytotoxicity and sister chromatid exchange induction by a chemical carcinogen and by a diesel particulate extract in V79 hamster cells. Cancer Lett. 22:77.

Poster A14

The MTT *In Vitro* Cytotoxicity Test: Correlation with Cutaneous Irritancy in Two Animal Models

D.A. SWISHER, M.E. PREVO, and P.W. LEDGER

ALZA Corporation
950 Page Mill Road
Palo Alto, CA 94303

INTRODUCTION

In recent years there has been a great increase in the characterization and exploitation of in vitro assays for cytotoxicity (1). Objective evaluations and comparisons of tests have been published (2,3) and attempts have been made to correlate in vitro cytotoxicity measurements with in vivo irritancy data (4).

Among those attributes of cytotoxicity tests commonly considered to be advantageous are their suitability for the screening of numerous materials at a range of concentrations, and the generation of an objective endpoint measurement. Achievement of these features has been greatly aided by the widespread introduction of multi-well cell culture plates and scanning spectrophotometers ('ELISA readers').

As part of a program of research on the biology and biochemistry of the skin, we have made much use of a modification of the MTT (3-(4,5-dimethylthiazol-2-yl)-2,5-diphenyltetrazolium bromide) assay. Initially introduced by Mosmann (5) for use in determining proliferation or survival of cells in bioassays, this assay depends on the fact that MTT (which is yellow in aqueous solution at neutral pH) is metabolized by mitochondria of living cells to a blue formazan dye. When used as a cytotoxicity assay, spectrophotometric quantitation of the formazan generated by cells after their incubation with a toxic agent gives an indication of the number and/or metabolic activity of surviving cells.

Our modification of the MTT assay (6) uses normal human keratinocytes as target cells. The use of these cells in cytotoxicity assays has been proposed previously (7), but in our system the use of feeder layers has been obviated. The present study compares the relative in vitro toxicities of a range of compounds with their acute primary skin irritancy in the rabbit and the guinea pig.

METHODS

Cell culture. Keratinocytes were prepared from human facial skin by trypsinization of 0.3 mm split thickness sections. Cells were established in culture by seeding into collagen coated tissue culture plates in MCDB 153 (8) containing 5% fetal bovine serum (FBS). The following day, non-adherent cells were removed and medium was changed to serum-free MCDB 153.

At 50% confluency, cultures were passaged by trypsinization. After 3 or 4 passages on collagen, cultures were expanded in non-coated dishes and passaged into 96-well plates for MTT assay.

MTT assay. Our modification of the method of Mosmann has been described in detail elsewhere (6). Briefly, medium was removed from 96-well plates and 100 ul of medium (MCDB 153 + 5% serum) or medium containing dilutions of the agent being investigated were added to wells. Some wells were maintained in medium throughout the incubation; these served as 100% viability controls. Another series treated with 10 mM iodoacetamide (which inhibits all MTT metabolism) acted as a positive control. Peripheral wells were not used in the assay because they introduced considerable heterogeneity to the results (presumably because of evaporation). During incubations these were filled with sterile PBS. After 18 h, culture medium was removed and replaced with medium containing MTT at 0.5 mg/ml and the plates were returned to the incubator for a further 4 h. Plates were then flicked to remove medium and 200 ul of 0.04 M HCl in isopropanol was added to each well. Dissolution of the formazan which had been deposited in and around the keratinocytes was accelerated by agitating the plates on a mechanical shaker. MTT metabolism (generation of formazan) was quantitated on a 96-well plate spectrophotometer using a test wavelength of 540 nm. The spectrophotometer was linked to data reduction software which transformed absorbance values into percent absorbance obtained for negative control wells (live cells).

Cutaneous irritancy. Acute primary skin irritation tests were performed on both Hartley guinea pigs and albino rabbits. Animals were shaved on the dorsal surface the day before application of test materials. In most cases there were six sites per concentration of test material. In the rabbit, half of the sites were intentionally abraded by scraping with the tip of an 18 gauge needle. Materials were dissolved in aqueous vehicle, ethanolic vehicle or mineral oil (100 ul) and applied for 24 h under occlusion at different concentrations (0.01 - 10%). Skin sites were scored on a 1 to 4 scale for erythema and edema (9) at 2 h and 48 h after removal of the test material. The primary irritation index (PII) for a each concentration of test material was derived using the following formula:

$$PII = \frac{\text{Total score (erythema + edema)}}{\text{Number of sites x number of observations (2h and 48 h)}}$$

To facilitate comparison between irritation and cytotoxicity it was necessary to normalize PII scores. The molar concentration of agent applied to the skin was divided by the PII obtained at that concentration. This yielded the hypothetical concentration necessary to give a PII of one. Results were transformed to log values; linear regressions were performed and correlation coefficients were determined.

RESULTS AND DISCUSSION

Over 50 materials have been screened in our laboratory using the MTT assay. Of these, acute primary skin irritancy data have been determined for 12 materials in the rabbit and 13 (mostly different materials) in the guinea pig. *In vitro* cytotoxicity (MI50) and cutaneous irritancy for these compounds are given in Tables I and II. Values are plotted and the linear regression shown in Figs 1 and 2. A correlation coefficient of 0.668 was obtained for the rabbit correlation and 0.677 for the guinea pig.

The *in vitro* and *in vivo* studies described here were not originally performed with the intention of determining the correlation between the two. Because of this, the materials investigated have a wide range of pharmacological and physicochemical properties), very different permeation

Table I: In vitro cytotoxicity and cutaneous irritancy in the rabbit

#	Material	Cytotoxicity [MI50 (M)]	Cutaneous Irritancy [concentration (M)/PII]
1	permeation enhancer A	3.2e-4	3.0e-2
2	propranolol	4.7e-4	8.0e-2
3	therapeutic agent A	6.2e-4	1.1e-1
4	n-decylmethyl sulfoxide	6.2e-4	8.7e-2
5	formaldehyde	7.8e-4	8.3e-1
6	therapeutic agent B	1.0e-3	6.2e-1
7	permeation enhancer B	2.1e-3	1.5e-2
8	therapeutic agent C	2.9e-3	7.0e-2
9	permeation enhancer C	4.2e-3	1.3e 0
10	therapeutic agent D	4.6e-3	1.8e-1
11	permeation enhancer D	1.1e-2	3.3e-1
12	ethanol	1.0e 0	5.7e-0

Table II: In vitro cytotoxicity and cutaneous irritancy in the guinea pig

#	Material	Cytotoxicity [MI50 (M)]	Cutaneous Irritancy [concentration (M)/PII]
1	therapeutic agent E	2.0e-5	5.1e-2
2	therapeutic agent F	2.8e-4	7.0e-3
3	therapeutic agent G	3.2e-4	5.3e-2
4	therapeutic agent H	4.0e-4	5.3e-2
5	therapeutic agent I	7.7e-4	5.9e-2
6	therapeutic agent J	9.5e-4	5.9e-2
7	therapeutic agent K	1.0e-3	1.1e-1
8	therapeutic agent L	1.9e-3	1.8e-2
9	clonidine	3.9e-3	5.3e-1
10	therapeutic agent D	4.6e-3	3.8e-1
11	therapeutic agent M	6.5e-3	2.3e-3
12	scopolamine	2.4e-2	4.3e-1
13	ethanol	1.0e 0	2.6e+1

Tables I & II: In vitro cytotoxicity concentrations and corresponding cutaneous irritancy values for a range of materials in the rabbit (I) and the Guinea pig (II). Cytotoxicity is measured as concentration of agent lowering MTT metabolism to 50% of control values. Cutaneous irritancy is the concentration (molarity) of agent divided by the irritation score at that concentration.

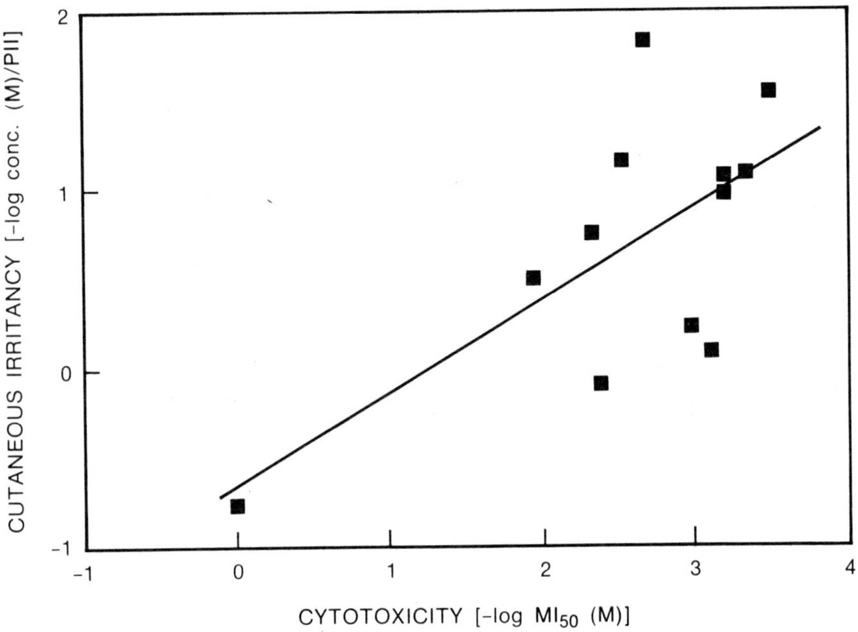

Fig. 1. Correlation between in vitro cytotoxicity towards human keratinocytes and cutaneous irritancy in the rabbit. The linear regression (fitted to log values) has a correlation coefficient (r) of 0.668.

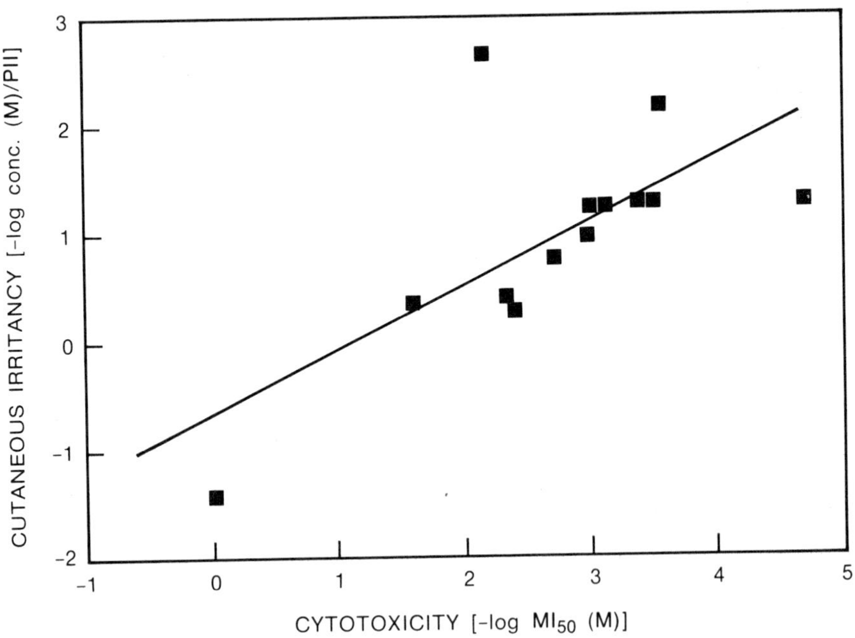

Fig. 2. Correlation between in vitro cytotoxicity towards human keratinocytes and cutaneous irritancy in the guinea pig (r = 0.677).

characteristics and potentially induce toxic/irritant reactions by different mechanisms. Consequently, the degree of correlation observed was considered surprisingly good. In our hands the MTT assay has proved particularly useful in determining the relative toxicities of compounds within a class, and for verifying the viability of cells after in vitro pharmacological investigations. Our present results suggest that this assay might also merit inclusion in any battery of assays designed to predict acute primary skin irritancy.

REFERENCES

1. Williams, G.M., Dunkel, V.C. and Ray, V.A. (Eds.) (1983) Cellular sytems for toxicity testing. Ann. N.Y. Acad. Sci. 407.

2. Riddell, R.J., Clothier, R.H. and Balls, M. (1986) An evaluation of three in vitro cytotoxicity assays. Fd Chem. Toxic. 24:469-471.

3. Know, P., Uphill, P.F., Fry, J.R., Benford, J.and Balls, M. (1986) The FRAME multicenter project on in vitro cytotoxicity. Fd Chem. Toxic. 24:457-463.

4. Hockley, K. and Baxter, D. (1986) Use of the 3T3 cell-neutral red uptake assay for irritants as an alternative to the rabbit (Draize) test. Fd Chem. Toxic. 24:473-475.

5. Mosmann, T. (1983) Rapid colorimetric assay for cellular growth and survival: Application to proliferation and cytotoxicity assays. J. Immun. Meth. 65:55-63

6. Swisher, D.A., Cormier, M., Johnson, J. and Ledger, P.W. A cytotoxicity assay using normal, human keratinocytes: Characterization and applications. Accepted for publication in Models in Dermatology Vol. 4. H.I. Maibach and N.J. Lowe (Eds.) Karger, Basel.

7. Mol, M.A.E., van Genderen, J. and Wolthius, O.L. (1986) Cultured human epidermal cells as a tool in skin toxicology. Fd Chem Toxic. 24:519-520.

8. Boyce, S.T. and Ham, R.A. (1985) Cultivation, frozen storage and clonal growth of normal human epidermal keratinocytes in serum-free medium. J. Tissue Cult. Methods 9:83-92

9. Draize, J.H., Woodward, G. Calverg, G. and Herbert, O. (1944) Methods for the study of irritation and toxicity of substances applied topically to the skin and mucous membranes. J. Pharmac. exp. Ther. 82:377-389.

Poster A15

Trans-Epithelial Permeability of Fluorescein *In Vitro* as an Assay to Determine Eye Irritants

RUY TCHAO

Department of Pathology
Medical College of Pennsylvania
3300 Henry Avenue
Philadelphia, PA 19129

ABSTRACT

An early effect of an injurious agent in the eye is increased permeability of the corneal epithelium. Normally, the epithelium maintains low permeability through tight junctions between the cells. Monolayer cultures of many established cell lines, including the Madin-Darby Canine Kidney (MDCK) cell line have tight junctions and exhibit permeability characteristics as observed in-vivo. We have grown MDCK cells as a monolayer on a filter in a special chamber, Millicell (Millipore Corp., Bedford, MA). for toxicity testing. We have shown that intact confluent MDCK monolayers will not allow the passage of Na-Fluorscein across the monolayer, whereas mechanically damaged or Na-Laural Sulfate treated cultures allowed the diffusion of Na-Fluorescein from one side of the epithelium to the other. We have tested several polyoxyethylene sorbitan (Tween compounds) in this new assay system, in contrast to other in-vitro cytotoxicity assays, we have shown that Tween 20, Tween 40 and Tween 60 are not toxic in this assay, and Tween 80 is mildly toxic. These results correspond well with the known Draize test results of these Tween compounds. We have also tested a variety of chemicals and commercial products in this assay, the results show that this is a dose dependent and quantitative assay. The degree of toxicity has also been correlated with the appearance in the scanning electron microscope of treated and untreated MDCK cultures. It is suggested that this in-vitro test system represent a suitable alternative for the Draize Rabbit Irritancy Test.

INTRODUCTION

The intregrity of trans-epithelial permeability is a major function of an epithelium such as the cornea and the skin. Trans-epithelial permeability is controlled by various epithelial junctions. The zonular occludens or tight junctions, which form a seal at the apical side of the epithelium and effectively prevent the passage of most molecules except water and some inorganic ions. The maculae adherens or desmosomes provide the strength in cell to cell connection as well as permeability barriers.

The corneal epithelium has both tight junctions and desmosomes (1). When an irritant or a toxic agent interacts with the cornea, one of the first physiological events is the loss of the permeability barrier. The tight junctions are disrupted and desmosomal junctions separate, leading to loss of cell contact and evetually to cell detachment (2,3,). The development of corneal opacity after sodium dodecyl sulfate (SDS) treatment is thought to be the permeation of SDS across the epithelium and reacting with the stroma (4).

Epithelial cells in culture such as MDCK, of dog kidney origin, also develop functional tight junctions and desmosomes. (see review by Cereijdo,(5)). In confluent monolayers of these cells grown on impermeable substrates such as glass or plastic, the sheet of cells engages in transepithelial transport of fluid, and "domes" develop in the monolayer (6). The mechanism of transepithelial fluid transport by MDCK cells have been studied extensively (7,8,9).

An accurate and direct measurement of transepithelial transport activity is the electrical potential and resistance across the epithelium. There are however, significant limitations; measurements can be made only on one membrane at a time. The equipment and chambers are not readily available. Therefore we have developed a rapid and quantitative method of assaying the MDCK transepithelial permeability in response to toxic agents. In this method, irritants as well as non-irritants, according to the Draize Eye test, can be tested. This report will describe the methodology of this assay and the testing of a series of Tween compounds that have caused difficulties in other in-vitro assays. This new assay system has the potential to be a suitable in-vitro alternative to replace the Draize Eye Test.

MATERIAL AND METHODS

MDCK cell line has been routinely cultured in T-75 flask in our laboratory since 1972. The culture medium is MEM supplemented with 10% fetal bovine serum and gentamycin (1ug/ml). The stock culture is passed at weekly interval using trypsin-versene. For toxicity assay, we are using the recently developed Millicell insert by Millipore Corp., Bedford, MA. This insert cylinder is 12 mm in diameter with a HATF (surfactant free) filter membrane sealed to one end. The inserts are then placed in a 24-well culture plate, each well contains 0.5 ml medium. By seeding $1.5x10^5$ MDCK cells in each insert, a confluent monolayer of MDCK cells covers the filter surface in 3 days which can be varified by examining stained fixedcultures. The cultures are fed daily by changing the medium inthe inserts and in the wells. A 24-well plate allows testing a compound at 6 concentrations with 4 replicates of each. When the cultures are confluent, the medium in each insert is removed and the cells rinsed with buffered Hanks Balanced Salt Solution (HBSS). Each insert is then placed in a fresh 24-well plate and 0.5 ml HBSS buffer containing a specific amount of the test agent is added to each insert. After 15 minutes incubation at 24° without shaking, the contents of the insert is decanted off and the insert gently rinsed 3 times, each with 1 ml of buffer. 0.5 ml buffer containing 0.02% Na-Fluorescein is added to each insert which is placed in a fresh 24-well plate, each well containing 0.5 ml buffer. After incubating for 30 minutes at 24°, the inserts are removed and the amount of Na-fluorescein in each well is diluted to 3 ml. for measurement in a spectrophotometer at 490 nm absorbance. Membranes after the diffusion assay are fixed for examination with light and electron microscopy.

For scanning electron microscopy the Millicell insert is fixed for 1 hour in 2.5% glutaraldehyde in 0.1 M cacodylate buffer at pH 7.2. After dehydration with graded alcohols, the insert is immersed in hexamethyldisilazane for 10 minutes and air dried. The dried filter is then cut out of the insert and mounted on a metal stud using silver paint or double-sided Scotch-tape, with the cell-side facing up. The specimen is coated with carbon and then gold/palladium in a Denton Vacuum evaporator, model DV-502 and viewed in a Hitachi model S450 SEM.

SDS,Tween compounds are bought from Sigma Chemical Co.,St.Louis, MO. The light duty cleaner is Windex.

RESULTS

An experiment to demonstrate the feasibility of using Millicell is shown in table 1:

TABLE 1

	Permeability to 0.02% Na-Fluorescein Measured at 490 nM at 20 minutes
Control, confluent MDCK culture	0.007
Culture 1/2 removed mechanically	0.582
Culture treated with 1% SDS for 2 mins. (no cells remained on filter)	1.123

This experiment shows that by removing partially or completely the cells grown on the filter, Na-Fluorescein diffusion across the filter is considerably facilitated. The data also showed that intact confluent layer of MDCK would not allow Na-Fluorescein to pass from the Millicell insert to the outside well.

The diffusion rate of Na-Fluorescein across a filter without cells has been studied. By 60 minutes, the Na-Fluorescein in the Millicell has equilibrated completetly with the buffer in the outside well. At 30 minutes, about 80-90% equilibration is reached.

The next series of experiments show that permeability of a monolayer of MDCK to Na-Fluorescein is dependent on the length and conditions of SDS treatment and the dose of SDS.

Fig.1 shows that permeability increased with increase in time of SDS treatment. A linear relationship of increased permeability with time was obtained from 10 minutes to 20 minutes of treatment, therefore an incubation time of 15 minutes was selected for this study.

The effect of shaking on a gyratory shaker at 100 rpm has been examined. Shaking the plate containing Millicell insert without cells increased the diffusion of Na-Fluorescein by 10-20%. When cells have been grown on the filter, in control cultures, there is no increase in the

FIGURE 1

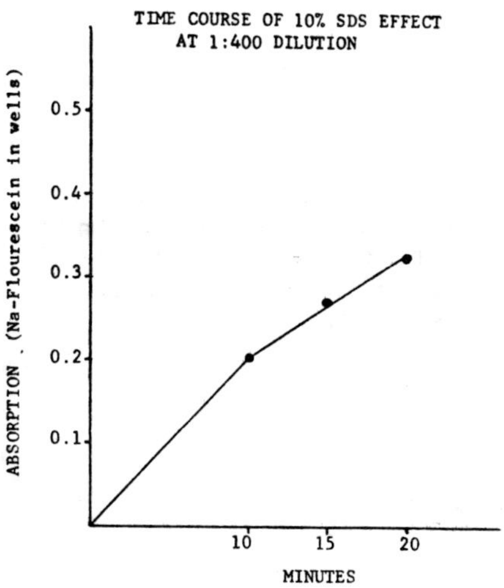

FIGURE 2

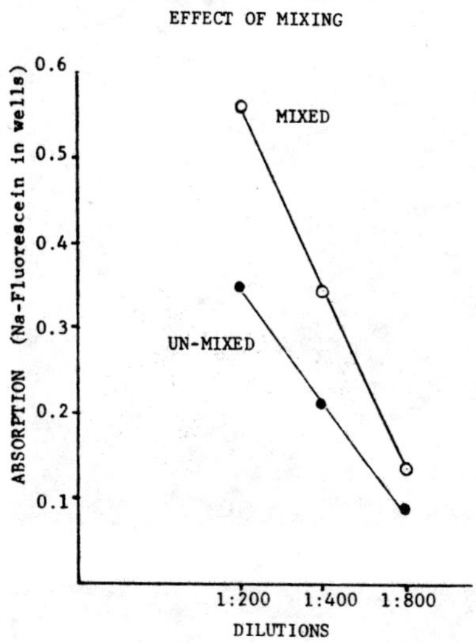

FIGURE 3

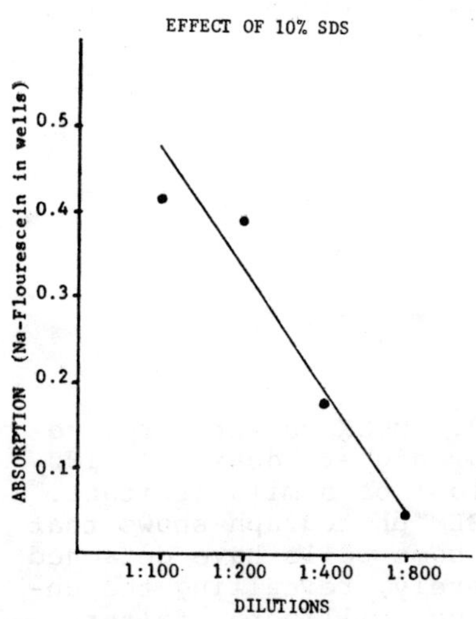

FIGURE 4

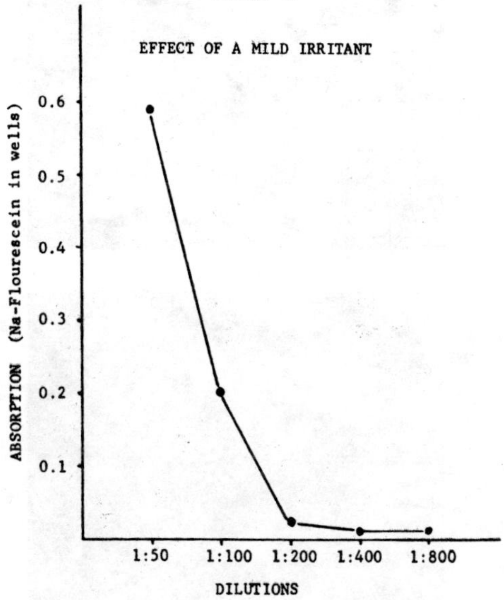

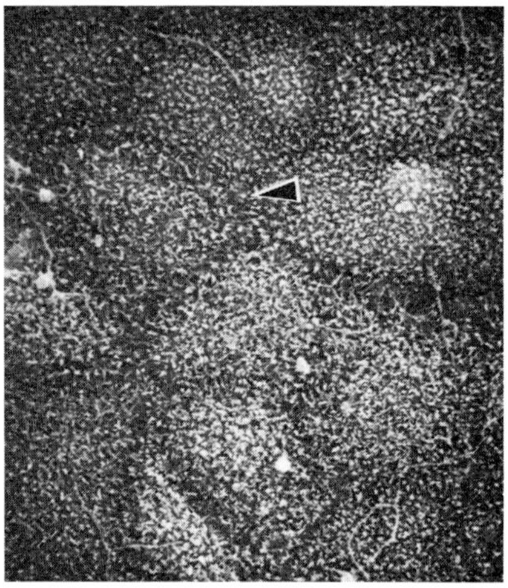

Fig. 5 SEM photograph of control MDCK culture showing good cell to cell junctions, (indicated by an arroehead), X 1100.

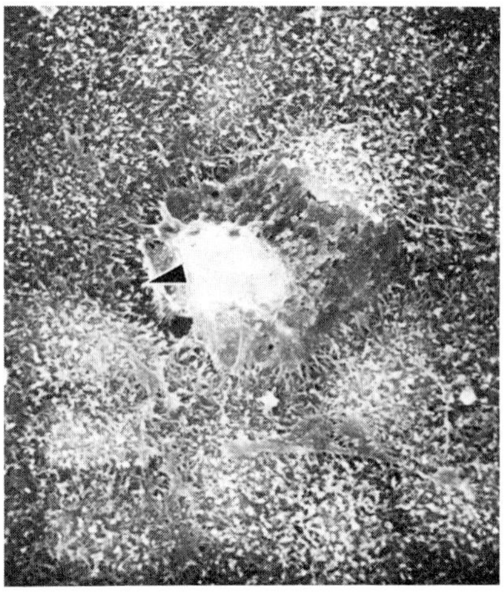

Fig.6. MDCK culture treated with a low dose (1:200 dilution) of a mild irritant. This SEM photograph shows one cell detached from its neighbors, the cell junctions (indicated by an arrowhead), are damaged. X1100

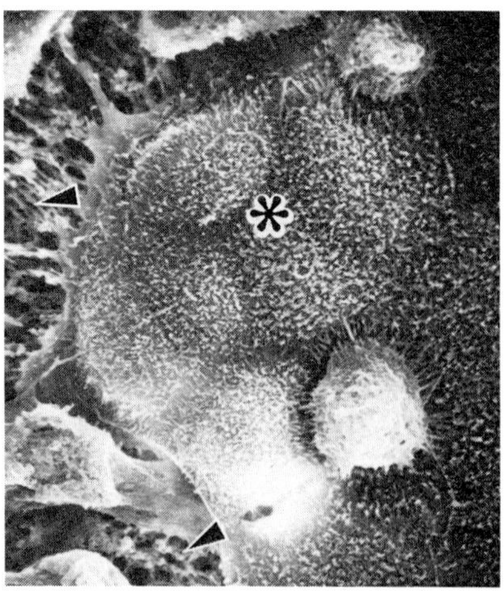

Fig. 7. MDCK culture treated with a higher dose (1:100 dilution) of a mild irritant. This SEM photograph shows that while some cells have detached completely, revealling the underlying Millipore filter, (indicated by arrowheads),many cells seem to be undamaged, (indicated by a star). X1100

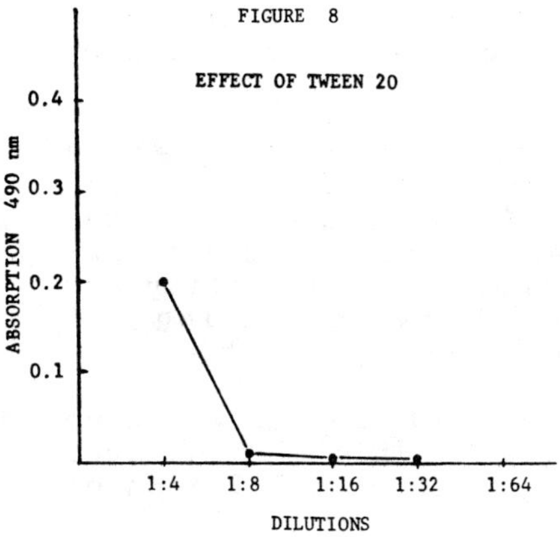

FIGURE 8

EFFECT OF TWEEN 20

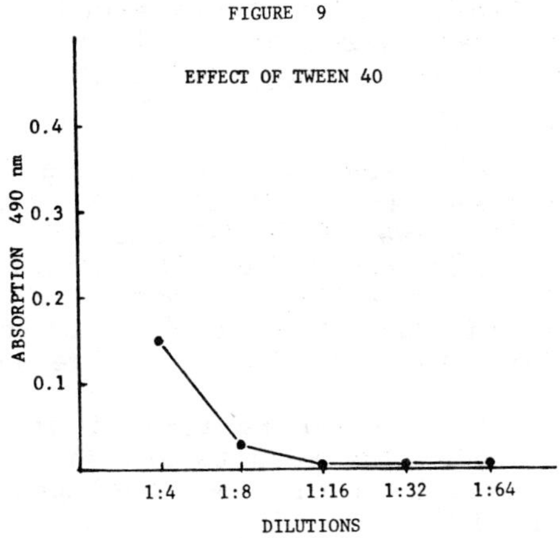

FIGURE 9

EFFECT OF TWEEN 40

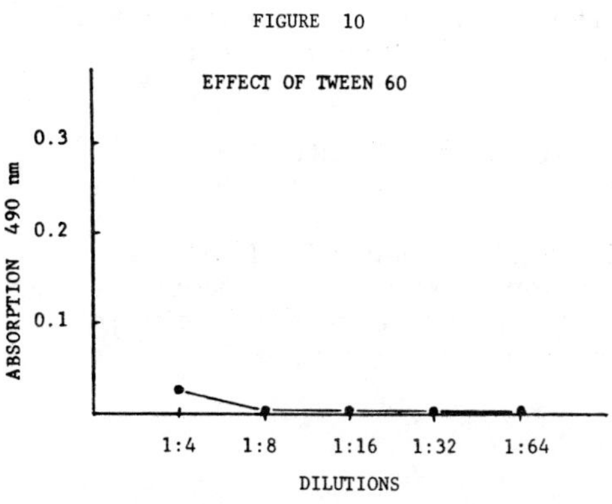

FIGURE 10

EFFECT OF TWEEN 60

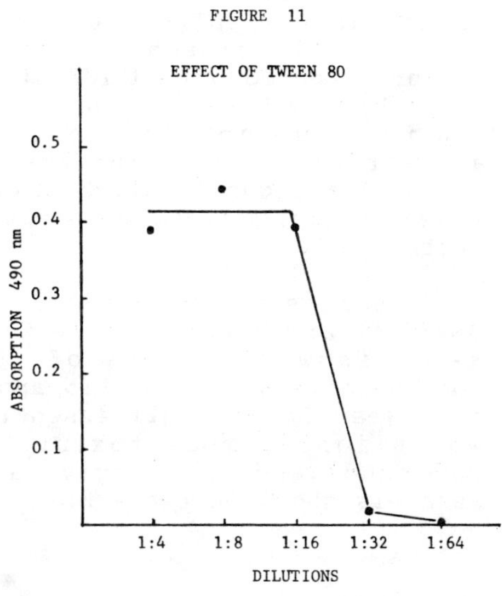

FIGURE 11

EFFECT OF TWEEN 80

diffusion of Na-Fluorescein, but in treated cultures the increase was significant as shown in fig.2. This increased permeability may represent enhanced detachment of cells by shaking.

Fig.3 shows a semi-log plot of permeabilityversus concentration of SDS. At 1:800 dilution of 1% SDS (125 ug/ml) the increased permeability of the epithelium to Na-fluorescein was barely detectable. At 1:200 dilution (500 ug/ml) distinct damage to the epithelial permeability was observed. A linear relationship between the $\log_n$ of concentrations in this range and permeability was obtained.

A mild irritant, a light duty liquid cleaner was then tested. The results are shown in fig.4. This mild irritant caused an increase in permeability only at a dilution of 1:100.

Morphologic appearances of cultures treated with irritants have been examined in the SEM. Figures 5,6,7, show representative fields of treated cultures, all fixed immediately after Na-Fluorescein diffusion experiment. Fig. 5 shows a control culture, the cells form a continuous sheet, sealing the filter mambrane from the passage of Na-Fluorescein solution. Fig.6 shows a culture treated with a 1:800 dilution of a light duty cleaner. It shows focal damage in the epithelium of a few cells, and the loss in cell to cell attachment in a few foci. Fig 7 shows a culture treated with 1:100 dilution of the same agent. Many cells have detached, revealing the underlying filter. With vigorous shaking the cell detachment process could be accelerated. It is interesting to not that damage to an epithelium began focally. Even with many cells detached, as shown in fig.7, there were apparently undamaged cells in the epithelium.

A series of non-ionic detergents ,Tween 20, Tween 40, Tween 60 and Tween 80 were tested in this system. Figures 8-11 show the plots of permeability versus $\log_2$ of concentrations tested. It appears that Tween 20, Tween 40, and Tween 60 were all essentially non-toxic while Tween 80 was slightly more toxic. The concentrations of these compounds and SDS to give a comparable response in this assay is shown in table 2.

TABLE 2

	Concentration causing a similar increase in the diffusion of Na-Fluorescein across the MDCK epithelium
SDS	25Ø ug/ml (*)
Tween 2Ø	>27Ø mg/ml (#)
Tween 4Ø	>27Ø mg/ml (#)
Tween 6Ø	>275 mg/ml (#)
Tween 8Ø	45 mg/ml

(*) At this level, it will be judged as a mild irritant

(#) The syrupy nature of Tween compounds prevented testing at concentrations higher than that indicated

DISCUSSION

In recent years there has been increased need for developing new and better in-vitro techniques for the evaluation of the safety of commercial products. The impetus have come from both societal pressure and scientific need for improvement (1Ø). Among all the animal tests, the Draize rabbit eye irritancy test (11,12) has received most attention fordeveloping suitable alternatives. Sharpe(13) has discussed succinctly the motivation for an alternative to the Draize test. Detailed critiques of the Draize test have been presented (14,15,16).

Alternatives to the Draize Eye irritancy test have been considered since 1956 when Shapiro used isolated corneas from rabbits to study the effect of sodium hydroxide on corneal swelling (17). Burton et al. (18) demonstrated good correlation between in-vivo and in-vitro irritancy testing on a number of chemicals. The use of cultured corneal cells for irritancy testing was developed by North-Root et al. (19). Using cytotoxicity and colony formation as an end point, they found good rank correlation between in-vitro and in-vivo irritancy of a number of surfactants. Recently a number of in-vitro culture systems have been developed using a variety of cell types. Many different end points have been used: cytotoxicity, such as that described by Borenfreund et al. (2Ø), cell proliferation by North-Root et al. (19,21), altered cellular membrane permeability and cellular metabolism by Scaif (22), and Shopsis and Sathe (23), and cell motility by Simmons et al. (24). Frazier et al. (16) has reviewed comprehensively in-vitro techniques that have been applied as alternatives to animal toxicity testing. One of the problems of in-vitro test system is its correlation with in-vivo observations of some chemicals, for example,Tween 2Ø and other non-ionic surfactants have always been rated as moderate to severe irritants in in-vitro tests whereas Tween 2Ø is a non-irritant in the Draize rabbit eye test.

Frazier et al. (16) in "A critical evaluation of alternatives to acute ocular irritation testing" have commented that there are very few methods using the tissue physiology of an epithelium as a model for toxicity testing. The study described here represent a new approach, using a functional expression of epithelial tissue, namely trans-epithelial permeability, for testing toxic and irritating compounds. Permeability of many epithelia respond sensitively to toxic substances. For example, bronchial epithelial permeability of both guinea pig (25, 26) and human (27) increase after exposure to cigarette smoke for 1/2 hour. However, there is no morphological alteration of tight junctions at this time (28). The recovery of epithelial permeability is rapid in the bronchial epithelium after injury with cigarette smoke (26,29) and in regenerating rabbit cornea after mechanical and chemical injury (3Ø). The development of corneal opacity after SDS treatment is thought to be the permeation of SDS across the epithelium and reacting with the stroma (4). We have selected to use Na-Fluorescein diffusion to detect permeability of the epithelium because it is routinely used in the examination of the eye and its diffusion across the cornea is well studied (31). Its molecular weight is 376 and is soluable in aqueous solution and is non-toxic. The concentration of Na-Fluorescein in a solution is easily measured in a spectrophotometer.

Our results demonstrate that this assay is quantitative and is dose dependent on the toxic agent applied. The concentration of SDS that causes measurable increase inMDCK trans-epithelial permeability compares well with other in-vitro assays and the CAM assay (32). The very encouraging results with the series of Tween compounds suggest that this assay could be very useful in distinguishing mild irritants from non-irritants.

An interesting observation is that in a confluent monolayer there appears to be heterogeneity in sensitivity of cells to the action of detergents. Since the MDCK monolayer has cells in various phases of the cell cycle, it may be that sensitivity to detergents is related to the cell cycle. Experiemtns using synchronized cells are under way. This may have application in-vivo, as tissue undergoing repair may respond differently to toxic agents (24,30).

Acknowledgment: The author wishes to thank Judy Verdone for technical assistance. This study is supported by grants from The International foundation for Ethical Research, The Ben-Franklin Partnership Program of the Commonwealth of Pennsylvania and, The American Fund for Alternative to Animal Research.

REFERENCES

1. Beridge, M.J. and Oschman, J.L. (1972), In "Transporting Epithelia". p.72, Academic Press, New York
2. Marshall, W.S. and Klyce, S.D. (1983), Cellular and paracellular pathway resistances in the tight Cl_ secreting epithelium of the rabbit cornea. J. Memb. Biol. 73: 275.
3. Maurice, D.M. (1984), "Cornea and Sclera", 1-158, in "The Eye", H.Davson (ed.). vol. 1 B, Academic Press.
4. Igarashi,H.(1986). With which componentof the bovine isolated cornea does Sodium Lauryl Sulphate react to produce opacity? Toxicology Letters, 32: 249.
5 Cereijido, M. (1984), Electrical properties of Madin-Darby canine kidney cells. Fed. Proc. 43: 2230.
6. Leighton,J.,Brada, Z.,Estes, L.W.and Justh, G. (1969), Secretory activities and oncogenicity of a cell line (MDCK) derived from canine kidney. Science (Washington) 158: 472.
7 Valentich, J., Tchao,R.and Leighton, J. (1979), Hemicyst formation stimulated by cyclic AMP in dog kidney cell line MDCK. J. Cell Physiol. 100: 291.
8. Rabito, C.A. and Tchao,R. (1980), ^{3}H-Ouabain binding during the monolayer organization and cell cycle in MDCK cells. Am. J. Physiol. 238: C43.
9. Handler, J.S. (1983), Use of cultured epithelia to study transport and its regulation. J. Exp. Biol. 106: 55.
10. Goldberg, A. M. (1985), An approach to the development of invitro toxicological methods. Fd.Chem. Tox. 23: 205.
11. Draize J.H., Woodward, G.and Calvery, H.O. (1944), Methods for the study of irritation and toxicity of sub-

stances applied topically to the skin and mucous membranes. J. Phamacol. Exp. Ther. 82: 377.
12. Friedenwald, J. S., Hughes, W. F. and Herman, H. (1944), Acid-base tolerance of the cornea. Arch. Ophthalmol. 31: 279.
13. Sharp,R.,(1985), The Draize Test - motovation for change Fd. Chem. Toxic. 23: 139.
14. Goldberg, A. M. (1983), in "Alternative Methods in Toxicology" vol.2, Acute toxicity testing: Alternative approaches. Goldberg,A.M. (ed.) Mary Ann Liebert Inc..
15. Alternative Methods in Toxicology, vol.3, In Vitro Toxicology: A progress report from the Johns Hopkins Center for Alternatives to Animal Testing. Goldberg, A. M. (ed.) Mary Ann Liebert Inc.. 1985.
16. Alternative Methods in Toxicology,vol 4. A critical evaluation of alternatives to acute ocular irritation testing. Frazier,J.M.,Gad, S.C.,Goldberg, A.M.and McCulley, J.P. (ed.). Mary Ann Liebert Inc.. 1987.
17. Shapiro, H., (1956), Swelling and dissolution of the rabbit cornea in alkali. Am. J. Ophthalmol. 42: 292.
18. Burton,A.B.G.,York,M.and Lawrence R.S. (1981), The in-vitro assessment of severe eye irritant. Fd. Cosmet. Toxicol. 19: 471.
19. North-Root, H., Yackovich, F. Demetrulias, J. Gacula, M. Jr. and Heinze, J. G. (1982), Evaluation of an invitro cell toxicity test using rabbit corneal cells to predict the eye irritation potential of surfactants. Toxicol. Lett. 14: 207.
20. Borenfreund, E., Shopsis, C., Barrero, O. and Sathe, S. (1983), In vitro alternative irritancy assays: Comparison of cytotoxic and membrane transport effects of alcohols. Ann. N.Y. Acad. Sci. 407: 416.
21. North-Root,H.,Yackovich, F.,Demetrulias, J., Gacula, M. Jr.. and Heinze, J. E. (1985), Prediction of the eye irritation potential of shampoos using the in-vitro SIRC cell toxicity test. Fd. Chem. Toxic. 23: 271.
22. Scaife, M. C. (1985), An in vitro cytotoxicity test to predict the ocular irritation potential of detergents and detergent products. Fd. Chem. Toxic. 23: 253.
23. Shopsis, C. and Sathe, S. (1984), Uridine uptake inhibition as a cytotoxicity test : Correlations with the Draize test. Toxicology 29: 195.
24. Simmons, S., Jumblatt, M. M. and Neufeld, A. H. (1987) Corneal epithelial wound closure in tissue culture; an in-vitro model of ocular irritancy. Toxicol. Appl. Pharmacol. 88: 13.
25. Simani, A. S., Inoue, S. and Hogg, J. C. (1974), Penetration of the respiratory epithelium of guinea pigs following exposure to cigarette smoke. Lab. Invest. 31: 75.
26. Hulbert, W.C., Walker, D.C., Jackson, A. and Hogg, J.C. (1981), Airway permeability to horse radish peroxidase in guinea pigs: the repair phase after injury by cigarette smoke. Am. Rev. Respir. Dis. 123: 320.
27. Jones, J. G., Minty, B. D., Lawler, P., Hulands, G.,

Crawley, J. C. W. and Veall, N. (1980), Increased alveolar epithelial permeability in cigarette smokers. Lancet 1: 66.

28. Walker, D.C., Mackenzie, A., Wiggs, B.R., Hulbert, W.C., and Hoggs, J.C. (1984), The structure of tight junctions in the tracheal epithelium may not correlate with permeability. Cell Tissue Res. 235: 607.
29. Minty, B.D., Jordan, C. and Jones, J.G. (1981), Rapid improvement in abnormal pulmonary epithelial permeability after stopping cigarettes. Brit. Med. J. 282: 1183.
30. Thoft, R.A. and Friend, J. (1975) Permeability of regenerated corneal epithelium. Exp. Eye Res. 21: 409.
31 Maurice D.M. (1967) The use of fluorescein in ophthalmological reseach. Invest. Ophthalmol. 6: 464.
32. Leighton, J., Nassauer, J. and Tchao, R. (1985) The chick embryo in toxicology: an alternative to the rabbit eye. Fd. Chem. Toxic. 23: 291.

Poster A16

In Vitro Cytotoxicity Test Using Primary Cells Derived from Rabbit Eye Is Useful as an Alternative for Draize Testing

MASAMI WATANABE,[1] KIMIKO WATANABE,[1]
KEIJI SUZUKI,[1] OSAMU NIKAIDO,[2] TSUTOMU SUGAHARA,[3]
IZUMI ISHII,[4] and HIROAKI KONISHI[4]

[1]*Division of Radiation Biology, School of Medicine*
Yokohama City University, Yokohama 236, Japan
[2]*Pharmaceutical Sciences, Kanazawa University, Kanazawa 920, Japan*
[3]*Health Research Foundation, Kyoto 606, Japan*
[4]*Biochemical Research Laboratory*
Nihon Menado Cosmetic Corporation, Gifu 505, Japan

ABSTRACT

We used cells freshly isolated from rabbit cornea to determine cytotoxicity based on colony forming ability to 14 chemicals. The results showed that the cationic detergents, such as Stearyl trimethyl- and Alkyl benzyl dimethyl-ammonium chloride, were the most toxic. The anionic detergents showed moderate toxicity. POE(10) mono laurate, 2- Alkyl- N-carboxymethyl- N-hydroxyethyl imidazoline betaine and acetone were nonirritating in vivo and they were ranked accordingly. There was a close correlation between the relative toxicity in rabbit corneal cells in vitro and the relative eye irritation in a Draize test was seen in response to treatment with 14 chemicals. The degree of correlation between the in vivo and in vitro systems described here is excellent despite the wide variety of surfactants which was evaluated. This sensitive and reproducible assay lend themselves to a screening procedure of potential toxicants which can help reduce the use of animals for toxicity testing.

INTRODUCTION

The Draize eye irritation test has been primary method used to assess the potential eye irritation of most chemicals and consumer products 1) . Over the year, this method is received much criticism due to lack of interlaboratory consistency and limited correlation with human experience ; however, it is considered useful for screening potentially severe eye irritants. Unfortunately, the testing of chemicals may cause pain to the animals, as well as severe and ,in some instances, permanent damage to the eye. For these reasons, recently, interest has been expressed in supplementing or replacing the Draize test with one or more in vitro tests designed to predict ocular irritancy. Ideally, such test systems would be quantitative, cost effective and humane, as well as productive of even mild ocular irritancy.

Several in vitro tests have been developed to predict, by analogy, ocular irritancy. These include tests based on changes in enzyme secretion by cultured ocular cells [2], cytotoxicity in cultured ocular cells [3,4], and the inability of dead and damaged cells to take up the dye neutral red [5,6]. Although, at this time, it seems neither prudent nor feasible to replace in vivo testing, a concerted effort to develop sensitive and meaningful short-term in vitro assays seems appropriate. Among the criteria to be met by such in vitro tests are sensitivity, dose response, ease of manipulation and scoring, reproducibility, cost effectiveness and good correlation with the considerably more complex in vivo system. Therefore, an in vitro test based on colony forming ability of cultured ocular cells would be appropriate. Usually, investigators have tried to use established ocular cells [3,4]. However, cells maintained in continuous culture are generally lack of functioning organ complete with structural components.

Therefore, This study was designed to determine whether primary rabbit corneal cells are essential for an in vitro Draize rabbit eye irritancy test replacement.

MATERIALS AND METHODS

Cells: Primary rabbit corneal cells were used in this experiments. The corneas from a Japanese white rabbit were rinsed with phosphate-buffered saline without calcium and magnesium (PBS) containing 100 units/ml penicilin and 100 µg/ml kanamycin. Then corneas were minced with scissors and trypsinized at 37 °C for 20 min to make a cell suspension. An appropriate number of cells was delivered into 75 cm^2 culture flask and incubated at 37 °C in CO_2 incubator for 3-5 days. Primary cultures were established and grown to confluence in complete medium composed of Eagle's MEM with 10% fetal bovine serum, penicilin (50 units/ml) and kanamycin (50 µg/ml). Primary confluent cultures were tripsinized briefly, suspended in culture medium containing 10% DMSO and stocked in liquid nitrogen until use. Cells were subcultured every 5 days at 10^6 cells per 75 cm^2 flask. Although cells freshly isolated from grew at a high rate at passage 1-3, then the growth rates declined gradually up to passage 10. The cloning efficiency of these cells before passage 5 ranged 80-100 %, but declined gradually thereafter. Thus only cells between passage 2 and 5 were used in cytotoxicity tests.

Cytotoxicity test: Cells from exponentially growing cultures were trypsinized briefly, suspended in culture medium, and plated at cloning density (i.e., 50-100 cells per 60-mm diameter dish, 3-6 dishes per dose). After 6 to 12 h, the cells were treated with chemicals for 20 min at 37 °C ,then washed twice with 5ml PBS, and allowed to form colonies in the original dishes. Chemicals listed in table 1 were dissolved in PBS, ethanol or DMSO on a weight/weight basis, sterilized with filter and put into medium directly with micro-pipettes. The percent survival was determined from the cloning efficiency of treated and untreated cells.

Table 1. List of chemicals used in this study.

Chemicals	Abbreviation
Nonionic detergent	
1. POE(10) mono laurate	MYL-10
2. POE(9) lauryl ether	BL-9EX
3. POE(10) nonylphenyl ether	NP-10
Anionic detergent	
4. Sodium polyoxyethylene(2) lauryl ether sulfate	Emal
5. Sodium tetradecenesulfonate	-AOS
6. Sodium lauryl sulfate	SDS
Cationic detergent	
7. Stearyl trimethyl ammonium chloride	Kotamin
8. Alkyl benzyl dimethyl ammonium chloride	Sanisol
9. Penta ethoxy stearl ammonium	KS-5
10. Dimethyl distearyl ammonium chloride	DSAC
Amphoteric detergent	
11. Lauryl dimethylaminoacetic acid betaine	Amphitol
12. 2-Alkyl-N-carboxymethyi-N-hydroxyethyl imidazoline betaine	Miranol
Others	
13. Formalin	Formalin
14. Acetone	Acetone

Animal test: Japanese white rabbits of both sexes were used. The animals were assigned randomly to treatment groups and 3-6 animals comprised a treatment group. Corneal, iris and conjunctival responses were evaluated using the scale described by Draize et al.[1]. Scoring was done at 1, 3, 6, 24, 96 and 168 h following application of each chemical. Fluorescein stain was used to aid in determining the extent of corneal damage.

RESULTS

Table 2 shows the LD_{50} value, i.e. the chemical concentration allowing 50% cell survival, obtained for each of 14 chemicals in vitro

Table 2. In vitro LD50 values and surfactant concentrations predicted to cauze Draise scores od 20.

Surfactants	LD_{50} values (w/w%)	Surfactant concentration predicted score of 20. (w/w%)
Nonionic detergent		
1. MYL-10	27 ($\times 10^{-3}$)	85
2. BL-9EX	1.8	4
3. NP-10	5	5
Anionic detergent		
4. Emal	12	8
5. α-AOS	10	12
6. SLS	2.2	4
Cationic detergent		
7. Kotamin	1	2.2
8. Sanisol	1	2.0
9. KS-5	2	6
10. DSAC	3.5	16
Amphoteric detergent		
11. Amphitol	11	5.8
12. Miranol	30	30
Others		
13. Formalin	8	8
14. Acetone	35	45

testing using the rabbit corneal cells and the concentration of each chemical predicted to cause a Draize score of 20 in the rabbit eye in vivo. Using the data in table 1, a rank correlation analysis was performed and the results are depicted graphically in figure 1. The concentration (w/w%) of each chemical predicted to cause a Draize score of 20 in vivo was plotted as the relative toxicity value in vivo and LD $_{50}$ of each chemical multiplied with 10 was used as the relative toxicity value in vitro. The cationic detergents, such as Stearyl trimethyl- and Alkyl benzyl dimethyl-ammonium chloride, were the most toxic both in vivo and in vitro. The anionic detergents, Sodium polyoxyethylene(2) lauryl ether sulfate, Sodium tetradecenesulfonate and Sodium lauryl sulfate, showed moderate toxicity. POE(10) mono laurate, 2- Alkyl- N- carboxymethyl- N- hydroxy- ethyl imidazoline be-taine and acetone were nonirritating in vivo and they were ranked accordingly in vitro.

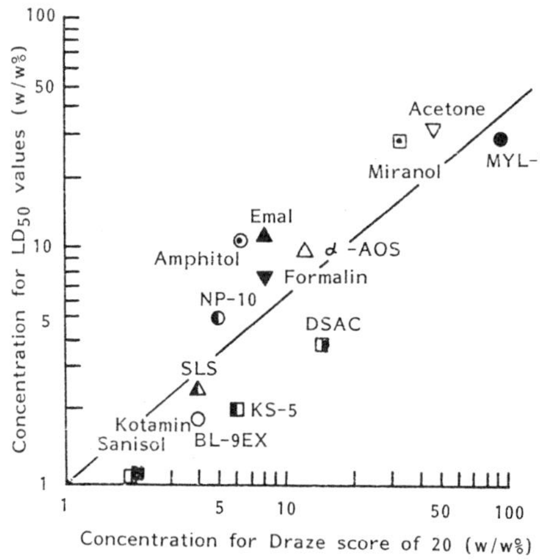

Figure 1. Correlation between the relative toxicity value in vitro and the relative toxicity value in vivo.

DISCUSSION

In vitro cytotoxicity test based on colony-forming assay has been developed for predicting relative eye irritation by measuring cell toxicity in rabbit. In these studies, investigators usually used continuously growing cells [3,4]. However, cells maintained in continuous culture are generally lack of a functioning organ complete with structural components. Therefore, we tried to use cells freshly isolated from rabbit cornea in this study. The growth, structural morphology and biochemical properties of these cells were found to be comparable to those in vivo [7]. These cells grew at a high growth rates at early passage after culturing and cloning efficiency of these cells at passage 2-4 were 80-100 %, but declined thereafter. The rate of tetraproid cells in culture of rabbit corneal cells increased up to 55% at passage 8, then decreased gradually.

We used these cells to determine cytotoxicity based on colony forming ability to 14 chemicals. The results indicate a strong correlation between the relative toxicity in vitro and the relative toxicity in vivo. Our observation that cationic surfactants are more potent than those with anionic or non-ionic chemical structure is in agreement with the ranking reported previously [3,4]. Draize rabbit eye irritancy scores also indicate that of the surfactants commonly present in shampoos and cosmetics, the cationic are most irritating in vivo, the anionic intermediate, and the non-ionic least irritating [8]. Thus, the data presented in this reports indicate that mammalian cells propagated in vitro can be successfully used for preliminary screening and range finding of toxic concentrations of potentially irritant compounds. These assays are economical, easy to execute and can reduce the number of animals required for in vivo testing.

REFERENCES

1. Draize, J., Woodard, G. and Calvery, H., (1944), Methods for the study of irritation and toxicity of substances applied topically to the skin and mucous membranes. J. Pharm. Exp. Ther. 82: 377-390.
2. Chan, K.Y., (1985), An in vitro alternative to the Draize test. Altern. Methods. Toxicol. 3: 405-422.
3. Borenfreund, E. and Borrero, O., (1984) In vitro cytotoxicity assays. Potential alternatives to the Draize ocular irritancy test. Cell Biol. and Toxicol. 1: 55-65.
4. North-Root, H., Yackvich, F., Demetrulias, J., Gacula, M. Jr. and Heinze, J.E., (1982), Evaluation of an in vitro cell toxicity test using rabbit corneal cells to predict the eye irritation potential of surfactants. Toxicol. Lett. 14: 207-212.
5. Borenfreund, E. and Puerner, J.A., (1985), Toxicity determined in vitro by morphological alterations and neutral red absorption. Toxicol. Lett. 24: 119-124.
6. Hockley, K. and Baxter, D., (1986), Use of the 3T3 cell-neutral red uptake assay for irritants as alternative to the rabbit (Draize) test. Fd. Chem. Toxic. 24: 473-475.
7. Chan, K., Haschke, R. and Burg, A., (1980), Culture of corneal cells using a new isolation technique. Invest. Ophthalmol. Vis. Sci. (Suppl.): 25.
8. Grant, M.E., (1974), Toxicology of the eye. 2nd ed., C.C. Thomas (ed.), Springfield, IL.

Poster A17

Evaluation of Organic Nephrotoxins Using Rabbit Renal Cortical Slices

G.H.I. WOLFGANG,[1] A.J. GANDOLFI,[1] C.L. KRUMDIECK,[2] and K. BRENDEL[1]

[1]*Department of Pharmacology and Toxicology*
University of Arizona
Tucson, AZ 85724
[2]*Department of Nutritional Science*
University of Alabama
Birmingham, AL 35294

ABSTRACT

Our past studies have shown the usefulness of precision-cut rabbit renal cortical slices (RCS) in studying the in vitro toxicity of acute direct acting toxins. This RCS system can also be used to evaluate the toxicity of organic compounds requiring transport/accumulation or biotransformation to express their toxicity. RCS from adult male New Zealand White rabbits were incubated (serum free DME/F12 medium, 95:5 O_2/CO_2, 25° C) for up to 24 hr with the test compounds and monitored for intracellular potassium, LDH, PAH/TEA accumulation, and histopathology. Cephaloridine (10^{-3} M) causes an S_3 lesion within 12 hr of incubation. Higher doses (5 x 10^{-3} and 10^{-4} M) decrease the time to lesion formation, however, the lesion is still limited to the S_3 segment. Gentamicin (5 x 10^{-3} and 10^{-2} M), initially causes an S_3 lesion, however, the lesion later encompasses all proximal tubules. Hexachlorobutadiene (10^{-4} M) and dichlorovinylcysteine (5 x 10^{-5} M) produce a lesion within 8 hr that is localized in the S_3 segment. Increased doses shorten the time to lesion appearance and at later time points all segments of the proximal tubules are affected. All of these toxins cause a dose- and time-related decrease in the biochemical parameters. Decreases in intracellular potassium and changes in transport precede any lesion development; alterations in LDH release are concurrent with lesion development. The precision-cut rabbit renal cortical slice system is applicable to a wide range of toxins including those that produce toxicity via transport/accumulation and/or biotransformation. This further substantiates the validity of this system and its usefulness for evaluating potential nephrotoxins in vitro.

INTRODUCTION

Cephaloridine, gentamicin, hexachloro-1-3-butadiene (HCBD) and S-(1-2-dichlorovinyl)-L-cysteine (DCVC) are four organic compounds commonly used to induce proximal tubular damage in experimental animals. Cephaloridine is a broad-spectrum cephalosporin antibiotic, gentamicin is an aminoglycoside; both compounds are selectively transported and accumulated within the proximal tubule, the site of damage (1,2). HCBD and DCVC are halogenated hydrocarbons which require bioactivation to become toxic (3,4,5). In vivo all of these compounds cause necrosis of the proximal tubules (6,7,8,9).

Cephaloridine is believed to cause proximal tubular damage as it is actively transported into the proximal tubule via the organic anion system and accumulates in these cells since secretion across the luminal membrane to the tubular lumen is minimal (1,10). The high concentration of drug in these cells correlates with the pathological lesion which manifests as extensive damage to all portions of the proximal tubule with the exception of the first few convolutions (6).

Gentamicin apparently undergoes a multistep uptake process on the apical side of proximal tubules resulting in gentamicin uptake and concentration within lysosomes (11). Resulting alterations include phospholipidosis of the proximal tubular cells (2) and subsequent necrosis (7).

The proposed mechanism for HCBD toxicity is that of enzymatic conjugation with glutathione followed by renal metabolism to a cysteine conjugate (3). The enzyme, β-lyase, is then responsible for the cleavage of cysteine, leaving a postulated reactive thiol product. In vivo HCBD produces damage initially to the straight portion (S_3 segment) of the proximal tubule (8).

DCVC is a model cysteine conjugate which is metabolized by β-lyase to form a reactive thiol, pyruvate and ammonia (5). This potent nephrotoxin causes selective (S_3) proximal tubular necrosis when administered in vivo (9,12).

It is useful to have a model in which both biochemical and histological status can be assessed and yet mechanistic studies can still be performed. In vitro systems allow the innate cellular responses to chemical agents to be investigated independent of physiological parameters, however, in vitro events must parallel in vivo events in order for mechanistic studies to be legitimate (13). Past in vitro studies have shown the usefulness of precision-cut rabbit renal cortical slices in studying the toxicity of acute direct acting toxins (14). Here, time- and dose-responses were determined using renal cortical slices exposed to several organic nephrotoxins. Validation of this system will allow mechanistic studies to be performed in the future.

METHODS

Slice preparation and incubation

Kidneys from male New Zealand White rabbits (1.5 - 2.0 kg, Blue Ribbon Ranch, Tucson, AZ) were excised, decapsulated, and cored along their cortical-papillary axis. Positional renal cortical slices were prepared using a modified version of a mechanical tissue slicer (15). Slices were collected and stored in ice cold Kreb's Hepes buffer prior to experimental exposure. The prepared slices were incubated with appropriate toxicants in serum-free DME/F12 medium (95/5, O_2/CO_2) for up to 24 hr at room temperature.

Toxin Exposure

Slices exposed to cephaloridine (Sigma Chemical Company, St. Louis, MO), gentamicin (Sigma Chemical Company, St. Louis, MO) and DCVC (synthesized by the method of McKinney et al, 16) were incubated in an open slice support system (15, 17). Appropriate concentrations of these compounds were prepared in DME/F12 medium and added to incubation vessels. Slices exposed to HCBD (Aldrich Chemical Company, Milwaukee, WI) were incubated in a closed roller culture system (17, 18) due to the volatility of the compound. Dimethylsulfoxide (<1%) was used as a carrier in HCBD-exposed slices as well as in concurrent control vessels. Slices were removed at designated time points for measurement of intracellular potassium (K^+), intracellular lactate dehydrogenase (LDH), organic ion transport and histopathology.

Structural and Biochemical Analysis

Samples for histology (1 slice per time point) were fixed in a phosphate-buffered 4% formaldehyde, 1% glutaraldehyde solution (19). After fixation slices underwent serial dehydration and embedding in methacrylate plastic (Polyscience Incorporated, Warrington, PA.). 2 um sections were cut and stained with 1% toluidine blue. Areas of the proximal tubule were anatomically defined according to Kaissling and Kriz (21). Slices for K^+, LDH and DNA analysis were blotted, placed in 0.5 ml deionized water and homogenized. K^+ and LDH were measured by flame photometry (20) and a kinetic assay (Sigma Kit 228-10) respectively. DNA content was measured by a fluorometric assay (22) and was used to normalize K^+ and LDH values. Organic anion (para-aminohippurate, PAH) and cation (tetraethylammonium, TEA) accumulation were assessed with ^{14}C-labeled substrates (New England Nuclear, Boston, MA). Slices were incubated in DME/F12 media and subsequently transferred to vessels containing Krebs-Hepes buffer, ^{14}C-labeled substrate, and ^3H_2O (ICN, Irvine, CA) as a volume marker. After 40 min, slices and buffer aliquots were removed and counted by liquid scintillation spectroscopy. The organic ion accumulation is expressed as the slice ($^{14}C/^3H$) to medium ($^{14}C/^3H$) ratio.

Statistics

Values were pooled from several experiments and results were analyzed by ANOVA and treatment differences were identified by Newman-Keuls multiple comparison tests. A 0.05 level of probability or less was used as criteria of significance.

RESULTS

All compounds exhibited concentration- and time- dependent decreases in biochemical and functional indices. This is demonstrated by the changes in K^+ (Fig. 1-2) Other biochemical or functional changes are shown as end-point data although time-dependent alterations were also evident (Table 1). Histopathology of control slices was maintained throughout 24 hr (Fig. 3) thus allowing site-specific necrosis to be detected in experimental slices.

Cephaloridine caused a selective lesion to the straight segment of the proximal tubules (Fig. 4A). While 10^{-4} M cephaloridine had no effect, 10^{-3} - 10^{-2} M cephaloridine all caused an S_3 lesion; however, higher doses caused the lesion to appear earlier (8 hr vs 12 hr). The selective lesion is reflected in the biochemical results as an incomplete loss of K^+, LDH, and organic ion transport (Fig. 1A, Table 1). This is expected as collecting ducts, distal tubules and glomeruli appear to remain healthy.

Gentamicin caused a more non-specific necrosis of the proximal tubule, although S_3 segments appeared to be most susceptible. The necrotic lesion took longer to develop than with any other compound; necrosis was not evident until 12 hr with the highest dose of gentamicin (Fig. 4B). At 24 hr some distal tubules (ascending thicks) also appeared damaged. While 10^{-3} M gentamicin had no effect, 5 x 10^{-3} M appeared to cause some identifiable damage (Fig. 1B, Table 1) by 24 hr. Again, incomplete inhibition of biochemical parameters reflects selective necrosis within the cortex.

10^{-4} M HCBD caused site-specific necrosis of the S_3 segments between 4 and 8 hr (Fig. 4C). By 12 hr all proximal tubule segments were affected. 10^{-3} M HCBD followed a similar profile; a S_3 lesion was evident by 4 hr , however the lesion encompassed all proximal tubules by 8 hr. 10^{-5} M HCBD had no effect structurally or biochemically. The functional parameters of PAH and TEA (Table 1), were completely inhibited as would be expected from a lesion to all proximal tubular segments, the regions responsible for transport. Biochemical parameters were significantly declined (Fig. 2A, Table 1), however complete inhibition was not observed as collecting ducts, distal tubules and glomeruli remain viable.

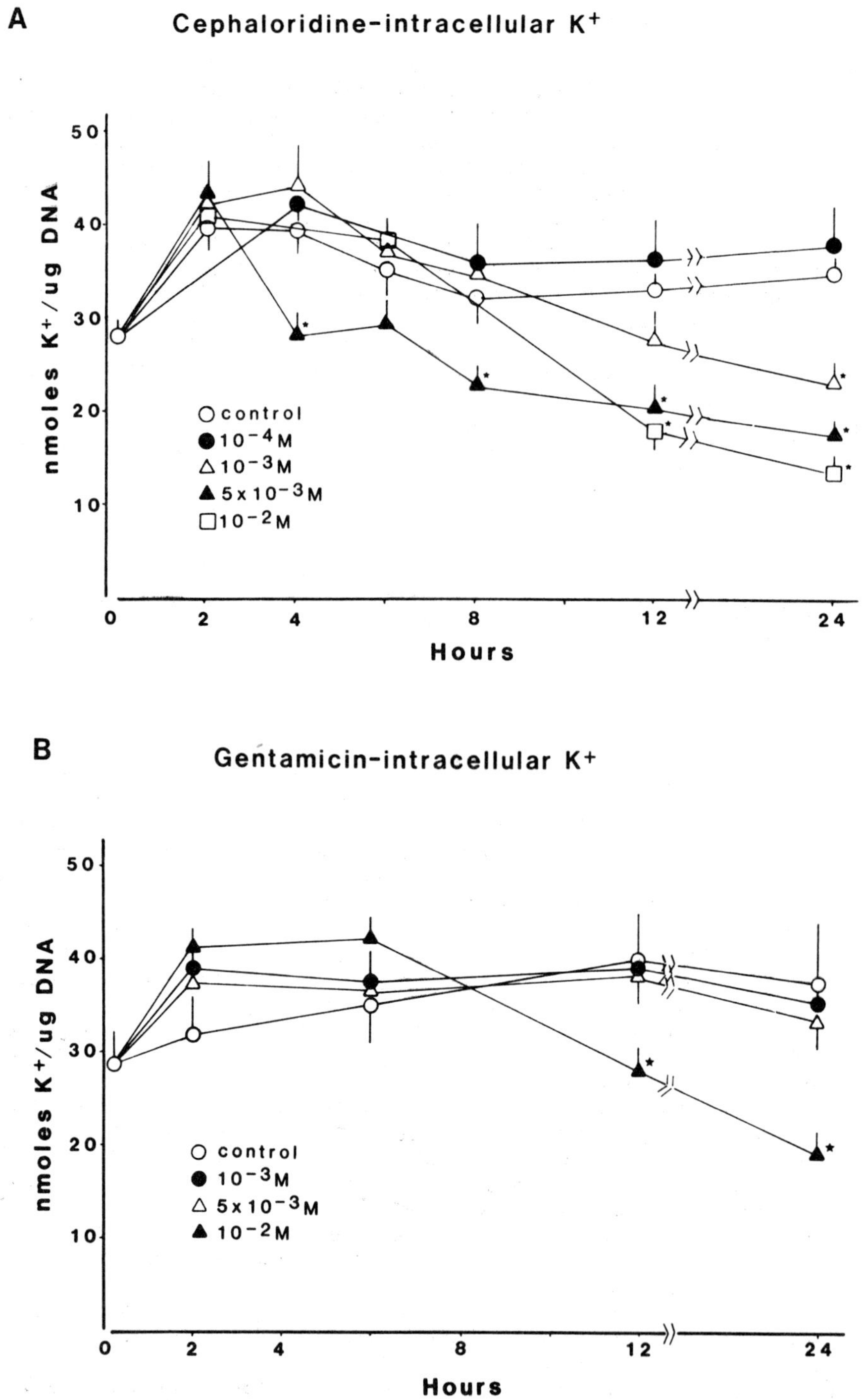

Figure 1. In vitro effects of cephaloridine (A) and gentamicin (B) on intracellular K^+ measured in rabbit cortical slices. Each time point represents $\bar{x} \pm$ SE of 8 or more observations. Stars indicate a significant difference from control at the same time point.

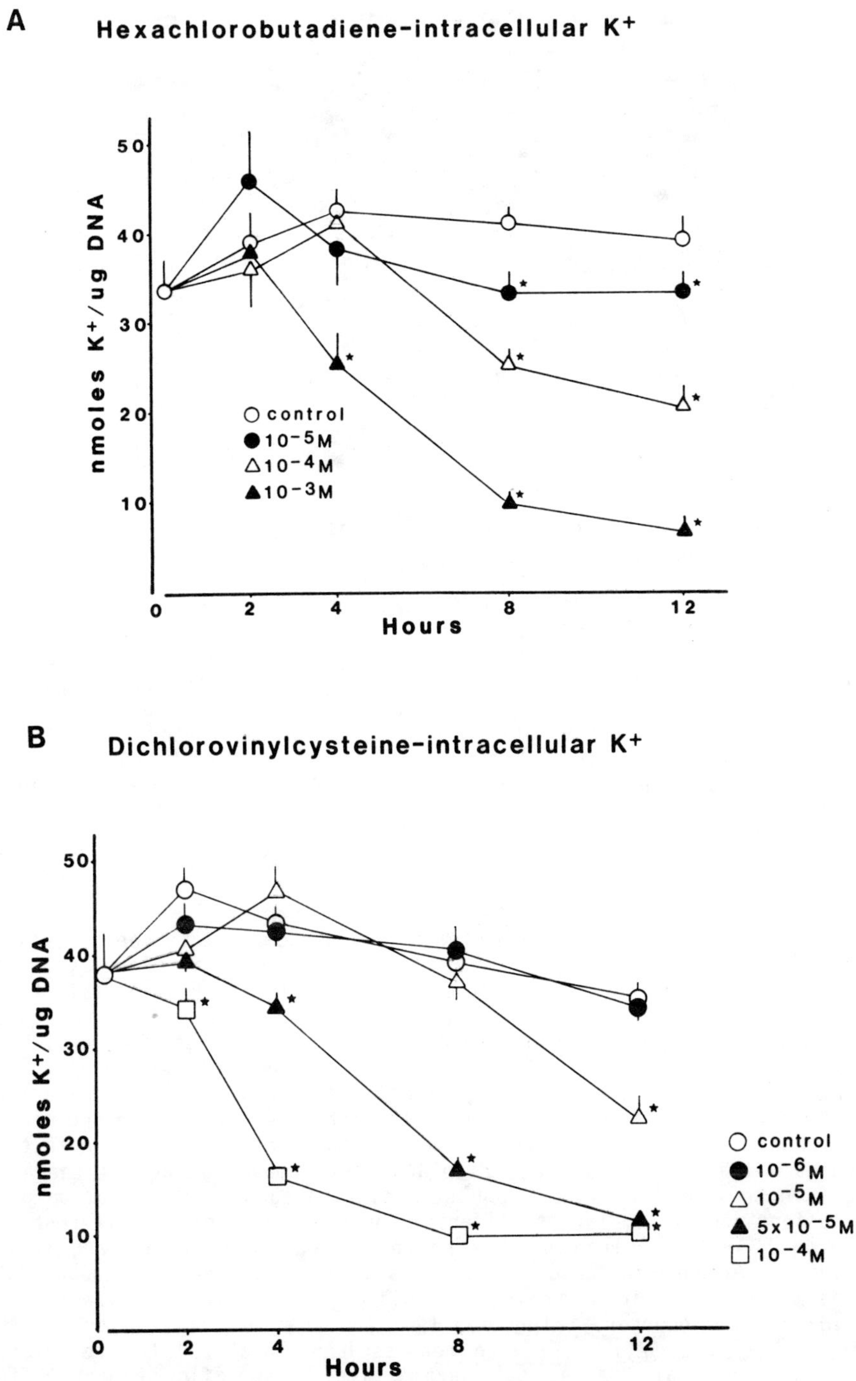

Figure 2. In vitro effects of HCBD (A) and DCVC (B) on intracellular K^+ measured in rabbit cortical slices. Each time point represents $\bar{x} \pm$ SE of 8 or more observations. Stars indicate a significant difference from controls at the same time point.

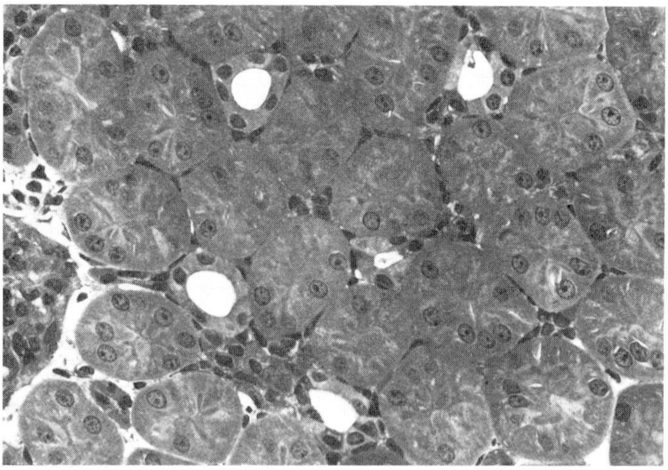

Figure 3. Precision-cut rabbit renal cortical slice incubated for 24 hr under control conditions. (toluidine blue, x100)

DCVC proved to be the most potent toxin of the four examined. Although 10^{-6} M DCVC had no effect, 10^{-5} M DCVC produced a site-specific lesion between 8 and 12 hr (Fig. 4D). Although higher doses (5×10^{-5} M and 10^{-4} M) produced an S_3 lesion early (4-8 hr), at later time points all proximal tubular segments were affected. Similar to HCBD, DCVC produced complete inhibition of functional parameters and significant alterations in biochemical parameters (Table 1, Fig. 2B). Throughout the studies, alterations in K^+, PAH and TEA accumulation preceded evidence of a necrotic lesion, however LDH proved to be a less sensitive indicator.

DISCUSSION

The precision-cut renal slice system allows us to evaluate nephrotoxins both biochemically and structurally. All four compounds exposed in vitro demonstrated histopathological lesions similar to those found in vivo. Biochemical (K^+, LDH) and functional (PAH, TEA) parameters could be maintained in control cultured slices allowing dose- and time-dependent responses to be obtained with various nephrotoxins.

Cephaloridine transport into the proximal tubule has been well characterized (1,10). Cephaloridine is actively transported into the cell by the organic anion carrier mechanism located on the apical side. Cephaloridine is unique in that it concentrates within the tubule and displays little movement across the luminal membrane into the tubular fluid. Our studies also suggest accumulation plays a role as lesions appear similar at different doses but develop at different rates. In addition, PAH accumulation is affected as early as 4 hr by 5×10^{-3} M cephaloridine. Although anionic transport is greatest in the S_2 segment (23) our lesion was most evident in S_3 segments. This may be explained by the effects of cephaloridine on mitochondrial function (24) and the fact that mitochondria are fewer in S_3 segments (21). In vivo reports have localized the cephaloridine lesion to the proximal tubule, but have varied in specific segments affected (6,25,26). Renal cortical slices may be used to clarify the susceptible cell population and the mechanism of cephaloridine toxicity.

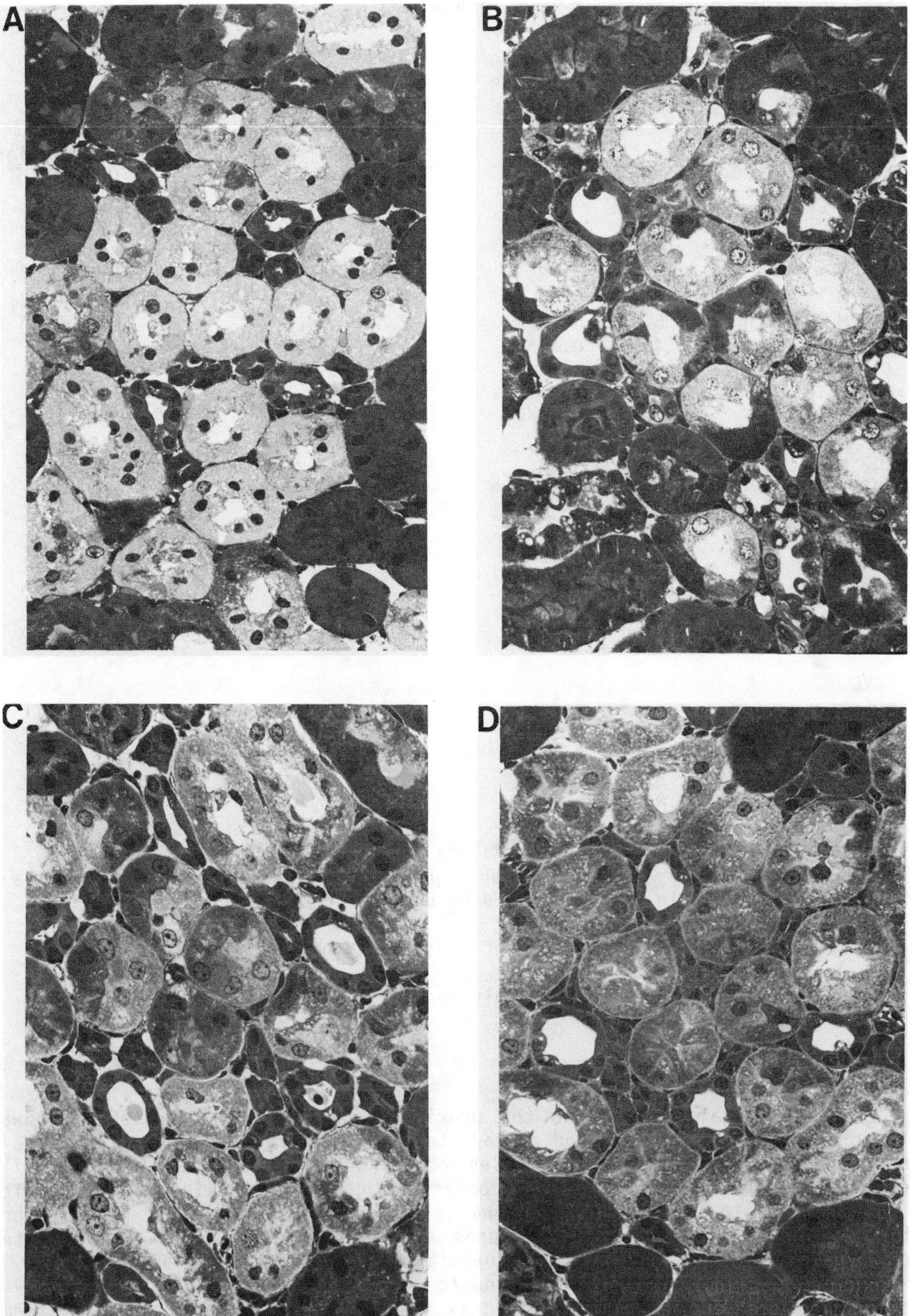

Figure 4. Histopathology of rabbit cortical slices (toluidine blue, 100x) exposed to: A. 5×10^{-3} M cephaloridine, 12 hr, B. 10^{-2} M gentamicin, 12 hr, C. 10^{-4} M HCBD, 8 hr and D. 10^{-5} M HCBD, 12 hr.

Table 1

Biochemical and functional alterations due to *in vitro* exposure to organic nephrotoxins

	Intracellular LDH (U LDH/mg DNA)	PAH accumulation (S/M ratio)	TEA accumulation (S/M ratio)
Cephaloridine			
Control	9.87 ± 0.52	3.64 ± 0.10	5.21 ± 0.13
10^{-4}M	10.68 ± 1.28	4.12 ± 0.14	5.21 ± 0.09
10^{-3}M	7.79 ± 0.94	2.47 ± 0.17*	3.39 ± 0.15*
5×10^{-3}M	5.85 ± 0.52*	2.07 ± 0.17*	2.65 ± 0.14*
10^{-2}M	4.67 ± 0.42*	1.81 ± 0.06*	N.D.
Gentamicin			
Control	10.13 ± 0.62	N.D.	N.D.
10^{-3}M	11.07 ± 0.71	N.D.	N.D.
5×10^{-3}M	8.67 ± 0.66	N.D.	N.D.
10^{-2}M	5.21 ± 0.41*	N.D.	N.D.
HCBD			
Control	9.60 ± 0.88	3.59 ± 0.26	4.85 ± 0.11
10^{-5}M	8.97 ± 1.25	3.78 ± 0.13	5.02 ± 0.20
10^{-4}M	6.78 ± 0.53*	1.18 ± 0.09*	3.10 ± 0.10*
10^{-3}M	3.09 ± 0.67*	0.88 ± 0.0.3	0.90 ± 0.02*
DCVC			
Control	8.76 ± 0.34	3.14 ± 0.08	4.53 ± 0.17
10^{-6}M	9.44 ± 0.39	3.31 ± 0.10	4.69 ± 0.12
10^{-5}M	8.14 ± 0.41	1.78 ± 0.16*	3.52 ± 0.21*
5×10^{-5}M	6.15 ± 0.28*	N.D.	N.D.
10^{-4}M	5.91 ± 0.46*	1.03 ± 0.20*	0.94 ± 0.01*

All data are expressed as end-point values of dose- and time response curves. With the exception of LDH values for cephaloridine and gentamicin (24 hr) all data is from a 12 hr *in vitro* exposure to chemical.

n≥ 8 slices per time point except gentamicin where n=4.

* Significantly different from controls ($p<0.05$).

N.D. not determined.

Gentamicin gains access to the proximal tubule by an endocytotic pathway primarily on the apical side and appears to localize within lysosomes (2). The *in vivo* production of myeloid bodies occurs prior to tubular necrosis (7). Necrosis of the proximal tubule was observed in the renal slices by 12 hr with 10^{-2} M gentamicin, however alterations in K^+ and LDH were minimal until 24 hr. The development of longer term cultures in the future will allow us to better investigate mechanisms of sub-acute toxicity such as that caused by gentamicin.

HCBD has been demonstrated to undergo glutathione conjugation in the liver and subsequent metabolism in the kidney (3). Incubation *in vitro* with renal cortical slices indicates that the kidney may be able to solely biotransform HCBD to a toxic metabolite. Previous *in vitro* studies (27,28) have had mixed success in producing toxicity by HCBD. Kluwe (27) found high doses of HCBD decreased K^+, PAH accumulation and O_2 consumption, however Lock (28) found no effect of HCBD in renal cortical slices. Our studies show 10^{-4} M HCBD produced substantial changes in all parameters measured. A site-specific S_3 lesion was observed between 4 and 8 hr, similar to that seen *in vivo* (8). This system can thus be used to investigate the role of metabolism in the production of a site-specific lesion by HCBD.

DCVC has been used as a model cysteine conjugate in numerous *in vitro* nephrotoxicity studies (29,30). The metabolism of DCVC by β-lyase has been demonstrated to play a significant role in the toxicity of this compound (4,31). Our system demonstrates substantial decreases in K^+, PAH and TEA accumulation when slices were exposed to DCVC. Effects on LDH were less dramatic, probably due to higher concentrations of this enzyme in distal tubules (32) which are unaffected by DCVC treatment. Recent studies show the brush border enzymes gamma-glutamyl transpeptidase and alkaline phosphatase are much earlier and more severely affected by DCVC treatment (unpublished). The site-specific S_3 lesion produced *in vitro* and the progression to all proximal tubules being affected is similar to the chronology observed *in vivo* (9). The renal slice system has proven effective in studying the transport and biotransformation of this compound (33) allowing mechanistic studies to be undertaken.

All of the compounds investigated demonstrated a selectivity for the S_3 segment of the proximal tubule. This susceptibility has been postulated to be dependent on concentration of a compound by passive diffusion, ischemia due to altered renal hemodynamics, local metabolism of compounds or selective accumulation by S_3 segments (8). The first two postulates can be ruled out by virtue of an *in vitro* system, concentration is not occurring along tubular segments and incubation under 95/5 O_2/CO_2 conditions prevents ischemic damage. Accumulation has been shown to be greater in S_2 segments (23) although accumulation does occur along S_3 segments. Both cephaloridine and gentamicin toxicity appear to be dependent on an accumulation mechanism for the resultant S_3 toxicity although further research is needed. Local metabolism of HCBD and DCVC by β-lyase could explain the regional toxicity of either compound. β-lyase has as yet not been localized to specific nephron segments although subcellular location has been investigated (4,34). One also can not rule out the accumulation of these compounds and the innate cellular susceptibility of this region.

The precision-cut rabbit renal cortical slice system has proven to be applicable to a wide range of nephrotoxins, inorganic (14) and organic. This further substantiates the validity of this system and its usefulness for evaluating potential nephrotoxins *in vitro*.

REFERENCES

1. Tune, B.M., Fernholt, M., and Schwartz, A., (1974). Mechanism of cephaloridine transport in the kidney. J. Pharmacol. Exp. Ther. 191:34-317.

2. Kaloyanides, G.J., (1984). Aminoglycoside-induced functional and biochemical defects in the renal cortex. Fundam. Appl. Toxicol. 4:930-943.

3. Nash, J.A., Wing, L.J., Lock, E.A., and Green, T., (1984). The metabolism and deposition of hexachloro-1-3-butadiene in rat and its relevance to nephrotoxicity. Toxicol. Appl. Pharmacol. 73:124-137.

4. Lash, L.H., Elfarra, A.A., and Anders, M.W., (1986). Renal cysteine conjugate β-lyase, bioactivation of nephrotoxic cysteine S-conjugates in mitochondria outer membrane. J. Biol. Chem. 216(13):5930-5935.

5. Anderson, P.M. and Schultze, M.O., (1965). Cleavage of S-(1,2 dichlorovinyl)-L-cysteine by an enzyme of bovine origin. Arch. Biochem. Biophys. 111:593-602.

6. Silverblatt, F. and Turck, M., and Bulger, R., (1970). Nephrotoxicity due to cephaloridine: A light- and electron microscopic study in rabbits. J. Infect. Dis. 122:33-44.

7. Houghton, D.C., Hartnett, M., Campbell-Boswell, M., Porter, G. and Bennett, W., (1976). A light and electron microscopic analysis of gentamicin nephrotoxicity in rats. Am. J. Pathol. 82:589-612.

8. Ishmael, J., Pratt, I., and Lock, E.A., (1982). Necrosis of the pars recta (S_3 segment) of the rat kidney produced by hexachloro 1:3 butadiene. J. Pathol. 138:99-113.

9. Hassall, C.D., Gandolfi, A.J., and Brendel, K., (1983). Correlation of the in vivo and in vitro renal toxicity of S-(1,2-dichlorovinyl)-L-cysteine. Drug Chem. Toxicol. 6:507-520.

10. Tune, B.M. and Fernholt, M., (1973). Relationship between cephaloridine and p-aminohippurate transport in the kidney. Am. J. Physiol. 225:1114-1117.

11. Saito, H., Inui, K. and Hork, R., (1986). Mechanisms of gentamicin transport in kidney epithelial cell line (LLC-PK_1). J. Pharmacol. Exp. Ther. 238:1071-1076.

12. Terracine, B. and Parker, V.H., (1965). A pathological study on the toxicity of S-dichlorovinyl-L-cysteine. Cosmetic Toxicol. 3:67-74.

13. McLean, A.E.M. and NuHall, L., (1978). An in vitro model of liver injury using paracetamol treatment of liver slices and prevention of injury by some antioxidants. Biochem. Pharmacol. 27:425-430.

14. Ruegg, C.E., Gandolfi, A.J., Nagle, R.B., and Brendel, K., (1987). Differential patterns of injury to the proximal tubule of renal cortical slices following in vitro exposure to mercuric chloride, potassium dichromate or hypoxic conditions. Toxicol. Appl. Pharmacol. 90:261-273.

15. Ruegg, C.E, Gandolfi, A.J., Nagle, R.B., Krumdieck, C.L., and Brendel, K., (1984). Preparation of positional renal slices for study of cell-specific toxicity. J. Pharmacol. Methods 17:111-123.

16. McKinney, L.L., Picken, J.C., Jr., Weakley, F.B., Eldridge, A.C., Campbell, R.E., Cowan, J.C., and Biester, H.E., (1959). Possible toxic factor of trichloroethylene-extracted soybean oil meal. J. Am. Chem. Society 81:909-915.

17. Wolfgang, G.H.I., Ruegg, C.R., Gandolfi, A.J., and Brendel, K., (1986). Comparison of renal cortical slices incubated in two in vitro systems. Mountain West Society of Toxicology, Tucson, AZ.

18. Smith, P.F., Gandolfi, A.J., Krumdieck, C.L., Putnam, C.W., Zukoski, C.F., Davis, W.M., and Brendel, K., (1985). Dynamic organ culture of precision liver slices for in vitro toxicology. Life Sci. 36:1367-1375.

19. McDowell, G.M. and Trump, B.F., (1976). Histologic fixatives suitable for diagnostic light and electron microscopy. Arch. Pathol. Lab. Med. 100:405-414.

20. Stacey, N.H., (1978). Toxicity of halogenated volatile anesthetics in isolated rat hepatocytes. Anesthesiology 48:17-22.

21. Kaissling, B and Kriz, W., (1979). Structural analysis of the rabbit kidney. Adv. Anat. Embryol. Cell. Biol. 56:1-123.

22. Kissane, J.M. and Robins, E., (1958). The fluorometric measurement of

deoxyribonucleic acid in animal tissue with special reference to the central nervous system. J. Biol. Chem. 233:184-188.

23. Woodhall, P.B., Tisher, C.C., Simonton, C.A., and Robinson, R.R., (1978). Relationship between para-aminohippurate secretion and cellular morphology in rabbit proximal tubules. J. Clin. Invest. 61:1320-1329.

24. Tune, B.M., Wu, K.Y., Fravert, D., and Holtzman, D., (1979). Effect of cephaloridine on respiration by renal cortical mitochondria. J. Pharmacol. Exp. Ther. 210:98-100.

25. Kuo, C., Maita, K., Sleight, S.D., and Hook, J.B., (1983). Lipid peroxidation: A possible mechanism of cephaloridine-induced nephrotoxicity. Toxicol. Appl. Pharmacol. 67:78-88.

26. Hook, J.B. and Smith, J.H., (1985). Biochemical mechanisms of nephrotoxicity. Transplant. Proc. 17, Suppl. 1:41-50.

27. Kluwe, W.M., Harrington, F.W., and Cooper, S.E., (1982). Toxic effects of organohalide compounds on renal tubular cells in vivo and in vitro. J. Pharmacol. Exp. Ther. 220:597-603.

28. Lock, E.A. and Ishmael, J., (1979). The acute toxic effects of hexachloro-1:3-butadiene on the rat kidney. Arch. Toxicol. 43:47-57.

29. Lash, L.H. and Anders, M.W., (1986). Cytotoxicity of S-(1,2-dichlorovinyl) glutathione and S-(1,2 dichlorovinyl)-L-cysteine in isolated rat kidney cells. J. Biol. Chem. 261:73076-73081.

30. Stevens, J., Hayden, P., and Taylor, G., (1986). The role of glutathione conjugate metabolism and cysteine conjugate B-lyase in the mechanism of S-cysteine-conjugate toxicity in LLC-RK1 cells. J. Biol. Chem. 261:3325-3332.

31. Elfarra, A.A., Jakobson, I., and Anders, M.W., (1986). Mechanism of S-(1,2-dichlorovinyl)glutathione-induced nephrotoxicity. Biochem. Pharmacol. 35:283-288.

32. Price, R.B., (1982). Urinary enzymes, nephrotoxicity and renal disease. Toxicology 23:99-134.

33. Wolfgang, G.H.I., Gandolfi, A.J., And Brendel, K., (1987). Regioselective toxicity by dichlorovinylcysteine in rabbit renal cortical slices. In vitro to in vivo extrapolations in renal toxicology. In press.

34. Stevens, J.L., (1985). Cysteine conjugate β-lyase activities in rat kidney cortex: Subcellular localization and relationship to the hepatic enzyme. Biochem. Biophys. Res. Commun. 129:499-504.

Poster A18

A Rapid and Reliable Acute Toxicity Test for Hepatotoxic Agents Using Only a Single Animal

URI WORMSER and DANIEL CALP

Department of Pharmacology
The Hebrew University–Hadassah Medical School
P.O.B. 1172, 91010 Jerusalem, Israel

ABSTRACT

A simple method for rapid and reliable assessment of hepatotoxic agents is described. One rat liver was sliced into many small pieces, and washed with Krebs Ringer Hepes (KRH) medium. Each group of slices was incubated in this medium, with different concentrations of carbon tetrachloride (CCl_4). This resulted in leakage of liver enzymes into the medium in a dose dependent manner. Accumulation of aspartate and alanine aminotransferases (AST, ALT), could be quantitatively detected 15, 30 and 60 minutes after exposure to CCl_4. The level of these enzymes in the control slice system remained unchanged during the experiment. Similar results were obtained with acetaminophen (APAP) but the kinetics of enzyme leakage was slower i.e. ALT could be measured in the slice medium only 30 minutes after application of the hepatotoxin. Additional studies have shown that mouse liver slices were more sensitive to APAP than those of the rat. These findings demonstrate that the liver slice system provides the same type of information about hepatotoxins that is usually obtained by the use of acute <u>in vivo</u> tests on large number of animals. It can be used to compare the relative toxicity of different substances and may demonstrate differences in the kinetics of their toxic activities. A variety of potential hepatotoxic substances can be tested on the liver of a <u>single animal</u> in a wide range of concentrations. In conclusion, the tissue slice methodology may provide a rapid reliable <u>in vitro</u>, acute toxicity test with a marked reduction in the use of experimental animals.

INTRODUCTION

The routine experimental procedure for acute hepatotoxicity test requires large number of animals of several species. The ethical as well as economic problems associated with such experiments emphasize the urgent need for replacement of experimental animals by <u>in vitro</u> methods in the routine toxicological screening (2). In recent years intensive research has been carried out in order to develop a hepatocyte culture technique as a suitable alternative for the in vivo procedures (3, 4). Although the cell culture methodology is of great value in acute toxicity tests, the dispersed hepatocytes do not always have the same characteristics as those in the intact organ. Consequently, the results obtained by this methodology are, in some cases, not well correlated with those of the classic in vivo experiments. Moreover, liver cell culturing technique is time consuming and requires expensive equipments and materials. Therefore it would be of great importance to develop additional in vitro tests which will address the problems of the current assays. In the present study, the liver slice system has been developed as a quantitative acute toxicity test for hazard assessment of hepatotoxic agents.

METHODS

Preparation of tissue slice system

Male rat or mouse was sacrificed by blow on the head after light ether anesthesia. Liver lobes were removed, sliced into small pieces and washed several times with KRH (Krebs Ringer Hepes) medium. The slices were divided into small portions and suspended in KRH medium as described by Wormser et al. (1). APAP (Sigma, St. Louis, USA) and CCl_4 (Merck, Darmstadt, FRG) were dissolved in propylene glycol and applied to the slices. At the indicated time intervals aliquots (100µl) were removed for enzyme analysis. AST and ALT were determined by commercial kits (Raichem™, San Diego, USA).

Animals and treatment

Male rats or mice were injected intraperitoneally with APAP (dissolved in propylene glycol 20% in saline). Animals were sacrificed 24 hours following exposure and serum analysis has been carried out. In another type of experiments mice were treated with APAP and after 10, 20, 30 and 40 minutes serum hepatotoxin level was determined by a commercial kit (Sigma, St. Louis, USA).

RESULTS AND DISCUSSION

The liver slice system offers a possible solution for the current problems of the in vitro hepatotoxicity assays. The APAP concentration required for liver damage in the in vivo and in vitro systems was identical. It was shown that the maximal serum APAP level in mice treated with the hepatotoxin (500 mg/kg) was 6.8 mg/ml (Table 1) and the same APAP concentration resulted in hepatocellular damage in the mouse slice system (Fig. 1). This close relationship between in vitro and in vivo liver toxicity was also found in another species, the rat, but a higher concentration of APAP (13.5 mg/ml) was needed to cause enzyme leakage in this species (Fig. 2, Table 1). Mouse slices responded at a concentration of 6.8 mg/ml (Fig. 1, Table 1).

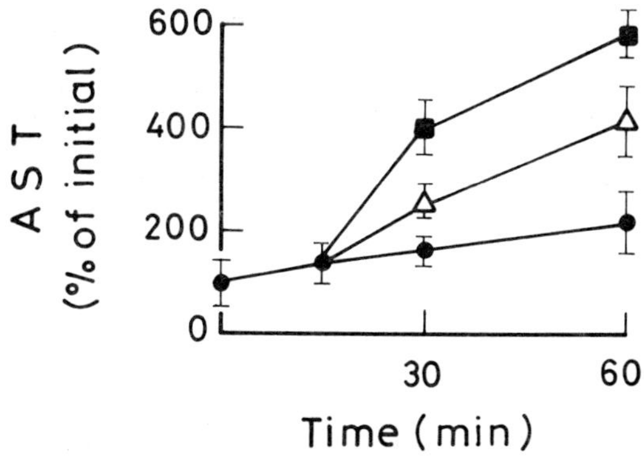

Fig. 1: AST leakage from mouse liver slices following in vitro APAP exposure.
Liver slices were prepared and suspended in 2ml of physiological medium. APAP (dissolved in propylene glycol) was applied at final concentrations of 6.8 (△) and 13.5 (■) mg/ml. The control system (●) received 200µl of the vehicle. At the indicated time intervals aliquots (100µl) of slice medium were removed for enzyme analysis.

Similar results were obtained in in vivo intoxication i.e. treatment of mice with APAP at a dose of 500 mg/kg resulted in marked elevation of serum AST while rats were not affected by this dose level of hepatotoxin (Table 1). Such interspecies differences cannot be easily obtained by cell culture because of availability of the appropriate system. Moreover, the liver slice system provides information about the differences in the toxico-kinetics of hepatotoxic agents namely, aminotransferase leakage from rat slices was observed 15 minutes after CCl_4 application (Fig. 3) whereas APAP caused such an effect only 30 minutes following exposure (Fig. 1, 2). This kind of information could be obtained by using only a single animal since one rat or mouse liver can provide tens of slice systems with which toxicity of various substances in a wide range of concentrations can be

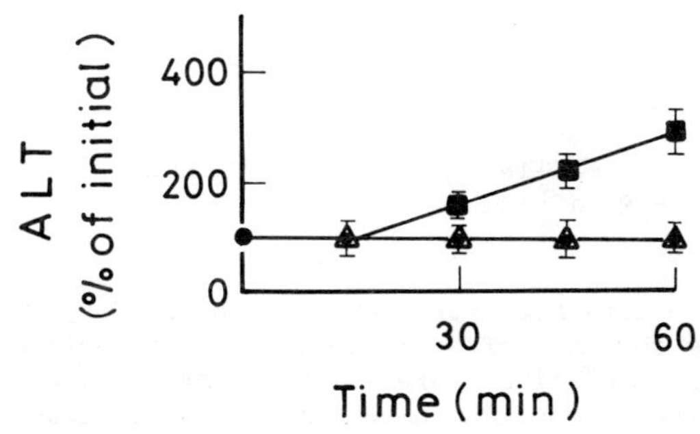

Fig. 2: ALT leakage from rat liver slices following in vitro APAP exposure.
Liver slices were prepared and suspended in 2ml of physiological medium. APAP (dissolved in propylene glycol) was applied at final concentrations of 6.8 (△) and 13.5 (■) mg/ml. The control system (●) received 200µl of the vehicle. At the indicated time intervals aliquots (100µl) of slice medium were removed for enzyme analysis.

assessed. In addition, slice systems of other organs (from which cell cultures are not available) from the same animal can serve as in vitro assays for toxicity assessment of a variety of substances, and also as an experimental system for investigation of toxicity mechanism of hazardous substances. The simple and quick preparation of the slices as well as its low cost can provide a good alternative to the classical acute toxicity test.

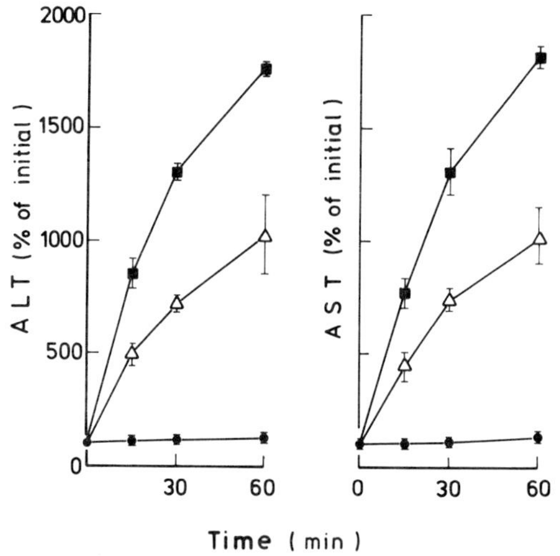

Fig. 3: Enzyme leakage from rat liver slices following in vitro CCl_4 exposure. Liver slices were prepared and suspended in 2ml of physiological medium. CCl_4 (dissolved in propylene glycol) was applied at final concentrations of 0.1% (△) and 0.25% (■). The control system (●) received 200µl of the vehicle. At the indicated time intervals aliquots (100µl) of slice medium were removed for ALT (left) and AST (right) analysis.

Table 1: APAP induced hepatocellular damage: comparison between the slice system and the intact animal.

IN VITRO			IN VIVO		
APAP concentration (mg/ml)	enzyme increase in slice medium (% of control)		APAP dose (mg/kg)	serum AST increase (% of control)	
	rat	mouse		rat	mouse
3.4	0	0			
6.8*	0	73±16	500*	0	455±75
13.5	78±9	155±36	1000	90±17	ND

In vitro: Results were obtained from Figures 1 and 2. Enzyme increase was calculated for values obtained after 30 minutes of incubation with APAP.
In vivo: Male rats and mice were injected intraperitoneally with APAP (dissolved in propylene glycol 20% in saline) at the indicated doses. The animals were sacrificed 24 hours following exposure and blood analysis was carried out.

*In a separate experiment mice were injected with APAP (500 mg/kg) and the maximal hepatotoxin level in serum was achieved 30 min after injection and it was shown to be 6.8 mg/ml. The same APAP concentration caused hepatocellular damage in the in vitro mouse liver slice system.

ND: not determined; The animals died within 1 hour post injection.

REFERENCES

1) WORMSER, U., CHOREV, M., GILON, C., LAUFER, R., FRIEDMAN, Z. Y. and SELINGER, Z. (1984) Substance P degrading systems of rat parotid and hypothalamus. Biochim. Biophys. Acta. 798: 28-36

2) STENBERG, K. (1986) Cellular methods for measuring drug toxicity in vitro. Trends Pharmacol. Sci. 7: 218-220

3) KISO, Y., TOHKIN, M. and HIKINO, H. (1983) Assay method for antihepatotoxic activity using galactosamine-induced cytotoxicity in primary cultured hepatocytes. J. Nat. Prod. 46: 841-847.

4) VONEN, B. and MORLAND, J. (1984) Isolated rat hepatocytes in suspension: Potential hepatotoxic effects of six different drugs. Arch. Toxicol. 56: 33-37.

B. Commercial Poster Presentations

Poster B1

The EYTEX-MPA System: An *In Vitro* Method for the Evaluation of Ocular Safety

V.C. GORDON and H.C. BERGMAN

National Testing Corporation
888 Research Drive
Palm Springs, CA 92262

ABSTRACT

The standard EYTEX* System is a chemical method for the evaluation of ocular safety with demonstrates a high correlation with results obtained *in vivo* for chemicals and and mixtures which can be solubilized in aqueous medium. However, there are many samples of great interest which can not be evaluated at significant concentrations due to insolubility, sample opacity or other limiting factors. The Membrane Partition Assay (MPA), a two phase assay system which proceeds for eighteen hours, has been developed and evaluated to address these problems. The EYTEX-MPA permits the classification of most test samples at 100% or close to 100%.

We evaluated the effectiveness of the EYTEX-MPA for a wide variety of chemicals, mixtures and product formulations by comparing results obtained *in vitro* with *in vivo* test results reported in the scientific literature and by manufacturers and independent testing laboratories. Out of 67 tests employing independent samples, 61 resulted in the same irritancy classification; six were within one Draize irritancy classification *in vitro* and *in vivo*. These results demonstrate a correlation of 96%. Only five materials (8%) of the sixty four evaluated required testing at concentrations below 50%. No ocular irritants were classified as non-irritants and no non-irritants were classified as ocular irritants. These results indicate the applicability of the EYTEX-MPA procedure for screening chemicals and formulations for ocular safety.

INTRODUCTION

National Testing Corporation has developed a chemical method for determination of ocular safety of materials and formulations; the trade name of this product is EYTEX (1). The advantages to this product include:

1. Simple procedure: Can be performed by technicians with limited training and experience.
2. Quantitative results: Spectrophotometric measurments are compared to standard curve; no subjectivity.
3. Rapid: All measurments require less than two hours of technician time; compared to several days or weeks for in vivo testing.
4. Reproducible: All reagents, calibrators and controls are supplied; within assay coefficients of variation range from 5% for samples with low irritancy to approximately 2% for high irritancy samples.
5. Cost effective: Cost per test is less than 10% that of *in vivo* method.

* EYTEX is a Trademark of National Testing Corporation: U.S. Patent No. 4,613,574

Extensive studies have been performed to compare results from the EYTEX method and from *in vivo* testing using the Draize procedure. A comparison of *in vitro* EYTEX results with *in vivo* Draize results demonstrated a 90% correlation. However, many samples of great interest could not be evaluated at significant concentrations due to insolubility, sample opacity or other limiting factors. The Membrane Partition Assay (MPA) has been developed and evaluated to address these problems and permit classification of many materials at close to 100%.

EXPERIMENTAL PRCEDURES

Materials. The EYTEX-MPA System includes the EYTEX-MPA Reagent Kit and EYTEX Supplies. It is intended to be used in conjunction with the EYTEX Laboratory to evaluate ocular safety of test samples. The EYTEX Laboratory includes a Jenway PC-01 Colorimeter with specialized filter, unique light source and modified optics to optimize and standardize laboratory measurements at 400nm. The EYTEX™ Reagent is a lyophilized powder containing proteins, glycoproteins, and macropolysaccharides, along with buffer salts. The powder is reconstituted by addition of distilled water.

Test Procedure. The procedure for evaluation of ocular safety using the EYTEX-MPA System consist of five stages.

STAGE ONE:

Sample Preparation. The solid samples are studied at 100% by adding 100mg of sample to each of the membrane cups. 100*ul* of diluent is added to conserve volumes and facilitate comparisons to liquid samples and blanks. The solid does not need to be solubilized. Liquid samples are studied at 100% by adding 100*ul*; of sample to the membrane cup. Dilutions can be prepared if concentrations of 100% do not qualify for EYTEX classification. Samples were obtained from standard commercial sources or individual manufacturers.

STAGE TWO:

Perform the Test. The actual test consist of three steps, the EYTEX reaction, the negative control test, and the positive control test.

The EYTEX Reaction: In the MPA, the sample is placed in cup formed by the membrane which is permeable to molecules of molecular weight 16,000 or below, which separates the sample from the cuvette chamber. The EYTEX Reagent or diluent is added to the cuvette. The membrane cup and sample are placed in the cuvette, and are sealed with a cap. The capped system is mixed by rotation for 18 hours. (Important: During incubation, temperature must be maintained at 22 to 28°C). Low molecular weight materials can diffuse between the sample and reagent compartments, and chemical irritants which are solubilized by the buffer can interact with the EYTEX Reagent to produce opacity just as in the standard EYTEX procedure. The EYTEX reaction is measured in optical density units on the Jenway PC-01, at 400nm. The EYTEX response is calibrated using a set of special MPA Calibrators, which consist of varying amounts of a known chemical irritant in opaque liquid. The MPA Calibrators are provided in the EYTEX-MPA Kit. All samples and calibrators must have a corresponding sample blank run in parallel.

Next, the **Negative Control Test** is performed by adding Negative Control Reagent to sample mixtures; incubating and then measuring optical densities. This test identifies sample concentrations which inhibit or saturate the response of the EYTEX Reagent.

The third step is the **Positive Control Test**. Add Positve Control Reagent to sample and blank mixture after incubation. Then optical densities are measured. This test identifies sample concentraions producing opacity wihich is unrelated to chemical irritancy.

STAGE THREE:
DATA ANALYSIS: CALCULATE THE FOLLOWING THREE QUANTITIES.

$\triangle$EYTEX: The net opacity produced by mixing the sample with EYTEX Reagent, after correction for the intrinsic opacity of the sample (as measured by the blank optical density). This quantity is also termed the net EYTEX Response.

$\triangle$N: The net increase in opacity produced by addition of the Negative Control Reagent, which contains a known chemical irritant.

$\triangle$P: A calculated quantity obtained by subtracting two times the opacity remaining after addition of Positive Control Reagent from the △EYTEX value. If △P is greater than zero, then the Positive Control Reagent, which contains an inhibitor of the EYTEX reaction, reduced the net EYTEX Response by greater than 50%.

STAGE FOUR: DATA QUALIFICATION: EVALUATE THE FOLLOWING THREE QUANTITIES

The three criteria to qualify the results are based on these three calculated quantities; the rationale of these tests is as follows:

EYTEX Response: the net opacity should always be equal to or greater than zero. Some slightly negative values may be obtained, due to pipetting or measurement errors; these values can be taken as zero. However, △EYTEX values of -0.050 or lower indicate a possible artifact and so not qualify.

Negative Control: Addition of the Negative Reagent to EYTEX Reagent alone will induce a large increase in opacity, resulting in an optical density greater than 0.6 O.D. When the Negative Control Reagent is added to a mixture of sample and EYTEX Reagent, a substantial increase in the opacity (△N) should be observed. If not, and if the △EYTEX is low, then the sample has inhibited the ability of the EYTEX Reagent to aggregate in response to a chemical irritant. If the △EYTEX was large, and △N was small, then the sample has saturated the aability of the EYTEX Reagent to aggregate in response to a chemical irritant. Since either phenomena can lead to underestimation of chemical irritancy, do not evaluate any result where △N < 0.1.

Positive Control: Addition of Positive Control Reagent to a mixture of a chemical irritant and EYTEX Reagent will cause a substantial decrease in opacity; usually by greater than 75%. If addition of Positive Control Reagent to a mixture of a sample and EYTEX Reagent does not reduce the opacity, then the apparent net EYTEX response probably resulted from an artificial aggregation of the EYTEX Reagent unrelated to the chemical irritancy of the sample. This phenomena can lead to an overestimation of chemical irritancy. If, however, the △EYTEX is small, experimental errors can lead to rejection of valid data. therefore, this criterion is only applied if the EYTEX Response is greater than optical density of the first calibrator.

STAGE FIVE:

Determine the Ocular Safety Classification. Each sample dilution must pass criterion described for the EYTEX Response and the negative and positive controls to qualify for safety classification. the net sample opacity can then be compared to the calibrator results to determine the safety classification.

INVESTIGATIONAL PROCEDURE

The efficacy of the EYTEX method for *in vitro* determination of ocular safety classifications was evaluated by comparison with results obtained by the *in vivo* Draize procedure. Tests were performed on a wide variety of individual chemicals and formulations from the following classes of materials: organic solvents, laboratory chemicals, pharmaceuticals, preservatives and antiseptic chemicals and formulations, detergent formulations, cosmetic formulations, and household products. Ten Samples were analyzed for ocular irritancy at two concentrations, and the results compared to values obtained using the Draize procedure. The Draize values were either taken from literature or from testing performed by independent laboratories.

CALCULATIONS

A correlation was calculated in the following manner: the results of EYTEX and *in vivo* testing were compared whenever there was at least one result with the Draize method at the same concentration for which there was no *in vitro* EYTEX result. A full correlation value of 1.0 was assigned when a test substance received an identical irritancy classification by the two methods. A partial correlation value of 0.5 was assigned when the EYTEX result was within one classification of the *in vivo* result. Results differing by more than one classification were assigned a correlation value of 0. Thus if the results are expressed as follows:

A = *Number of samples with full correlation,*
B = *Number of samples with partial correlation,*
C = *Number of samples with zero correlation;*

Then the percent correlation was calculated as: % Correlation = 100 x (A + 0.5 x B) / (A + B + C) = 96%

RESULTS

In the EYTEX-MPA the test samples in a membrane cup incubates with EYTEX Reagent containing biological macromolecules which bind chemicals potentially toxic to the eye. As illustrated in Figure 1, binding of chemical irritants to components of the EYTEX Reagent results in aggregation which can be measured optically.

The chemical irritancy of a test sample can be classified by the degree of opacity produced upon eighteen (18) hours incubation in the membrane cup with EYTEX Reagent. The opacity, and thus the optical density of the sample-reagent mixture increases with increasing chemical irritancy, which is also a function of the sample concentration. The net opacity is then compared to the opacities produced by known irritants with mild, moderate, and severe irritancy.

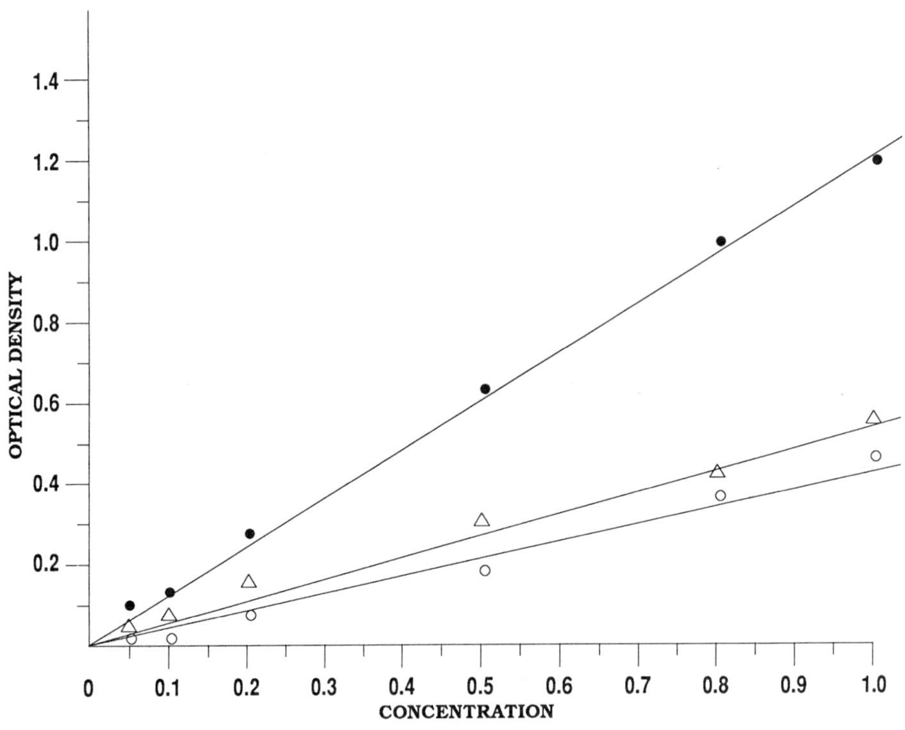

FIGURE 1. DOSE RESPONSE OF CHEMICAL IRRITANTS IN THE EYTEX-MPA
(•) Hydrochloric Acid, 0.05N to 1.0N,
(△) Granulated soap powder, 10mg to 100mg,
(○) Isopropanol, 10*ul* to 100*ul*

The results from testing of sixty-one different chemicals *in vivo* and *in vitro* are listed and summarized in Table 1. In several cases, data were available for more than one concentration; thus sixty-seven results were included in the correlation calculation. An overall correlation of 96% was obtained for all substances and concentrations tested. Of the five test substances which gave partial correlation results, all agreed with the Draize score within one classification.

TABLE 1.

CORRELATION OF EYTEX™ RESULTS WITH *IN VIVO* OCULAR IRRITANCY DATA

CHEMICAL	CONCENTRATION	EYTEX	IN VIVO RESULTS	REFERENCE
• ORGANIC SOLVENTS:				
Methanol	100ul	<mild	<mild	2
Glycerol	50ul	<mild	<mild	3
Tetrahydrofurfuryl Alcohol	100ul	<mild	mild	4
Butanol	50ul	moderate	moderate	3
n, Propanol	100ul	moderate	moderate	2
2,2 Ethoxy (ethoxyethanol)	100ul	<mild	<mild	2
Heptane	100ul	<mild	<mild	3
Acetonitrile	100ul	<mild	mild	3
N,N' Dimethyformamide	50ul	<mild	<mild	3
Formamide	100ul	<mild	<mild	3
Dimethylsulfoxide	100ul	<mild	<mild	5
Propylene Glycol	15ul	<mild	<mild	6
Ethylene Glycol	15ul	<mild	<mild	6
Isopropanol	100ul	mild	mild	2
Octanol	100ul	severe	severe	3
2, Phenoxyethanol	50ul	severe	severe	3
Ethanol	100ul	mild	mild	3
Ethanol	50ul	<mild	<mild	3
• PRESERVATIVES:				
Chloroform	100ul	<mild	<mild	2
• DISINFECTANTS & PRESERVATIVES:				
Hibiclens	100ul	moderate	moderate	7
Betadine	100ul	<mild	<mild	7
Chlorhexidine	20mg	moderate	severe	7
Tincture Iodide	100ul	severe	moderate	7
Tincture Iodine	100ul	moderate	moderate	7
Liquid Disinfectant	100ul	severe	severe	8
• SURFACTANTS				
Benzalkonium Chloride	100mg	severe	severe	3
Amphoteric Surfactant	10mg	<mild	<mild	8
Tween 80	10mg	<mild	<mild	3
Tween 20	10mg	<mild	<mild	3
• DRUGS				
Eye Drops	100ul	<mild	<mild	3
Ascorbic Acid	10mg	<mild	<mild	3
Aspirin	100mg	severe	severe	3

(table continues on the next page)

TABLE 1. (Continued)

• ACIDS & BASES:				
Ammonium Hydroxide	10ul	moderate	moderate	9
Acetic Acid	10ul	moderate	moderate	9
Trichloroacetic Acid	50mg	severe	severe	
Oxalic Acid	100mg	severe	severe	
Phenol	1mg	<mild	<mild	10
Phenol	5mg	<mild	<mild	10
Phenol	10mg	moderate	moderate	10
Triethanolamine	100ul	moderate	moderate	3
Citric Acid	50mg	severe	severe	3
Ethylenediamine	50ul	severe	severe	2
• INSECT REPELLENT:				
N, N' Diethyltoluamide	20ul	moderate	moderate	11
• CHEMICALS:				
Isoproplmyristate	100ul	<mild	<mild	3
Thymol	100mg	severe	severe	3
Polyethylene Glycol 200	100mg	<mild	<mild	3
• HOUSEHOLD PRODUCTS:				
Heavy Duty Laundry	60mg	moderate	moderate	8
Industrial Cleanser	100mg	moderate	moderate	8
Laundry Soap	100mg	moderate	moderate	8
Scouring Powder	100mg	severe	severe	8
• PERSONAL CARE PRODUCTS:				
Hair Spray	100mg	<mild	<mild	8
Skin Toner	100mg	<mild	<mild	8
Astringent Toner	100mg	<mild	<mild	8
Sun Screen	100mg	<mild	<mild	8
Lip Conditioner	100mg	<mild	<mild	8
Skin Lotion	100mg	<mild	<mild	8
Perfumed Skin Lotion	100mg	<mild	<mild	8
Men's Skin Lotion	100mg	<mild	<mild	8
Moisturizer	100mg	<mild	<mild	8
Baby Lotion	100mg	<mild	<mild	8
Baby Oil	100mg	<mild	<mild	8
• WAXES AND POLISHES:				
Furniture Polish	100ul	<mild	<mild	8
Floor Wax	100ul	<mild	<mild	8

Only five materials required EYTEX testing at concentrations below 50%. Materials must be tested at lower concentrations in the EYTEX System when results at higher concentrations do not qualify for evaluation. Results must pass three criteria to be qualified. First the EYTEX response, then △EYTEX or net opacity produced in the EYTEX System must be ≥0.05. △EYTEX below the reading are a result of interference with the EYTEX Reagent and can not be interpreted. The Negative Conctrol must also be passed. △N, the net increase in opacity, upon addition of a known irritant must be ≥0.1. This criteria ensures the EYTEX System is not inhibited or saturated. Finally, the Postive Control must be passed. △P, the difference between the EYTEX reading and the residual opacity after addition of the Postive Control, must be △P>0. This criteria ensures that the opacity produced by the test sample is due to the expected biological mechanism.

TABLE II.
SUMMARY OF CORRELATION

SAMPLE CATEGORY	SAMPLES TESTED	CORRELATION VALUE
Solvents	18	91.7%
Preservatives	10	91.7%
Surfactants	4	100.0%
Drugs	3	82.8%
Acids & Bases	10	100.0%
Household Products	5	100.0%
Personal Products	10	100.0%
Chemicals	3	100.0%
Insect Repellents	1	100.0%
Waxes & Polishes	2	100.0%
Test Samples	**67**	**96.0%**

DISCUSSION

There is a current and pressing need for alternatives to the Draize procedure for evaluation of ocular safety. The increasing number of chemicals introduced onto the market, the resulting requirements of protection of human health, the expense of animal testing, and the particular subjectivity of the Draize necessitate the development of rapid and reliable *in vitro* methods (12).

The EYTEX method for evaluation of ocular safety provides such an *in vitro* method. The EYTEX System is a chemical method, based on the ability of chemical irritants to aggregate the EYTEX Reagent, producing an opacity which can be measured optically.

The EYTEX Reagents is a concentrated solution of biological macromolecules with considerable intra- and intermolecular interactions based on hydrogen bonding and Van Der Waals forces. In this system, the chemical activity of water is much lower than that observed in dilute solutions, and a significant fraction of water molecules are bound to macromolecular solutes. These conditions are similar to those found *in vivo*; for example, the lens protein conformation is stabilized by protein-protein and protein-water interactions, which are essential to lens transparency (13). Chemical irritation results in a decreased transparency of the eye (14).

Irritant chemicals added to the reagent could disrupt the bonds between macromolecules, the intramolecular bonding necessary for secondary structure of macromolecules, and the bonds between macromolecules and water. Laser light scattering studies on the intact lens suggest that opacity results in changes in these short-range bonding interactions (15). Application of sodium lauryl sulfate results in opacification of the stromal layer, due primarily to precipitation of intra- and extracellular proteins (16). Similar precipitation producing opacity occurs when the chemical irritants bind to components of the EYTEX Reagent.

The results obtained in this study demonstrate the effectiveness of the EYTEX-MPA System. A high degree of correlation was obtained by comparison of EYTEX results with results obtained *in vivo*, using either the Draize procedure or its modifications. Over 96% of ocular safety classifications determined by the EYTEX-MPA method were identical to chemical irritancy classifications determined *in vivo*, and no results differed by more than one classification. The high percent correlation observed is particularly encouraging, considering that the Draize test is subjective in interpretation (17, 18) and yields variable results in the hands of individual technicians (19). Moreover, the Draize method itself does not correlate exactly with tests in humans, and authorites are in disagreement as to whether the rabbit eye is more or less sensitive than the human eye (20). The quantitative and reproducible nature of the EYTEX method would lead to more uniform results of tests performed at different locations or times.

Judicious substitution of the EYTEX test for the Draize procedure in these situations would allow a dramatic decrease in *in vivo* animal testing, resulting in a large cost reduction to industry. In addition, use of the EYTEX test could eliminate almost all of the animal suffering associated with Draize method, since chemicals identified as moderate to severe irritants *in vitro* would not require further *in vivo* testing. These factors, as well as the practical advantages of the EYTEX test, should encourage the use of this method for *in vitro* assessment of ocular irritancy.

REFERENCES

1. Gordon, V.C. and Bergman, H.C. (1987), in *In Vitro Toxicology: Approaches to Validation*. Goldberg, A.M. (ed), Mary Ann Liebert Inc., New York, p. 293.

2. Carpenter, C.P. and Smyth, H.F.(1976), Am. J. of Opth., **29:** 1963.

3. Grant, M.W. (1974), *Toxicology of the Eye*, Second Edition, Charles C. Thomas, Springfield, Illinois.

4. Results obtained from *in vivo* tests performed by Applied Biological Sciences Laboratory, Glendale, California.

5. Draize, J.H., Woodward, G., Calvery, H.O. (1944), J. Pharma. Exp. & Theory, **82:** 377.

6. Conquet, P., Durand, G., Laillier, J., and Plazonnet, B. (1977), Tox. Appl. Pharm., **39:** 129.

7. MacRae, S.M., Brown, B., and Edelhauser, H.E. (1944), Am. J. of Opth., **82:** 377.

8. Data supplied by manufacturer; testing performed by independent laboratories.

9. Murphy, J.C., Osterberg, R.E., Seabaugh, V.M. & Bierbouer, G.W. (1982), Toxicology, **23:** 281.

10. Hughes, W.F., Jr., Bull. Johns Hopkins Hosp. (1948), **82:** 338.

11. MacRae, S.M., Brown, B., Ubels, J.L., and Edelhauser, H.E. (1984), J. Tox. - Cut. & Oc. Tox., **3:** 17-30.

12. Swanson, D.W. (1983), in *Animals and alternatives to Toxicity Testing*, Balls, M., Riddell, R.J., and Worten, A.M., editions; Academic Press, London, United Kingdon, page 337.

13. Crompton, M., Rixon, K.C. and Harding, J.J. (1985), Exp. Eye Res., **40:** 297.

14. Clark, J.I., and Benedek, G.B. (1980), Invest. Opth. in Vis. Sci., **17:** 771.

15. Trokel, S., Invest. Opth. (1982), **1:** 495.

16. Jacaruso, R.B. (1985), J. Toxicol. Cut. & Oc. Toxicol., **4:** 49

17. Weil, C.S., and Scala, R.A. (1971), Tox. Appl. Pharm., **19:** 276.

18. Marzuli, F.N. & Ruggles, D.I. (1973), J. Am. Assoc. An. Chem., **56:** 905.

19. Northroot, H., Yackovich, F., Demetrolias, J., Gacola, M. and Heinze, J.E. (1982), Tox.Lett., **14:** 207.

20. Scaife, M.C. (1985), ATLA, **12:** 157.

Poster B2

External Evaluation of the Standard EYTEX System in Six Laboratories to Determine Intra- and Inter-Laboratory Accuracy and Precision

V.C. GORDON and H.C. BERGMAN

National Testing Corporation
888 Research Drive
Palm Springs, CA 92262

ABSTRACT

The EYTEX System has been developed as an *in vitro* chemical method for the evaluation of ocular safety. The standard EYTEX System consists of the EYTEX Reagent Kit and the EYTEX Laboratory, which contains all equipment and supplies required to perform the EYTEX procedure, thus allowing a standardized approach to ocular safety testing. Data obtained with the stand EYTEX System demonstrated a high correlation with *in vivo* Draize results. We have recently collaborated with six major industrial, governmental, and university laboratories to perform an external evaluation of the standard EYTEX System.

This external evaluation was designed to determine intra- and inter-laboratory accuracy and precision. Participating laboratories analyzed ten samples ranging in ocular irritancy from non-irritants to severe irritants. The test samples included a laundry soap, a hair spray, a surfactant, a germicide, a solvent, a cleanser, an eye rinse, a preservative, a skin toner, and a liquid dishwashing soap. Each sample was evaluated at two concentrations in three independent determinations. 90% of the results obtained in the six different laboratories were in agreement; 6% differed by only one safety classification. No ocular irritants were classified as non-irritants and no non-irritants were classified as irritants.

INTRODUCTION

National Testing Corporation has developed the EYTEX System, and *in vitro* chemical method for determination of ocular safety of materials and formulations. Extensive studies comparing in vitro EYTEX results with *in vivo* Draize results have demonstrated good correlation (1). The EYTEX System including EYTEX Reagent and supplies as well as the instrumentation and equipment, is a complete standardized method producing quantative and reproducible results. Technical staff can be trained to perform the EYTEX test using standardized procedures, straightforward report forms, and a detailed manual.

EXPERIMENTAL PRCEDURES

Materials. The EYTEX System includes the EYTEX Reagent Kit and EYTEX Supplies. It is intended to be used in conjunction with the EYTEX Laboratory to evaluate ocular safety of test samples. The EYTEX Laboratory includes a Jenway PC-01 Colorimeter with specialized filter, unique light source and modified optics to optimize and standardize laboratory measurements at 400nm. The EYTEX™ Reagent is a lyophilized powder containing proteins, glycoproteins, and mucopolysaccharides, along with buffer salts. The powder is reconstituted by addition of distilled water.

Test Procedure. The procedure for evaluation of ocular safety using the EYTEX-MPA SYSTEM consist of five stages.

STAGE ONE:

Sample Preparation. Solid samples and viscous liquids were studied at 5 and 10% by adding diluent to the samples. Two irritancy solids, in this study, were further diluted for analysis. Liquid samples were studied at 10% and 100%. Dilutions were prepared with diluent. These samples were obtained from commercial sources or industrial manufacturers.

STAGE TWO:

Perform the Test. The actual test consist of three steps, the EYTEX Reaction, the Negative Control Test, and the Positive Control Test.

The EYTEX Reaction: 100*ul* of the prepared dilution of test samples was added to the EYTEX Reagent. The EYTEX Reaction is measured in optical density units on the Jenway PC-01, at 400nm. The EYTEX Response is calibrated using a set of special Calibrators which consist of varying amounts of a known chemical irritant. The Calibrators are provided in the EYTEX Kit. All samples must have a corresponding sample blank in parallel.

Next, the **Negative Control Test** is performed by adding Negative Control Reagent to sample mixtures; incubating and then measuring optical densities. This test identifies sample concentrations which inhibit or saturate the response of the EYTEX Reagent.

The third step is the **Positive Control Test**. Add Positve Control Reagent to sample and blank mixture after incubation. Then optical densities are measured. This test identifies sample concentraions producing opacity wihich is unrelated to chemical irritancy.

STAGE THREE:

Data Analysis. In the data analysis process the following three quantities are calculated: $\triangle$EYTEX, $\triangle$N, and $\triangle$P.

STAGE FOUR:

Data Qualification. The EYTEX results are then qualified based on those these three quantities: $\triangle \text{EYTEX} \geq -0.05$, $\triangle N \geq 0.1$, $\triangle P > 0$ or $\triangle \text{EYTEX} \leq C_1$.

STAGE FIVE:

Determine the Ocular Safety Classification. Each sample dilution must pass criterion described for the EYTEX Response and the Negative and Positive Controls to qualify for safety classification. The net sample opacity can then be compared to the calibrator results to determine the safety classification.

INVESTIGATIONAL PROCEDURE

Six major laboratories representing governmental, industrial, and university laboratories were invited to participate in an external evaluation of the EYTEX System. Technical Staff attended a presentation, and six to eight hour training session in their laboratory with the EYTEX System in place.

The study was designed to optimize laboratory conditions; all equipment and instrumentation were standardized. Technical Staff was trained in test performance, data analysis and data interpretation.

Tests were performed on 10 individual chemicals and formulations from the following classes of materials: organic solvents, laboratory chemicals, pharmaceuticals, preservatives and antiseptics chemicals and formulations, detergent formulations, cosmetic formulations, and household products. Each sample was analyzed in triplicate for ocular irritancy at two concentrations, and the results compared to values obtained from other laboratories.

CALCULATIONS:

The reproducibility of the EYTEX System in six different laboratories was evaluated by empirical comparison of the results obtained in each laboratory.

STATISTICAL ANALYSIS:

Ocular safety classifications for each test sample were compiled by laboratory. Ocular safety classifications within two standard deviations of the calibrators were classfied between the two ocular safety classifications. A full correlation of 1.0 was assigned when a safety classification was identical to the consensus safety classification. A partial correlation of 0.75 was assigned when the EYTEX results was between the consensus classification and the next safety classification. A partial correlation of 0.5 was assigned when the EYTEX result was within one classification of the consensus classification. Finally, a partial correlation of 0.25 was assigned when the EYTEX result was between the second adjacent safety classification. A value of 0 was assigned when the results differed by two, safety classification.

A = Number of results with consensus classification,
B = Number of results within 0.5 classification,
C = Number of results within 1.0 classification,
D = Number of results within 1.5 classification,
E = Number of results within 2.0 or more classifications,

% Correlation = 100 x (A + 0.75B + 0.5C + 0.25D) / (A + B + C + D + E)

RESULTS

The results from testing ten test samples at two concentrations in six independent laboratories are presented in Figure I. If no result is presented, there was either a non-qualified result or incomplete data. EYTEX Responses within two standard deviations of an EYTEX calibrator optical density were designated between the two corresponding ocular safety classifications.

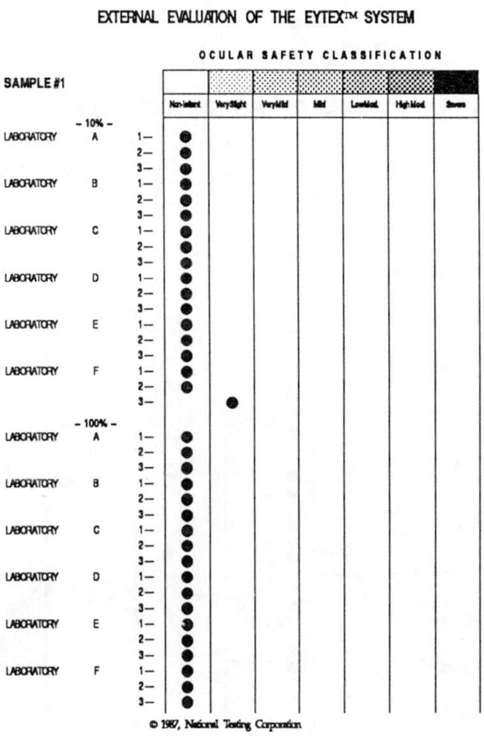

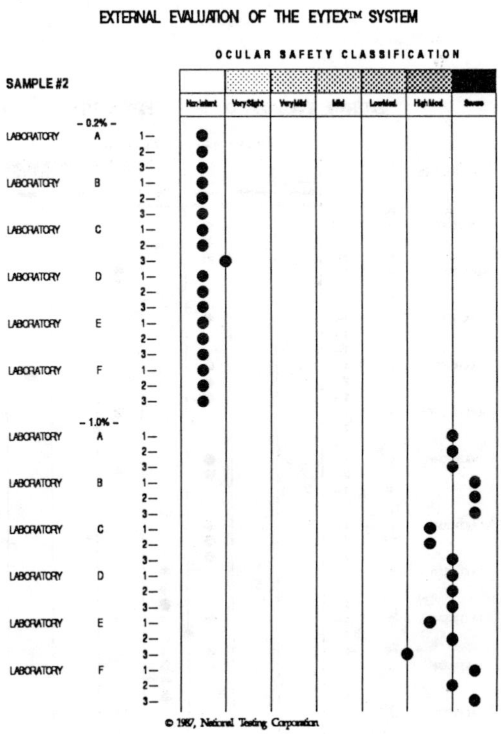

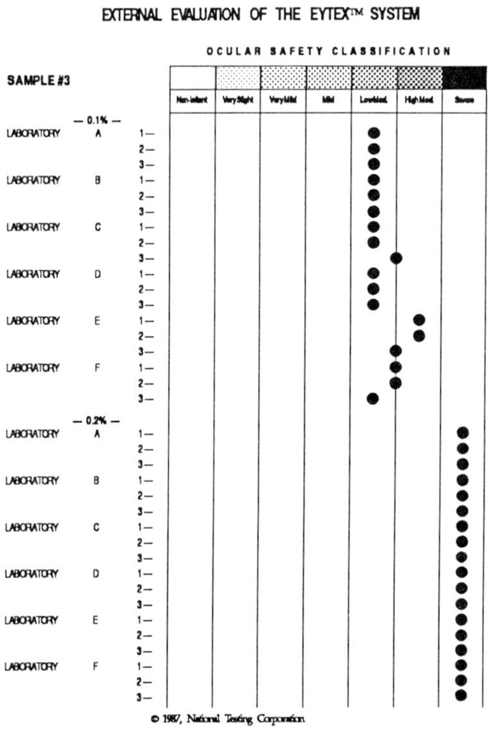
EXTERNAL EVALUATION OF THE EYTEX™ SYSTEM
OCULAR SAFETY CLASSIFICATION
SAMPLE #3
Non-irritant
Very Slight
Very Mild
Mild
Low Mod.
High Mod.
Severe
— 0.1% —
— 0.2% —
LABORATORY A
LABORATORY B
LABORATORY C
LABORATORY D
LABORATORY E
LABORATORY F
© 1987, National Testing Corporation

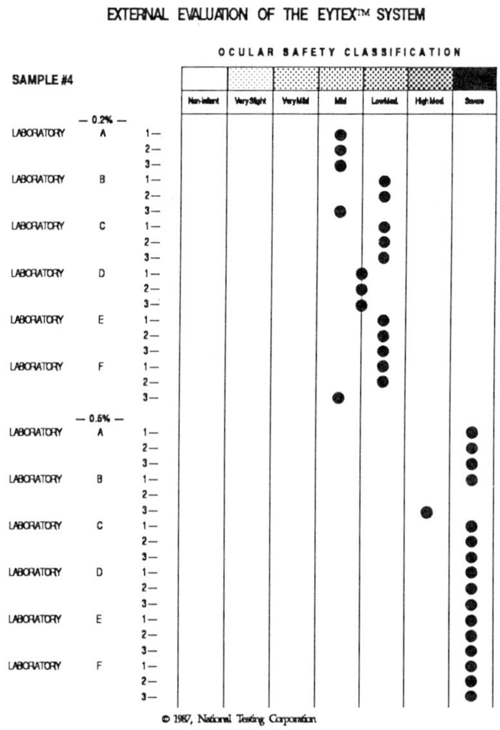
EXTERNAL EVALUATION OF THE EYTEX™ SYSTEM
OCULAR SAFETY CLASSIFICATION
SAMPLE #4
Non-irritant
Very Slight
Very Mild
Mild
Low Mod.
High Mod.
Severe
— 0.2% —
— 0.5% —
LABORATORY A
LABORATORY B
LABORATORY C
LABORATORY D
LABORATORY E
LABORATORY F
© 1987, National Testing Corporation

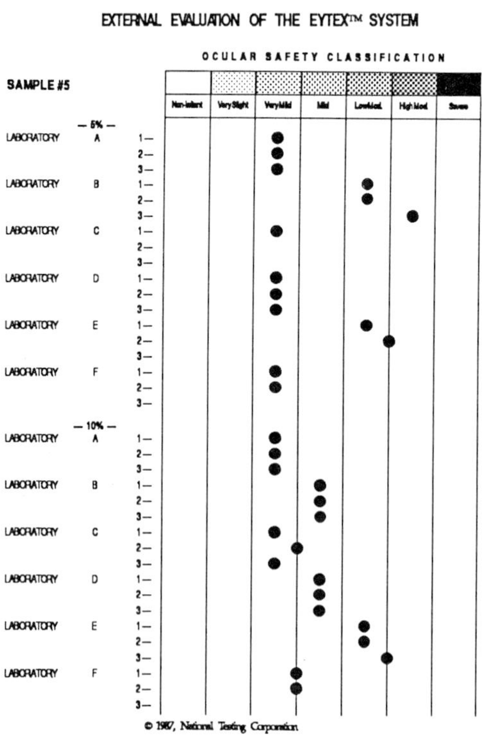
EXTERNAL EVALUATION OF THE EYTEX™ SYSTEM
OCULAR SAFETY CLASSIFICATION
SAMPLE #5
Non-irritant
Very Slight
Very Mild
Mild
Low Mod.
High Mod.
Severe
— 5% —
— 10% —
LABORATORY A
LABORATORY B
LABORATORY C
LABORATORY D
LABORATORY E
LABORATORY F
© 1987, National Testing Corporation

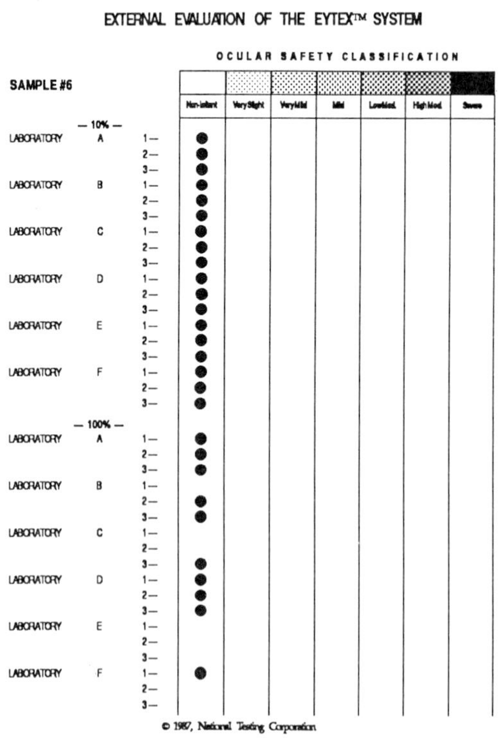
EXTERNAL EVALUATION OF THE EYTEX™ SYSTEM
OCULAR SAFETY CLASSIFICATION
SAMPLE #6
Non-irritant
Very Slight
Very Mild
Mild
Low Mod.
High Mod.
Severe
— 10% —
— 100% —
LABORATORY A
LABORATORY B
LABORATORY C
LABORATORY D
LABORATORY E
LABORATORY F
© 1987, National Testing Corporation

EXTERNAL EVALUATION OF THE EYTEX™ SYSTEM

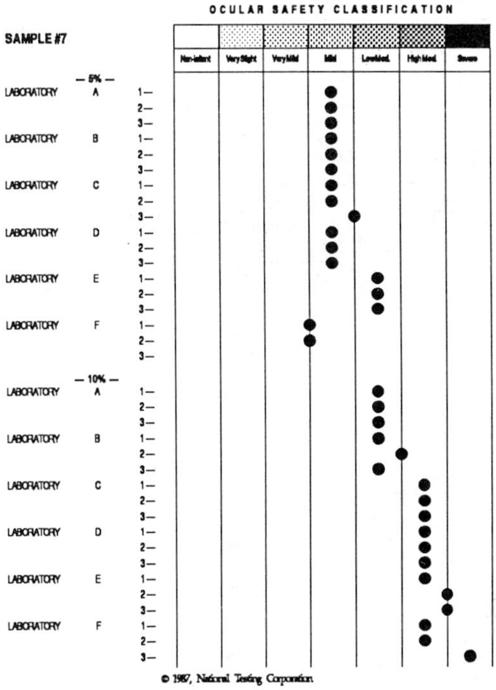

EXTERNAL EVALUATION OF THE EYTEX™ SYSTEM

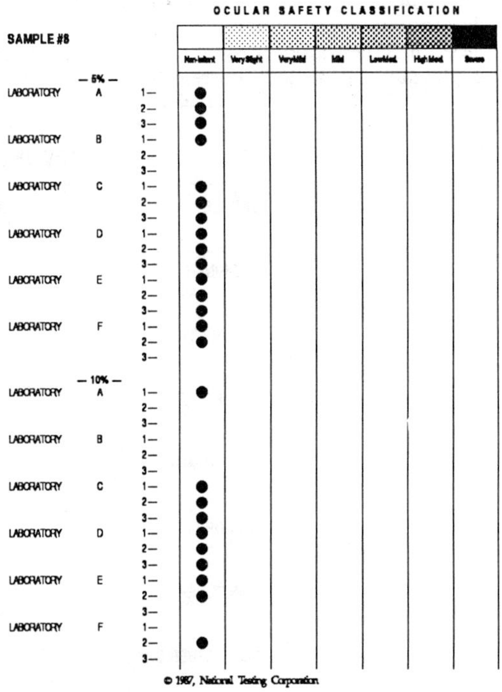

EXTERNAL EVALUATION OF THE EYTEX™ SYSTEM

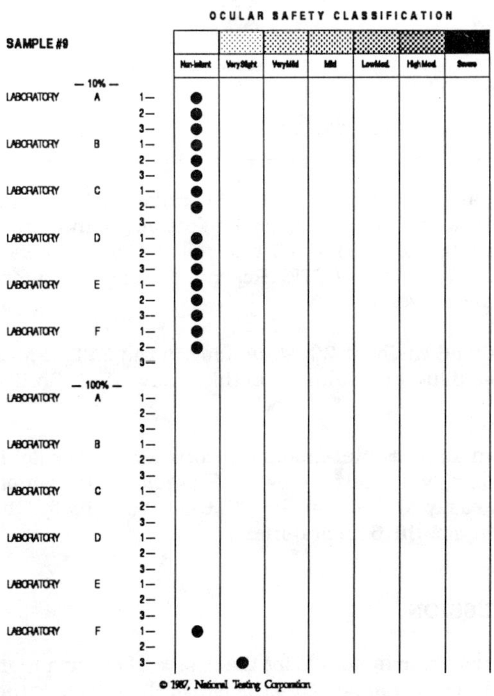

EXTERNAL EVALUATION OF THE EYTEX™ SYSTEM

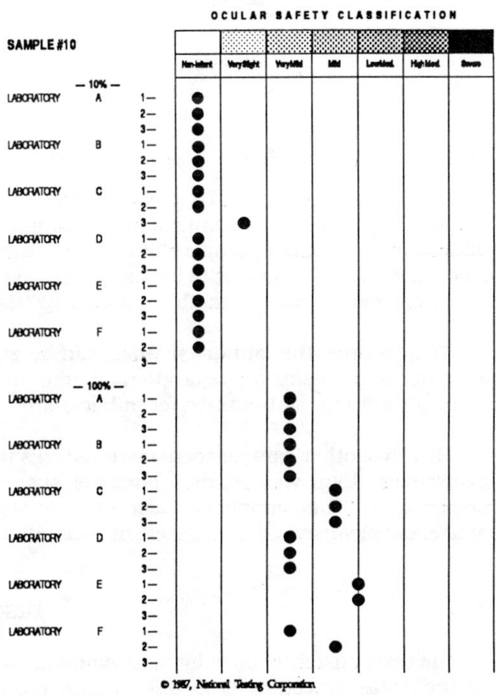

The summary of the results in Figure 1 is presented in Table I. This table illustrates the reproducibility between and within laboratories. The average interlaboratory correlation is 90%. the data represented in Figure 1 and summarized in Table 1, was collected from one to four technical personnel per laboratory. At least ten separate individuals submitted data, indicative of the significance of the 90% correlation.

TABLE I
SUMMARY OF CORRELATION DATA

SAMPLE	CONCENTRATION (%)	INTERLABORATORY CORRELATION
EYE RINSE	10.0	94.0%
	100.0	100.0%
DISINFECTANT	0.2	97.0%
	1.0	86.0%
PRESERVATIVE	0.1	89.0%
	0.2	100.0%
SURFACTANT	0.2	83.0%
	0.5	97.0%
LAUNDRY POWDER	5.0	53.0%
	10.0	63.0%
SKIN TONER	10.0	100.0%
	100.0	100.0%
DISHWASHER SOAP	5.0	87.0%
10.0	76.0%	
CREAM RINSE	5.0	100.0%
	10.0	100.0%
SOLVENT	10.0	89.0%
	100.0	94.0%
HOUSEHOLD CLEANSER	10.0	97.0%
	100.0	71.0%
		AVERAGE **90.0%**

Test sample #5, a laundry powder exhibits the largest variability. The data submitted for sample #5 demonstrated large variations in the sample blank. Since the sample blank is only a mixture of diluent and prepared sample dilution, the supernatant of sample #5 was not the same in each laboratory. The dilutions with low sample blanks exhibited lower EYTEX Response. Sample dilutions with high sample blanks exhibited higher EYTEX responses.

This sample, the laundry powder, can be analyzed easily at 20mg to 80mg in the EYTEX-MPA without the problems of preparation inherent in the dilutions evaluated in this study. (V.C. Gordon and H.C. Bergman, submitted for publication)

Only two other samples demonstrated less than an 83% inter-laboratory correlation. The liquid dishwasher soap was a thick aqueous suspension which also presented problems in sample preparation. This sample can also be evaluated easily at 100$u\ell$ in the EYTEX-MPA. Finally, the household cleanser exhibits excellent correlation in 5 of the 6 laboratories.

DISCUSSION

The tests currently used by most manufacturers to rate materials for the degree of eye irritation are the Draize procedure or modified Draize procedures. An important criticism of these tests is the demonstrated lack of reproducibility of the irritancy evaluation of materials within and between laboratories (2,3,4,5).

The present investigation was designed to determine the reproducibility of determining ocular safety classification in the EYTEX System. There are several major components of the EYTEX System essential to its standardization and reproducibility. The EYTEX Reagent a concentrated solution of biological macromolecules is subjected to stringent quality control procedures ensuring reproducible and quantitative calibration curves and reproducible responses to known irritants. The Jenway PC-01 is modified and standardized in conjunction with the EYTEX Reagent. Calibration curves on each instrument are in agreement within 3%. All supplied reagents, calibrators and controls produce within assay coefficients of variation of 5% to 10%.

The results in this study demonstrate good reproducibility of the ocular safety classifications of ten diverse materials at two different concentrations in six independent laboratories. Therefore, the EYTEX method can be performed in different laboratories by many different technical personnel to produce reproducible ocular safety classifications.

SUMMARY

1. The inter-laboratory comparisons demonstrated an average correlation of 90%.

2. The correlation within laboratories whether one or four technical personnel performed the assays was between 90% and 100%.

3. The experimentally observed range of classifications was uniform in all laboratories.

4. The largest variability was observed for opaque, insoluble materials which were difficult to prepare for analysis. These materials can easily and reproducibly be run in the EYTEX-MPA.

REFERENCES

1. Gordon, V.C. and Bergman, H.C., (1987), in *In Vitro* Toxicology: Approaches to Validation, Goldberg, A.M. (ed.) Mary Ann Liebert, Inc, N.Y.,N.Y.

2. Weil, C.S., and Scala, R.A., (1971), Toxicol. Appl. Pharmacol., **19**: 276-360

3. Marzuli, F.N., and Ruggles, D.I., (1972), J. Am. Assoc. Anal. Chem., **45**: 905-914

4. Russell, K.L., and Hoch, S.G., (1862), Proc. Sci. Sect. Toilet Goods Assoc., **37**: 27-32

5. Williams, S.J., Graepel, G.J. and Kennedy, G.L., (1982), Toxicol. Lett., **12**: 235-241

Poster B3

External Evaluation of the EYTEX and EYTEX-MPA Systems in Twelve Laboratories to Determine the Correlation of EYTEX Results with *In Vivo* Results

V.C. GORDON and H.C. BERGMAN

National Testing Corporation
888 Research Drive
Palm Springs, CA 92262

ABSTRACT

The EYTEX and the EYTEX-MPA System are *in vitro* chemical methods for the evaluation of ocular safety. Data obtained with the standard EYTEX and the EYTEX-MPA Systems has demonstrated high correlation with *in vivo* Draize results. We have recently collaborated with twelve major industrial, governmental, and university laboratories to perform an external evaluation of the adaptability of this system to a large variety of chemicals and mixtures unique to these twelve laboratories. We have correlated these results with Draize data obtained from each laboratory.

Each laboratory selected between 5 and 60 materials of particular interest to their laboratory evaluation in the EYTEX and EYTEX-MPA System. The materials evaluated included surgical scrubs, germicides, pesticides, cosmetics, personal care products, household goods, surfactants, preservatives and drugs. Comparison of results from these studies utilizing the EYTEX System with those of *in vivo* Draize test results demonstrated a strong correlation between the two methods. Depending on the type of materials evaluated, an overall correlation of 90% was obtained. These results indicate that the EYTEX System provides a reproducible, accurate, and transferable *in vitro* method for the evaluation of ocular safety of a wide variety of chemicals and mixtures.

INTRODUCTION

National Testing Corporation has developed the EYTEX System, a chemical method for determination of the ocular safety of materials and formulations. The system has demonstrated the capability to study diverse chemical formulations and products undiluted or at meaningful concentrations. The laboratory equipment and instrumentation provide accurate spectrophotometric measurements. All reagents, calibrators and controls are provided ensuring within assay coefficient of variation from 5% to 10%. The EYTEX test results correlate well with existing laboratory and literature Draize values.

An external evaluation of the EYTEX System in six laboratories was conducted to determine the reproducibility of the EYTEX System. The study demonstrated an inter-laboratory correlation of 90%. An expanded external evaluation of the capability of the EYTEX System was commenced in twelve major industrial, governmental and university laboratories. The twelve participating laboratories represented unique interests in diverse classes of materials, formulations and products.

EXPERIMENTAL PROCEDURES

Materials. The EYTEX System includes the EYTEX Reagent Kit and EYTEX Supplies. It is intended to be used in conjunction with the EYTEX Laboratory to evaluate ocular safety of test samples. The EYTEX Laboratory includes a Jenway PC-01 Colorimeter with specialized filter, unique light source and modified optics to optimize and standardize laboratory measurements at 400nm. The EYTEX™ Reagent is a lyophilized powder containing proteins, glycoproteins, and mucopolysaccharides, along with buffer salts. The powder is reconstituted by addition of distilled water.

Test Procedure. The procedure for evaluation of ocular safety using the EYTEX-MPA SYSTEM consist of five stages.

STAGE ONE:

Sample Preparation. Soluble and miscible liquids are evaluated in the standard system at 10% and 100%. If these concentrations do no qualify, lower concentrations can be evaluated in the standard system or the sample can be evaluated in the EYTEX-MPA System. Soluble solids are evaluated in the standard EYTEX System at 1% and 10%. If these concentrations do not qualify, the sample can be evaluated in the EYTEX-MPA. In the MPA, solid samples are studied neat by adding 100mg of sample to each of the membrane cups. 100 *ul* of diluent is added to conserve volumes and facilitate comparisons to liquid samples and blanks. The solid does not need to be solubilized. Liquid samples are studied neat by adding 100*ul* of sample to the membrane cup. Dilutions can be prepared if concentrations of 100% do not qualify for EYTEX classification. Samples were obtained from standard commercial sources or individual manufacturers.

STAGE TWO:

Perform the Test. The actual test consist of three steps, the EYTEX Reaction, the Negative Control Test, and the Positive Control Test.

The EYTEX Reaction: In the MPA, the sample is placed in cup formed by the membrane which is permeable to molecules of molecular weight of 16,000 or below, and which separates the sample from the cuvette chamber. The EYTEX Reagents or diluent is added to the cuvette. The membrane cup and sample are placed in the cuvette, and are sealed with a cap. The capped system is mixed by rotation for 18 hours. (Important: During incubation, temperature must be maintained at 22 to 28°C). Low molecular weight materials can diffuse between the sample and reagent compartments, and chemical irritants which are solubilized by the buffer can interact with the EYTEX Reagent to produce opacity.

In the standard EYTEX procedure, the sample is added directly to the EYTEX Reagent. The sample can interact to produce opacity.

The EYTEX Reaction is measured in optical density units on the Jenway PC-01, at 400nm. The EYTEX Response is calibrated using a set of special calibrators, which consist of varying amounts of a known chemical irritant. The calibrators are provided.

Next, the **Negative Control Test** is performed by adding Negative Control Reagent to sample mixtures; incubating and then measuring optical densities. The test identifies sample concentrations which inhibit or saturate the response of the EYTEX Reagent.

The third step is the **Positive Control Test**. Add Positive Control Reagent to samples and blanks after incubation. Then optical densities are measured. This test identifies sample concentrations producing opacity which is unrelated to chemical irritancy.

STAGE THREE:

Date Analysis: Calculate the following three quantities: $\triangle$EYTEX, $\triangle$N, and $\triangle$P.

STAGE FOUR:

DATA QUALIFICATION: Evaluate the following three quantities. The three criteria to qualify the results are based on these three calculated quantities; the rationale of these tests is as follows:

EYTEX Response: The net opacity should always be equal to or greater than zero. Some slightly negative values may be obtained, due to pipetting or measurement errors; these values can be taken as zero. However, $\triangle$EYTEX values of -0.050 or lower indicate a possible artifact and so do not qualify.

Negative Control: Addition of the Negative Control Reagent to EYTEX Reagent alone will induce a large increase in opacity, resulting in an optical density greater than 0.6 O.D. When the Negative Control Reagent is added to a mixture of sample the EYTEX Reagent, a substantial increase in the opacity ($\triangle$N) should be observed.

Positive Control: Addition of the Positive Control Reagent to a mixture of a chemical irritant and EYTEX Reagent will cause a substantial decrease in opacity; usually by greater than 75%. If addition of Positive Control Reagent to a mixture of a sample and EYTEX Reagent does not reduce the opacity, then $\triangle P>0$. Then , the sample does not qualify. This criterion is only applied if the EYTEX Response is greater than the optical density of the first calibrator.

STAGE FIVE:

Determine the Ocular Safety Classification. Each sample dilution must pass the criterion described for the EYTEX Response and the Negative and Positive Controls to qualify for safety classification. The net sample opacity can then be compared to the calibrator results to determine the ocular safety classification.

INVESTIGATIONAL PROCEDURE

Twelve major laboratories representing governmental, industrial, and university laboratories were invited to participate in an external evaluation of the EYTEX System. Technical Staff were introduced to the EYTEX System with a presentation and six to eight hour training session in their laboratory with the EYTEX System in place. The study was designed to optimize laboratory conditions. All equipment and instrumentation were standardized. Technical Staff were trained in test performance, data analysis and data interpretation. Each laboratory assayed ten materials at two concentrations to ensure experience with and technical knowledge of the EYTEX System. After this initial testing, test sample selection was made by each participating laboratory to reflect the particular interest and relevant formulations of the individual laboratory.

CALCULATIONS:

CORRELATION: 96% – Results obtained using the *in vitro* EYTEX Procedure were compared to *in vivo* results obtained by the Draize procedure. The sources for the Draize data were obtained from the literature or from individual laboratories indicated below. A correlation was calculated in the following manner: The results of EYTEX and *in vivo* testing were compared whenever there was at least one result with the Draize method at the same concentration for which there was an *in vitro* EYTEX result. A full correlation value of 1.0 was assigned when a test substance received an identical irritancy classification by the two methods. A partial correlation value of 0.5 was assigned when the EYTEX result was within one classification of the *in vivo* result. Results differing by more than one classification were assigned a correlation value of 0. Thus if the results are expressed as follows:

A = Number of samples with full correlation = 122
B = Number of samples with partial correlation = 8
C = Number of samples with zero correlation = 0

then the percent correlation was calculated as:

%Correlation = 100 x (A + 0.5 x B) / (A + B + C) = 100 x (122 + 0.5 x 8) / (130)) = 96%

SENSITIVITY: 95% – Sensitivity is the ratio of irritants which give a positive result to the number of irritants tested. In the EYTEX System, a positive result is defined as a test sample with an ocular safety classification of mild or greater. An irritant is defined as a test sample with a Draize classification of mild or greater.

a = Number irritants identified positive = 55
c = Number irritants not identified positive = 3
Sensitivity = a / a + c = 55 / 58 = 95%

SPECIFICITY: 99% – Specificity is the ratio of non-irritants which give a negative result to the total number of non-irritants tested. In the EYTEX System a negative result is defined as a test sample with an ocular safety classification of less than mild. A non-irritant is defined as a test sample with a Draize classification of less than mild.

d = Number non-irritants identified negative = 71
b = Number non-irritants identified positive = 1
Specificity = d / b + d = 71 / 72 = 96%

PREDICTIVE VALUE: 98% – The predictive Value is the ratio of the number of irritants identified positive to the total number of positive results. The Predictive Value is directly related to the prevalence value which is the ratio of the number of irritants tested to the total number of test. In this study, the prevalence is 45%.

Predictive Value = a /a + b = 55 / 56 = 98%

RESULTS

An excternal evaluation of the EYTEX System in twelve major industrial and governmental laboratories demonstrated a strong correlation between the EYTEX System and *in vivo* Draize results. The results correlated to date are presented in Table I.

TABLE I.
EXTERNAL EVALUATION OF THE EYTEX™ SYSTEM

		EYTEX SAFETY CLASSIFICATION	DRAIZE IRRITANCY CLASSIFICATION
A. ORGANIC SOLVENTS			
METHANOL	100.0%	less than mild	less than mild
GLYCEROL	100.0%	less than mild	less than mild
GLYCEROL	50.0%	less than mild	less than mild
TETRAHYDROFURFURYL ALCOHOL	100.0%	less than mild	mild
BUTANOL	50.0%	moderate	moderate
N-PROPANOL	100.0%	moderate	moderate
ETHOXYETHOXYETHANOL	100.0%	less than mild	less than mild
HEPTANE	100.0%	less than mild	less than mild
ACETONITRILE	100.0%	less than mild	mild
N, N'-DIMETHYLFORMAMIDE	50.0%	less than mild	less than mild
FORMAMIDE	100.0%	less than mild	less than mild
DIMETHYLSULFOXIDE	100.0%	less than mild	less than mild
PROPYLENE GLYCOL	15.0%	less than mild	less than mild
ETHYLENE GLYCOL	15.0%	less than mild	less than mild
ISOPROPANOL	100.0%	mild	mild
OCTANOL	100.0%	severe	severe
2-PHENOXY ETHANOL	50.0%	severe	severe
ETHANOL	100.0%	mild	less than mild
ETHANOL	50.0%	less than mild	less than mild
ETHANOL	10.0%	less than mild	less than mild
2-ETHOXY ETHANOL	100.0%	less than mild	less than mild
B. PRESERVATIVES			
CHLOROFORM	100.0%	less than mild	less than mild
FORMALDEHYDE	1.0%	less than mild	less than mild
THIMEROSAL	5.0%	less than mild	less than mild
METHYL PARABEN	0.04%	less than mild	less than mild
BIOBAN	0.5%	less than mild	less than mild
CHLOROBUTANOL	0.1%	less than mild	less than mild
DOWCIL 200	2.0%	less than mild	less than mild
GERMALL 115	10.0%	less than mild	less than mild
C. DISINFECTANTS & GERMICIDES			
HIBICLENS	100.0%	moderate	moderate
BETADINE	100.0%	less than mild	less than mild
CHLORHEXIDENE	20.0%	moderate	severe
TINCTURE OF IODIDE	100.0%	severe	moderate
TINCTURE OF IODINE	100.0%	moderate	moderate
LIQUID DISINFECTANT	100.0%	severe	severe
D. SURFACTANTS			
BENZALKONIUM CHLORIDE	100.0%	severe	severe
SODIUM DYODECYL SULFATE	0.5%	less than mild	less than mild
SODIUM DIOCYTYL SULFLOSUCCINATE	0.1%	less than mild	less than mild
SODIUM DIOCYTYL SULFLOSUCCINATE	0.5%	less than mild	less than mild

TRITON X-100	0.5%	less than mild	less than mild
AMPHOTERIC SURFACTANT	10.0%	less than mild	less than mild
TWEEN 20	10.0%	less than mild	less than mild
TWEEN 20	0.5%	less than mild	less than mild
TWEEN 80	10.0%	less than mild	less than mild
TWEEN 80	0.5%	less than mild	less than mild
CETYLTRIMETHYL AMMONIUM BROMIDE	1.0%	moderate	moderate
CETYLDIMETHYL AMMONIUM BROMIDE	1.0%	moderate	moderate
BENZETHONIUM CHLORIDE	100.0%	moderate	moderate
BENZETHONIUM CHLORIDE	0.1%	mild	mild
CETYLPYRIONIUM CHLORIDE	0.5%	moderate	moderate
E. DRUGS			
EYEDROPS	100.0%	less than mild	less than mild
ASCORBIC ACID	10.0%	less than mild	less than mild
ASPIRIN	100.0%	severe	moderate
PILOCARPINE	2.0%	less than mild	less than mild
DIBUCAINE HCI	0.1%	less than mild	less than mild
RESORCINOL	5.0%	lessa than mild	less than mild
NEOMYCIN SULFATE	0.5%	less than mild	less than mild
F. METAL SALTS			
NICKEL CHLORIDE	1.0%	less than mild	less than mild
ZINC CHLORIDE	0.2%	less than mild	less than mild
G. INSECT REPELLENT			
N, N-DIETHYLMETATOLUAMIDE	100.0%	moderate	moderate
N, N' DIETHYLMETHATOLUAMIDE	80.0%	moderate	moderate
N, N' DIETHYLMETHATOLUAMIDE	20.0%	moderate	moderate
N, N' DIETHYLMETHATOLUAMIDE	15.0%	moderate	moderate
N, N' DIETHYLMETHATOLUAMIDE	5.0%	less than mild	less than mild
H. CHEMICALS			
ISOPROPYL MYRISTATE	100.0%	less than mild	less than mild
THYMOL	100.0%	severe	severe
POLYETHYLENE GLYCOL 200	100.0%	less than mild	less than mild
THIOGYLCOLLIC ACID	100.0%	mild	mild
THIOGLYCOLLIC ACID	50.0%	less than mild	less than mild
PYRIDINE	100.0%	mild	mild
PYRIDINE	10.0%	less than mild	less than mild
AMMONIUM OXALATE	100.0%	severe	severe
PYROGALLOL	100.0%	severe	severe
I. ACIDS AND BASES			
AMMONIUM HYDROXIDE	50.0%	severe	severe
AMMONIUM HYDROXIDE	10.0%	moderate	moderate
AMMONIUM HYDROXIDE	2.0%	moderate	moderate
SODIUM HYDROXIDE	0.25%	less than mild	less than mild
SODIUM HYDROXIDE	0.5%	less than mild	less than mild
SODIUM HYDROXIDE	1.0%	less than mild	less than mild
ACETIC ACID	50.0%	severe	severe
ACETIC ACID	10.0%	moderate	moderate
ACETIC ACID	3.0%	less than mild	less than mild
TRICHLOROACETIC ACID	50.0%	severe	severe
OXALIC ACID	100.0%	severe	severe
CITRIC ACID	50.0%	severe	severe
PHENOL	1.0%	less than mild	less than mild

(table continues on next page)

PHENOL	5.0%	less than mild	less than mild
PHENOL	10.0%	moderate	moderate
TRIETHANOLAMINE	100.0%	moderate	moderate
ETHYLENEDIAMINE	50.0%	severe	severe
HYDROCHLORIC ACID	2.0N	severe	severe
HYDROCHLORIC ACID	1.0N	severe	severe
HYDROCHLORIC ACID	0.5N	moderate	moderate
HYDROCHLORIC ACID	0.2N	mild	mild
HYDROCHLORIC ACID	0.1N	less than mild	less than mild
$^{\gamma}$ RESORCYLIC ACID	100.0%	moderate	moderate
$^{\beta}$ RESORCYLIC ACID	100.0%	severe	severe
SULFOSALICYLIC ACID	100.0%	severe	severe

J. HOUSEHOLD PRODUCTS

HEAVY DUTY LAUNDRY POWDER	60.0%	moderate	moderate
INDUSTRIAL CLEANSER	100.0%	moderate	moderate
COLD WATER DETERGENT	10.0%	less than mild	less than mild
SOAP FLAKES	1.0%	less than mild	less than mild
HOUSEHOLD BLEACH	50.0%	less than mild	less than mild
LAUNDRY SOAP	100.0%	moderate	moderate
SCOURING POWDER	100.0%	severe	severe
SHAMPOO 1	1.0%	less than mild	less than mild
SHAMPOO 2	80.0%	moderate	moderate

K. PERSONAL CARE PRODUCTS

HAIR SPRAY	100.0%	less than mild	less than mild
SKIN TONER	100.0%	less than mild	less than mild
ASTRINGENT TONER	100.0%	less than mild	less than mild
COLOGNE	100.0%	mild	mild
SUNSCREEN	100.0%	less than mild	less than mild
LIP CONDITIONER	100.0%	less than mild	less than mild
SKIN LOTION	100.0%	less than mild	less than mild
PERFUMED SKIN LOTION	100.0%	less than mild	less than mild
MEN'S SKIN LOTION	100.0%	less than mild	less than mild
MOISTURIZER	100.0%	less than mild	less than mild
BODY LOTION	100.0%	less than mild	less than mild
BODY LOTION PERFUMED	100.0%	less than mild	less than mid
BODY OIL	50.0%	less than mild	less than mild

L. WAXES AND POLISHES

FURNITURE POLISH	100.0%	less than mild	less than mild
FLOOR WAX	100.0%	less than mild	less than mild

M. INSOLUBLE METHACRYLATE COMPOUNDS

TEST SAMPLE #1	100.0%	less than mild	less than mild
TEST SAMPLE #2	100.0%	less than mild	moderate
TEST SAMPLE #3	100.0%	less than mild	less than mild
TEST SAMPLE #4	100.0%	mild	mild
TEST SAMPLE #5	100.0%	mild	mild
TEST SAMPLE #6	100.0%	mild	mild
TEST SAMPLE #7	100.0%	severe	moderate

The data in Table I is summarized by sample category in Table II. In thirteen diverse categories of materials the correlation of 130 EYTEX results with *in vivo* results ranged from 83% to 100%. Data was not included if *in vivo* data was not available at exactly the concentrations assayed in the EYTEX System. Results from both the EYTEX and the EYTEX-MPA are included in this summary. Samples were evaluated from 0.04% to 100%. Ninety-six of the hundred and thirty results were obtained at concentrations of at least 10%.

TABLE II.
SUMMARY OF CORRELATION

SAMPLE CATEGORY	NUMBER RESULTS	CORRELATION
Solvents	21	93.0%
Preservatives	8	100.0%
Germicides and Disinfectants	6	83.0%
Surfactants	15	100.0%
Drugs	7	93.0%
Metals	2	100.0%
Insect Repellents	5	100.0%
Chemicals	9	100.0%
Acids and Bases	26	100.0%
Household Products	9	100.0%
Personal Care Products	13	100.0%
Waxes and Polishes	2	100.0%
Methacrylates	7	86.0%
	130	96.0%

DISCUSSION

The objective for National Testing Corporation has been the development of an alternative for the Draize eye irritancy test. In order to determine if the EYTEX test is an acceptable alternative, a multi-laboratory study was undertaken. This study demonstrated the capability of the EYTEX System (1).

In 1979, Cooper (2) defined several critical indices for screening assays; sensitivity, specificity and predictive values. The sensitivity, or the ability of the assay to identify positive test materials, of the EYTEX System is 95%. Irritants are defined as materials with Draize classifications of mild or greater. The specificity is the ability of the assay to discriminate negative and positive responses based upon *in vivo* data and is 99% for the EYTEX System. A high predictive value of 98% for the EYTEX System, describes the capacity of this assay to correctly predict classification, of test samples.

The EYTEX System has also demonstrated the capability to discriminate correctly different levels of ocular safety classifications ranging from minimal or less than mild to mild, moderate, and severe. In this 130 test result study, the correlation of EYTEX Ocular Safety Classifications with *in vivo* Draize data was 96%. This is an excellent correlation for the number and diversity of materials and formulations evaluated. Many materials were assayed at concentrations of at least 50%. Only a small number of materials were analyzed at low concentrations due to limitations of the EYTEX System.

The results obtained in this study demonstrate the applicability and transferability of the EYTEX System. The system is particularly appropriate for screening new ingredients and formulations. The EYTEX Test rapidly identifies moderate and severe irritants which can be eliminated from further *in vivo* testing. Trial formulations can be optimized for safety using this method. Testing of raw materials and bulk products in manufacturing with the EYTEX method could identify alterations affecting ocular safety.

REFERENCES

1. Gordon, V.C. and Bergman, H.C., (1987), in *In Vivo* Toxicology: Approaches to Validation, Goldberg, A.M. (ed.) Mary Ann Liebert, N.Y., N.Y.

2. Cooper, J.A., II, Saraci, R. and Cole, P., (1979), British Journal Cancer, **39:** 87

Poster B4

Current Uses of Normal Human Epidermal Keratinocytes in Serum-Free Medium for *In Vitro* Toxicology

PAUL T. WEGENER

Clonetics Corporation
San Diego, CA 92123

ABSTRACT

The use of normal human epidermal keratinocytes in serum-free medium allows a range of effects to be assayed. Seven of these new assay systems are described. The topics reviewed include: the human endpoints, the name and address of the principal investigator, a summary protocol of the assay, and a discussion of the promise for the future of each system. A commercially available strain of normal human epithelial cells brings a new relevance to *in vitro* toxicological studies by improving reproducibility and reliability of the culture model, as well as making the most sophisticated cell culture technology accessible to all tissue culture laboratories in a convenient form.

INTRODUCTION

Keratinocytes make up 95% of the epidermal cell population. Besides providing the *stratum corneum* as a shield against the environment, the basal keratinocytes also actively absorb xenobiotics through the membrane and by phagocytosis. Then they metabolize and detoxify these compounds with their active P-450 enzyme systems (3,14). They release various cytokines (10) and metabolites (4,5) which mediate the local immune and inflammatory responses, and they participate in wound healing. This repetoire of responses can lead to several useful endpoints for *in vitro* toxicology. Several assays are presented below which show how keratinocyte responses *in vitro* can yield quantitative results on the toxicity of compounds.

It is very important to use serum-free medium to culture these cells. Clonetics Corporation's Keratinocyte Growth Medium (KGM), an enhanced MCDB-153, supports the growth of a uniform monolayer of basal morphology, which permits the reactions to be homogenous throughout the culture. This optimized medium permits the growth of the keratinocytes without the use of feeder layers or modified culture substrates. Virtually all the cells in the culture are proliferating, with a cycle time of 28 hours; this allows any cell-cycle-dependent toxicity to be determined with reasonable exposure times.

One example of the importance of using a serum-free medium: cells in these cultures have been shown to be full of Interleukin 1 (IL-1) and covered with IL-1 receptors; when IL-1 is added to the culture, it triggers both the absorption and downregulation of the IL-1 receptor and the release of the intracellular IL-1 to the medium. This effect had been masked in serum-containing cultures because the cells would release their IL-1 as they differentiated, so the entire culture was stimulated and the receptors downregulated (10).

SURVEY OF SEVERAL ASSAYS

These assays are currently undergoing active development and are sufficiently developed to be used in an industrial context for developing data inhouse.

Human endpoint: **Eye irritancy**

Developed by: Dr. Charles Shopsis
Lab Animal Research Center
Rockefeller University
New York City, NY 10021

Industrial Sponsor: Revlon

Outline of protocol: Measures inhibition of NHEK proliferation over 48 hours exposure in 96 well plates, using colorimetric measurment of total protein (11, 12).

Advantages: Simple to perform, semi-automated, inexpensive, correlation coefficient of 0.87 with Draize rabbit eye test for the 8 SDA compounds.

Disadvantages: No mechanistic basis.

Promise for the future: The simplicity of this assay allows rapid generation of data in any cell culture facility. Once a data set is generated inhouse for those compounds with existing animal test data, it could be used to screen new compounds and formulations for potential eye irritancy in a rapid and effective manner. As the chart below demonstrates, the assay is very effective at isolating irritating from mild compounds; a low irritation score would make it possible to proceed to human volunteer testing and bypass the rabbit test altogether.

Correlation of NHEK Eye Irritancy Assay to Draize Scores

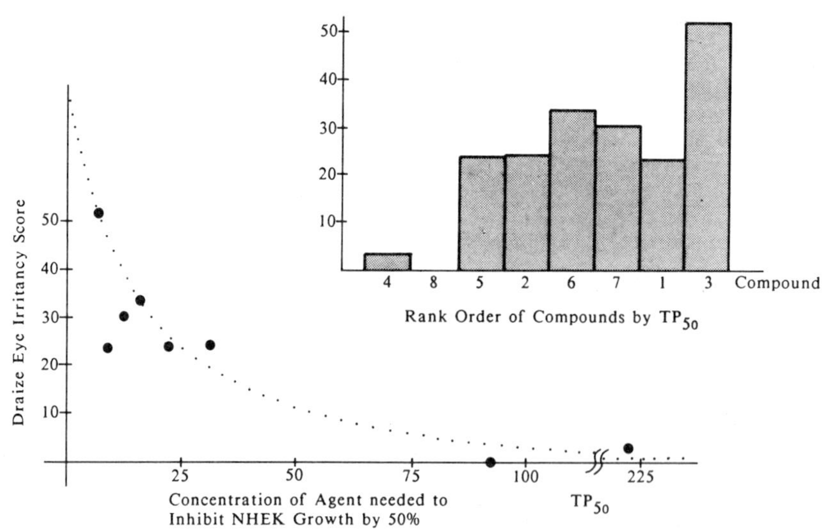

Human endpoint: **Skin irritancy**

Developed by: Dr. Vincent De Leo *et al*
Columbia University Dept. of Dermatology
New York City, NY 10032

Industrial Sponsor: Colgate-Palmolive

Outline of protocol: Measures release of labelled arachadonic acid from NHEK after exposure to irritants; specific prostaglandins may also be assayed by HPLC (4, 5).

Advantages: Good mechanistic basis.

Disadvantages: Requires use of radiolabelled compounds; limited data set.

Promise for the future: This assay shows promise in measuring the cause of "primary irritant reaction" or acute dermatosis, with a clear causal basis for the clinical condition being mimicked *in vitro*. This form of irritancy is difficult to measure convincingly in an animal model. The assay could be employed in the development of non-irritating formulations, as well as promote understanding of the underlying reactions in human skin.

Human endpoint: **Tumor promotion**

Developed by: Dr. James Trosko *et al*
Department of Ped. and Human Development
Michigan State University
East Lansing, MI 48824

Outline of protocol: Measures inhibition of the extensive gap-junctional intercellular communication of keratinocytes in serum-free medium in the absence of mitogens, by using scrape-loading to introduce a low-molecular-weight dye (6).

Advantages: Mechanistically interesting; uses target tissue; clear results from both known tumor promoters and mitogens; inexpensive.

Disadvantages: Mechanistically controversial; limited data set to date.

Promise for the future: Tumor promotion is only defined as a phenomenon in mouse skin and as a theoretical construct. In this assay tumor promoters exhibit a strong biological effect in a relevant human tissue. This assay deserves rapid application because of the expense and large numbers of animals needed in the mouse model; the assay is as promising and considerably simpler than the alternative V-79 metabolic cooperation assay and allows quantitative, dose-responsive measurement.

Other Endpoints of Interest

The following endpoints for keratinocytes have received various degrees of attention depending on the specific interests of the researchers involved; they may not have as widespread an application as the assays above, but should prove helpful in mechanistic studies.

Endpoints: **Metabolic activation**

Field of Interest: Pharmacology, toxicology

Outline of protocol: Exposure of agents to NHEK allows evaluation of metabolic products produced by P-450 monooxygenases and processed by detoxification enzymes (glutathione S transferases).

Advantages: Replaces use of hepatocytes which allows evaluation of toxicity over longer time frames; less variability in culture system; replaces animal use.

Disadvantages: P-450 is not as active as freshly isolated hepatocytes; not a relevant target tissue for hepatotoxicity; S-9 fractions give quicker results.

Promise for the future: Use of keratinocytes in cytotoxicity assays of all kinds is given additional confidence by the knowledge that they do contain a vigorous P-450 activation system; therefore these cells have been used in the investigation of:

Benzo(a)Pyrene metabolism and DNA adduct formation (3, 7).
Acetaminophen toxicity assay (2).
Chemoprevention assay of adduct formation (14).

Endpoints: **UV effects and phototoxicity**

Field of Interest: Pharmacology, cosmetics, photobiology

Outline of protocol: Keratinocytes grown in monolayer survive prolonged exposures to UV light in HEPES buffered saline solution.

Advantages: Unique model system for study of target tissue; melanocytes can be co-cultured in same medium.

Disadvantages: Protocols are unpublished.

Promise for the future: This model system is timely in light of the increased interest in UV effects on humans. Ability to culture a stratified keratinocyte culture *in vitro* (SKIN) will permit greater understanding of phototoxic effects as well as claims substantiation for sunscreens.

Endpoints: **Terminal differentiation**

Field of Interest: Pharmacology, developmental biology, cancer research, cosmetics

Outline of protocol: Increased calcium concentration in this serum-free medium induces terminal differentiation in a dose-responsive manner. Agents which enhance or antagonize this process, such as transglutimase inhibitors, can be assayed very simply in this novel system (1).

Advantages: Excellent differentiation model; simple to measure.

Disadvantages: Poorly characterized markers of differentiation; low data set to date.

Promise for the future: Control of differentiation is a key problem in many areas of modern biology. The use of this assay should isolate a number of probes of the process which will lead to its elucidation and allow therapies to be devised for some clinical differentiation malfunctions, as well as lend help in the area of aging.

Endpoints: **Transformation**

Field of Interest: Toxicology, mutagenesis, cancer research

Outline of protocol: Similar to the protocols developed by Yuspa *et al*; failure to differentiate and concomitant continued proliferation in the presence of elevated calcium is a sensitive marker of neoplastic transformation (8, 13).

Advantages: Allows malignant transformation to be assayed *in vitro* in a human system in a target tissue.

Disadvantages: Human cells are notoriously hard to transform *in vitro.*

Promise for the future: A good human cell transformation assay has yet to be developed to our knowledge; the ability to use the same endpoint as the mouse models may allow a comparison of carcinogens to be made across species lines.

Endpoints: **Mutational Assay**

Field of Interest: Toxicology, mutagenesis

Outline of protocol: Detection of mutation frequency by ability to survive selective media such as ouabain and growth of survivors at clonal densities.

Advantages: Human system; ability to grow keratinocytes at low density.

Disadvantages: Untested system; protocols poorly developed.

Promise for the future: A human cell mutagenesis assay would be very useful for answering a number of questions concerning carcinogenesis. As the assay is developed it should receive widespread attention.

BIBLIOGRAPHY

1. Boyce, S.T. and R.G. Ham. 1983. **Calcium-regulated differentiation of normal human epidermal keratinocytes in chemically defined clonal culture and free serial culture.** *J. Invest. Dermatol. 81, Supplement 1:33S-40S.*

2. Bush, L.F., P.A. Harper, D.N. Sauder and N.H. Shear, 1987. **Acetaminophen Toxicity to Keratinocytes In Vitro Assessed by a Novel Assay.** *JID 88/4 (abstract).*

3. Chang, M.J.W. 1987 Personal Communication.

4. De Leo, V.A., L.C. Harber, B. Kong and S. De Salva. 1985. **Surfactant-induced primary irritancy: an** ***in vitro*** **model.** *in "Alternative Methods in Toxicology"; Vol. 3, In Vitro Toxicology, pp 467-*481, *(Alan Goldberg, ed.); Mary Ann Liebert, NYC 1985.*

5. De Leo, V.A., L.C. Harber, B.M. Kong, and S.J. De Salva. 1987. **Surfactant-Induced Alteration of Arachidonic Acid Metabolism of Mammalian Cells in Culture.** *Society for Experim. Biology And Medicine 184:477-482, 1987*

6. El-Fouly, M.H., J.A. Trosko and C.C. Chang. 1986. **Scrape Loading and Dye Transfer.** *Experimental Cell Research. 1-9, 1986.*

7. Hukkelhoven, M.W.A.C., A.M. Bronkhorst, and A.J.M. Vermorken. 1985. **Covalent Binding of BP-Metabolites of Cultured Human Hair Follicle Keratinocytes.** *Arch Toxicol 57:6-12, 1985*

8. Kilkenny, A.E., D. Morgan, E.F Spangler and S.H. Yuspa. 1985. **Correlation of Initiating Potency of Skin Carcinogens with Potency to Induce Resistance to Terminal Differentiation in Cultured Mouse Keratinocytes.** *Cancer Res 45:2219.*

9. Kondoh, H., Y. Sato, and H. Kanoh. 1985. **Arachidonic Acid Metabolism in Cultured Mouse Keratinocytes.** *J. Invest. Dermatol. 85:64-69, 1985.*

10. Kupper, T. 1987 Personal Communication.

11. Shopsis, C. and G.J. Mackay. 1984. **A Semi-Automated Protein Assay for Cell Cultures.** *Analytical Biochemistry 140:104-107, 1985*

12. Shopsis, C. and B. Eng. 1985. **Rapid cytotoxicity testing using a semi-automated protein determination on cultured cells.** *Toxicology Letters 26:1-8, 1985*

13. Yuspa, S.H., P. Hawley-Nelson, B. Koehler and J.R. Stanley. 1980. **A Survey of Transformation Markers in Differentiating Epidermal Cell Lines in Culture.** *Cancer Research 40:4694*

14. Teel, R. 1987 Personal Communication.

Copies of all references available from Clonetics Corporation, 9620 Chesapeake Drive, San Diego, CA 92123.